Hepatic Metastases

Hepatic Metastases

Diagnosis and Management

David L. Morris MB ChB MD PhD FRCS FRACS Professor of Surgery, University of New South Wales, St George Hospital, Kogarah, Sydney, Australia

Colin S. McArdle MB ChB MD FRCS(Ed) FRCS(Eng) FRCS(Glas) Consultant Surgeon, University Department of Surgery, Royal Infirmary, Glasgow, UK

Gary M. Onik MD Visiting Professor, Department of Urology, University of Florida; Chairman, Department of Minimally Invasive Therapy, Princeton Hospital, Orlando, Florida, USA

BUTTERWORTH
HEINEMANN

Butterworth-Heinemann
Linacre House, Jordan Hill, Oxford OX2 8DP
A division of Reed Educational & Professional Publishing Ltd

A member of the Reed Elsevier plc group

OXFORD BOSTON JOHANNESBURG
MELBOURNE NEW DELHI SINGAPORE

First published 1996

British Library Cataloguing in Publication Data
Morris, David L.
Hepatic Metastases: Diagnosis and Management
I. Title
616.99434706

ISBN 0 7506 0879 X

Library of Congress Cataloguing in Publication Data
Hepatic metastases: diagnosis and management/[edited by] D. L. Morris, C. S. McArdle, G. M. Onik.
p. cm.
Includes bibliographical references and index.
ISBN 0 7506 0879 X
1. Liver—Cancer. 2. Colon (Anatomy)—Cancer—Complications. 3. Rectum—Cancer—Complications. 4. Metastasis. 5. Liver—Surgery. 6. Hepatic artery. I. Morris, David L. II. McArdle, C. S. (Colin Stewart) III. Onik, Gary, 1952–
[DNLM: 1. Liver Neoplasms—secondary. 2. Liver Neoplasms—diagnosis. 3. Liver Neoplasms—therapy. WI 735 H5267 1995]
RC280.L5H443
616.99′436—dc20
DNLM/DLC
for Library of Congress 95-7176
CIP

Photoset by Wilmaset Ltd, Birkenhead, Wirral
Printed in Great Britain by The Bath Press plc, Bath, Avon

Contents

List of contributors vii

Introduction ix

1 **The molecular basis of large bowel cancer metastasis** 1
I.R. Pickford and G.D. Birnie

2 **Imaging hepatic metastases** 21
Derek Glenn

3 **The detection of occult liver metastases: use of alternative techniques** 33
E. Leen and Colin S. McArdle

4 **Resection: how to do it** 45
Russell W. Strong

5 **Hepatic metastasis resection: results** 57
Glenn Steele Jr

6 **Intra-arterial chemotherapy: surgical approach** 67
Colin S. McArdle

7 **Results of systemic chemotherapy for the treatment of hepatic metastases from colorectal cancer** 73
Philip R. Clingan

8 **Regional cytotoxic therapy in patients with colorectal liver metastases** 85
Colin S. McArdle and D.J. Kerr

9 **Aspects of portal vein chemotherapy in the management of colorectal liver metastases** 95
I. Taylor

10 **Isolated liver perfusion** 101
K.R. Aigner

11 **Radiotherapy** 108
Bruce N. Gray and Mark A. Burton

12 **Cryotherapy**

I **Hepatic cryosurgery: technical considerations** 115
Gary M. Onik

II **Cryotherapy: mechanisms of action, scientific basis for current techniques** 133
David L. Morris and William B. Ross

III **Cryotherapy: patient selection, perioperative care, results** 137
David L. Morris and Angelo Preketes

13 **Physical methods of imaging-controlled destruction: percutaneous ethanol injections for hepatic metastases** 143
Tito Livraghi and Claudio Vettori

14 **Laser treatment of metastases** 148
Zahir Amin and Stephen G. Bown

15 **Hyperthermia** 160
Mark A. Burton and Bruce N. Gray

16 **Non-cytotoxic control of liver metastases from colon cancer** 166
David L. Morris

Index 171

Contributors

K.R. Aigner
Professor and Chief of Surgical Oncology, Krankenhaus Paulinenstift, Wiesbaden, Germany

Zahir Amin
National Medical Laser Centre, The Rayne Institute, London, UK

G.D. Birnie BSc PhD
Scientist, Beatson Institute for Cancer Research, Glasgow, UK

Stephen G. Bown
ICRF Professor of Laser Medicine and Surgery, Director, National Medical Laser Centre, The Rayne Institute, London, UK

Mark A. Burton
Department of Surgery, Royal Perth Hospital, Perth, Australia

Philip R. Clingan
Department of Medical Oncology, St George Hospital, Sydney and Wollongong, Australia

Derek Glenn
Chief Radiologist, The St George Hospital, Kogarah, Sydney, Australia

Bruce N. Gray
Professor of Surgery, Royal Perth Hospital, Perth, Australia

D.J. Kerr
Professor of Medical Oncology, University of Birmingham, UK

E. Leen
SHERT Research Fellow in Radiology, Royal Infirmary, Glasgow, UK

Tito Livraghi
Servizio di Radiologia, Ospedale Civile, Vimercate, Milan, Italy

Colin S. McArdle
Consultant Surgeon, Royal Infirmary, Glasgow, UK

David L. Morris
Professor of Surgery, The St George Hospital, Kogarah, Sydney, Australia

Gary M. Onik
Visiting Professor, Department of Urology, University of Florida; Chairman, Department of Minimally Invasive Therapy, Princeton Hospital, Orlando, Florida, USA

I. R. Pickford PhD FRCS
Department of Surgery, Victoria Infirmary NHS Trust, Glasgow, UK

Angelo Preketes
Research Fellow, St George Hospital, Sydney, Australia

William B. Ross
Senior Lecturer in Surgery, University of New South Wales, St George Hospital, Sydney, Australia

Glenn Steele Jr
Chairman, Department of Surgery, Harvard Medical School, New England Deaconess Hospital, Boston, USA

Russell W. Strong
Director of Surgery, Princess Alexandra Hospital, Brisbane, Australia

I. Taylor
Professor and Head of Dept of Surgery, UCL Medical School, London, UK

Claudio Vettori
Servizio di Radiologia, Ospedale Civile, Vimercate, Milan, Italy

Introduction

Colorectal cancer is the second commonest cancer in the Western world; the incidence is slowly increasing. In population based studies approximately half the patients are no longer amenable to cure at the time of initial presentation. Approximately one quarter of patients will have overt hepatic metastases; the remaining patients having locally advanced tumour or are unfit for surgery.

Furthermore, despite apparently curative resection, half the patients die within five years, the majority within the first three years with liver metastases. It is now clear that these patients have 'occult' hepatic metastases, that is metastases undetected by conventional imaging techniques or by the surgeon at laparotomy, at the time of initial presentation.

Overall therefore, approximately two thirds of patients who die of colorectal cancer have liver metastases at the time of death. It has been estimated that approximately one third of these would be suitable for treatment. However only a small proportion currently receive any form of therapy.

Patients with up to four metastases within the same segment may be suitable for resection. Survival of patients with resectable hepatic metastases now considerably exceeds that following resection of primary gastric, oesophageal and pancreatic cancer. Safety of liver resection has altered so that mortality is low and blood transfusion is only required in perhaps a third of patients. Hepatic artery perfusion, whilst not offering cure, does now considerably improve survival and can be undertaken with minimal morbidity.

This book seeks to be both very practical and to provide the data which establishes the value of such treatments which the reader may need to debate with more conservative colleagues. Chapters have been written by international experts, all with a specific interest in this area.

1

The molecular basis of large bowel cancer metastasis

I.R. Pickford and G.D. Birnie

Cancer of the colon and rectum is second only to lung cancer as the most frequent cause of death from malignant disease in the western world. Currently it accounts for 20 000 deaths per year in the UK (Seventh King's Fund Forum, 1990). In specialist centres in the UK the anticipated 5-year survival for patients with large bowel cancer is probably in excess of 50%. However, a prospective study of 645 patients with colorectal cancer in our own region, the West of Scotland, revealed a 5-year survival figure of only 27% (McArdle *et al.*, 1990). This depressing figure almost certainly reflects the average practice, at least in the UK. The reasons for surgical failure are twofold – tumour invasion locally and distant tumour metastasis. If it is accepted that surgeons who specialize in colorectal surgery can achieve resection rates for rectal cancer of over 90% and that the incidence of local tumour recurrence in the pelvis can be reduced to less than 5% following curative resection (Heald, 1988) then the next major goal in large bowel cancer surgery is the management and cure of patients with metastatic disease.

The impact of metastatic disease on outcome, following surgical resection of the primary tumour, has been conclusively demonstrated by Dukes. If at the time of operation the tumour is confined to the wall of the bowel, more than 90% of patients can be cured by surgery alone. Metastasis to the lymph glands draining the bowel significantly worsens the prognosis so that more than two-thirds of affected patients will die of recurrent disease within 5 years of operation. When liver metastases are present at the time of diagnosis, the majority of patients succumb within 2 years of surgery.

The metastatic process is complex. It involves the transfer of malignant cells from the primary growth across tissue barriers to distant organs, where tumour growth continues. The precise mechanisms which enable tumour cells to spread through the body and the host response to the metastatic process have yet to be defined and remain a matter of some debate. The aim in this chapter is to outline some of the more important biological and molecular mechanisms which are thought to be responsible for the secondary spread of tumours, with particular reference to the metastasis of large bowel cancer to the liver. To date this work has not had a significant influence on clinical practice, but things are likely to change rapidly. Although it is possible that some reduction in tumour metastasis will be achieved by earlier diagnosis of the primary tumour through screening, it is anticipated that molecular dissection of the metastatic process will ultimately lead to the development of more appropriate and more successful treatment for patients with disseminated cancer.

The seed and the soil

The mechanisms that enable tumour cells to spread through the body have still to be elucidated and remain largely a matter of speculation, though it should be borne in mind that all the properties attributed to the metastatic tumour cell, apart from tumorigenicity, are shared by a variety of normal cells. For example, the translocation of cells from one point in an organism to another occurs normally during embryogenesis, and in response to infection and injury. The precise translocation of cells during embryological development and the recognition that lymphocytes have regional specificity (lymphocyte homing) are now being explored as models to explain the pattern of tumour spread. The pattern of metastatic disease, that is, the sites affected by secondary tumour growth, is generally predictable for colorectal cancers with the liver and regional lymph nodes predominantly affected. The pattern of spread will also vary depending on the time at which the disease is staged. At presentation, as indicated above, we would expect metastasis from the large bowel to occur to regional lymph nodes, liver and occasionally lung. Analysis of postmortem data on the other hand would indicate that almost any organ can be a repository for metastatic large bowel cancer in patients dying of their disease. The liver is the organ most frequently affected (50–60%), followed by the lungs (25–40%), adrenals (14%), ovaries (14%), bone (5–10%). Metastatic lesions have also been detected in brain, kidney and spleen (Sugarbaker, 1981).

The frequent involvement of the liver in metastatic spread from the large bowel requires explanation. Anatomical constraints such as the tumour site and venous drainage, the environment of the affected tissues and tumour cell properties have all been implicated.

It is now more than 100 years since Paget, writing in the *Lancet*, posed the question: 'what is it that determines what organ shall suffer in a case of disseminated cancer?' (Paget, 1889). Based on his findings on the distribution of metastatic disease in 735 women dying of breast cancer, Paget concluded that the variability in involvement of the liver, lung, adrenals, bone, ovary and spleen was not a matter of chance but a reflection of the environment provided by each organ (the soil) as well as a property of the tumour cell (the seed). This has come to be known as the seed and soil hypothesis of metastasis. The various organ and tumour cell properties which might contribute to this organ pattern of metastasis will be reviewed subsequently. An alternative view is that, provided enough tumour cells enter an organ, irrespective of the 'soil', metastatic disease will ensue (Sugarbaker, 1981). Experimental animal models of metastasis indicate that millions of tumour cells are released into the circulation each day. If this reflects the situation in human large bowel cancer, then countless tumour cells are filtered out of the portal circulation in the liver, making metastasis almost inevitable.

The development of metastasis outside the organ of first encounter (the liver in large bowel cancer) also requires explanation. The development of systemic metastasis could occur simultaneously with the development of liver metastasis or, as some would suggest, subsequent to the establishment of hepatic metastasis. A proportion of disseminating cells, pehaps the most deformable variety, pass through the liver into the lungs with the possibility of producing lung metastasis. The number of viable cells traversing this capillary bed to enter the left heart and the systemic circulation would therefore be small, reducing the likelihood of metastases in the brain, spleen, ovaries, kidneys and adrenals. Weiss (1986) has argued that the number of cells entering the systemic circulation after passage through the liver and lungs renders it impossible for the surviving cells to give rise to systemic metastasis beyond the liver and lungs. He suggests a cascade process in which the liver, the organ of first encounter, succumbs to metastasis and then acts as a generalizing site for further metastasis into the lungs (Weiss, 1986; Weiss *et al.*, 1986). Such arguments are not simply of academic interest, but could have a significant effect on the approach to the treatment of metastatic disease from large bowel cancer. Acceptance of the cascade theory has already led to suggestions that treatment directed at the liver or liver and lungs prior to systemic metastasis will obviate the need for systemic therapy.

Model systems

Analysis of the metastatic behaviour of tumours poses a number of problems. The difficulties and limitations of experimental approaches to the study of human tumour metastasis are obvious. For example, it is still not possible, with any degree of certainty, to identify tumour cells in the circulation. Much of the clinical material is heterogeneous, and so-called studies of the natural history of colorectal cancer metastasis have been devalued by a variety of treatment regimens. We now suspect that even apparently routine clinical interventions, such as perioperative blood transfusion, affect the metastatic behaviour of malignant tumours perhaps through the host immune system. In an attempt to circumvent some of these problems a variety of animal models, using transplantable tumours, have been established to try to define the host and tumour cell properties responsible for secondary tumour spread. The experimental systems usually consist of an *in vitro* phase in tissue culture, permitting experimental manipulation of the tumour cells, and an *in vivo* phase when the tumour cells are introduced into animals to assay the expression of the metastatic phenotype. Animal models of metastasis are of two basic types:

1. Spontaneous metastasis assay – tumour cells are injected into the animal, usually subcutaneously or intramuscularly, to allow the formation of a tumour from which metastasis can occur.
2. Experimental metastasis assay – tumour cells are injected directly into the blood stream (usually via the tail vein) to produce colonies or metastases in distant organs.

This nomenclature is misleading. Both techniques are obviously experimental, but of the two, the latter is less likely to be representative of the whole metastatic process in humans. Nevertheless, the experimental metastasis assay is widely used to study metastasis. There is evidence that the 'metastatic' behaviour of tumour cells following intravenous injection does not necessarily parallel the metastasis behaviour of the same cells in a spontaneous metastasis assay, suggesting that these two tumour properties may represent two distinct phenotypes (Glaves, 1983; Stackpole, 1981, 1983). To avoid confusion, tumours produced in distant organs in a spontaneous metastasis assay should be described as metastases or secondaries (spontaneous metastasis assay) and tumours produced by direct injection into the blood stream should be referred to as colonies (colonization assay).

The animal most often used in these studies is the laboratory mouse. The metastatic phenotype of murine tumour cells can be assayed in syngeneic, inbred strains or immunodeficient animals. Assays of the metastatic behaviour of human tumour cell lines and human tumour xenografts are dependent on the use of immunodeficient animals. Although the athymic T-cell-deficient nude mouse supports the growth of human tumour cells metastasis is uncommon in these animals (Sharkey & Fogh, 1979; Hanna, 1982). The resistance of nude mice to experimental metastasis appears to be correlated with the levels of natural killer (NK) cells (see later) in these animals. Young nude mice have reduced levels of NK cell-mediated cytotoxicity and so most metastasis assays are carried out in young animals when the NK levels are low. It has also been demonstrated that the site of injection of human tumour cell lines and tumour xenographs may be an important variable in eliciting metastasis in the nude mouse (Kozlowski *et al.*, 1984; Fidler, 1986, 1991). The conditions required to elicit metastasis in the nude mouse have not yet been fully defined. It is possible that metastasis occurs late in these animals, with the result that many experiments are terminated before metastases have had time to develop (Sharkey & Fogh, 1979; Kozlowski *et al.*, 1984).

Although the lymphatic system is a major route of secondary spread for most of the common types of human tumours, there have been very few experimental studies of lymphatic metastasis. Almost all experimental models of metastasis are based on tumour dissemination via the blood stream, either from implanted cells or from the direct injection of cells into the blood. Because of the nature of the metastasis assays, the subsequent discussion will be confined almost entirely to the spread of tumour cells via the blood stream.

Attempts have also been made to study metastasis using *in vitro* assays of tumour invasion. The ability of tumour cells to invade a variety of substrates has been reported, including human amnion (Schultz *et al.*, 1988), chick chorioallantoic membrane (Chambers & Ling, 1984), deposits of collagen in tissue culture dishes (Vleminckx *et al.*, 1991), fragments of embryonic chick heart (Vleminckx *et al.*, 1991) and so-called reconstituted basement membrane consisting of layers of laminin, type IV collagen and type I collagen (Kleinman *et al.*, 1986; Terranova *et al.*, 1986). The relevance of these *in vitro* assays to metastasis is questionable; any extrapolation from such models to the full metastatic phenotype must be viewed with caution.

Multistep versus stochastic theories

For metastasis to occur, tumour cells must detach from the primary tumour mass singly or as clumps of cells, enter the venous circulation, embolize to and arrest in a capillary bed of a distant organ, and then possess the ability to grow within the tissue parenchyma. This appears to be an inefficient process since the proportion of tumour cells released into the circulation which go on to complete this complex series of events to form metastases is extremely small (Fidler & Kripke, 1977; Glaves, 1983; Weiss, 1986). Different interpretations of these observations have contributed to two essentially opposing theories of the metastatic process.

Multistep theory

In 1965, Zeidman suggested that the majority of tumour emboli were incapable of giving rise to metastases because 'only a particular mutant cell can yield a metastasis'. this statement was supported by experimental data showing that when lung colonies from the intravenous injection of B16 melanoma cells (of murine origin) were harvested and reinjected into syngeneic mice, they produced more lung metastases than the parent 'stock' cells. These studies were subsequently confirmed and extended by Fidler (1973), suggesting that some cells were expressing properties which provided an advantage for survival in the circulation and growth in the lungs of syngeneic mice.

A series of cell properties have been attributed to this particular mutant cell. It is argued that tissue invasion and penetration of lymphatics and blood vessels are achieved by cell movement and by the production of proteolytic enzymes which digest extracellular structures such as the basement membrane (Hart & Fidler, 1980; Wang *et al.*, 1980; Gullino & Liotta, 1981; Liotta *et al.*, 1983; Carlsen *et al.*, 1984; Zetter, 1990). Following penetration of the blood vessel wall and entry into the lumen, the metastatic cells then have to survive turbulence in the blood stream, attack from immune cells and arrest in the next capillary bed. The proponents of the multistep theory argue that the site of arrest is dependent on cell surface antigen expression and cell deformability (Hart & Fidler, 1980; Zetter, 1990; Hart & Saini, 1992). Following arrest the metastatic cells attach to the vascular endothelium, induce endothelial retraction and bind to glycoproteins (such as laminin) of the basement membrane by means of cell surface receptors (Liotta *et al.*, 1983; Zetter, 1990; Hart & Saini, 1992). Invasion of the tissue parenchyma is accomplished by the release of specific enzymes (for example, type IV collagenase) to degrade the basement membrane, and by cell migration (Liotta *et al.*, 1983; Liotta *et al.*, 1986; Liotta & Stetler-Stevenson, 1991). To summarize the multistep theory, metastasis is described as a non-random, genetically determined process which comprises a number of discrete steps, each of which must be completed for a cell to produce a secondary tumour deposit. It is argued that only a specialized subset of cells within a tumour population possess all the attributes required for metastasis.

Stochastic theory

An alternative view is that metastasis is a random process in which all malignant cells have a more or less equal ability to metastasize. The expression of metastatic behaviour by any individual cell is a matter of chance and is determined by local events (Giavazzi *et al.*, 1980; Alexander, 1983; Weiss, 1986). Experimental data from a number of studies have shown that cells derived from metastases are not necessarily more metastatic than the parent cell line – findings that are clearly at odds with the work of Fidler and others (Giavazzi *et al.*, 1980; Alexander, 1983; Weiss *et al.*, 1983; Ling *et al.*, 1985).

The necessity for tumour cells to possess the full complement of functions implied within the multistep theory has also been challenged. For example, the release of proteases from areas of tumour degeneration and from infiltrating leukocytes could facilitate local invasion. The basement membrane, which is generally considered to be a barrier to tumour cell dissemination, is frequently absent or discontinuous in tumour blood vessels and normal lymphatic capillaries, obviating the need for proteolytic enzyme activity to digest this structure (Carter, 1982; Liotta *et al.*, 1983). Clumping and aggregation of tumour and circulating host cells such as platelets and leukocytes in the circulation might be one mechanism by which tumour cells are protected against turbulence. Basement membrane is absent from normal liver sinusoids, so that tumour cells present in the portal blood have no requirement for enzymes capable of breaking down this structure during extravasation (Liotta *et al.*, 1983). It has also been argued that the arrest of tumour cell emboli in capillaries produces vascular occlusion, stasis and local thrombus formation, which in turn causes tissue ischaemia, infarction and disruption of local tissue barriers permitting escape of the disseminated cells into the tissue parenchyma. Although there are clear differences between these two theories there does seem to be a place for an intermediate model combining features from both. It is possible that the majority of malignant cells within a primary tumour have metastatic potential and that overexpression or abrogation of certain phenotypes will increase the likelihood of metastasis. From a clinical or therapeutic viewpoint this may appear to be a less satisfactory state of affairs since the stochastic or random elements are unpredictable and therefore less amenable to manipulation,

Invasion and extravasation

Invading tumour cells come into contact with a variety of extracellular molecules that constitute the extracellular matrix (ECM). The ECM not only provides support for tissues but also regulates the behaviour of cells which are in contact with it and also probably acts as a repository for enzymes and growth factors (Vlodavsky *et al.*, 1990). The ECM comprises fibrous proteins such as the collagens and adhesive proteins, examples of which are laminin and fibronectin, contained within a highly hydrated polysaccharide gel (Alberts *et al.*, 1983). One of the collagens, type IV, is a major constituent of basement membranes and is arranged in sheet form. Fibronectin, a glycoprotein, can be found in soluble form in the plasma, on the cell surface and as a component of the ECM. There are different domains on the fibronectin molecule, one of which binds to collagen, another to heparin and another to a receptor on the cell surface. The fibronectin receptor belongs to a super family of homologous matrix receptors known as integrins. The polysaccharides consist of long unbranched chains of repeating disaccharide units and are known as glycosaminoglycans (or GAGs). The GAGs are usually covalently linked to proteins to form proteoglycans; the exception is hyaluronic acid, which exists as a very long carbohydrate chain. Because of their molecular organization the GAG chains permit diffusion of water-soluble molecules and cell migration. Hyaluronic acid appears to be deposited in tissues in which there is active cell migration (for example, during development and wound repair). Laminin is another complex glycoprotein molecule, consisting of three polypeptide chains arranged in the shape of a cross, and is confined largely to the basement membrane (Liotta *et al.*, 1983). It has a number of functional domains, including binding sites for type IV collagen, heparan sulphate and the laminin receptor on cells.

Basement membrane is a specialized form of the ECM and is potentially of importance in the metastatic process. It is present as a thin sheet, which separates the vascular endothelium from the underlying connective tissue of the blood vessel wall. Although the precise composition of the basement membrane is highly variable, its constituents include type IV collagen, proteoglycans, fibronectin and laminin, with laminin providing attachment for the endothelial cells. The invasion by cells of the primary tumour into connective tissue containing blood and lymphatic vessels is clearly a prerequisite for tumour dissemination and metastasis. It is hypothesized that there are three stages to the invasion of the ECM by tumour cells:

1. Attachment through binding of cell surface receptors to molecules such as fibronectin and laminin.
2. Lysis of the ECM.
3. Movement of the cells through the ECM.

Following dissemination of the tumour cells and their lodgement in distant capillary bed, the same or related mechanisms might be expected to facilitate extravasation and tissue invasion.

Cell surface and metastasis

The role of cell adhesion molecules (CAMs) in tumour progression is a complex but highly topical subject. Much of the present impetus to study the CAMs of malignant cells has come from advances in the understanding of cell surface changes governing pattern formation in the embryo and of leukocyte behaviour during immune responses. A large number of adhesion systems are used by any one cell. There are at least four groups of receptors for cell adhesion which might play some part in the metastatic process, namely the immunoglobulin superfamily, the integrin superfamily, the cadherins and the Hermes/CD44 antigen family. It is likely that a combination of different types of molecule, as well as the surface density and distribution on the cell of these adhesion receptors, determines the affinities between cells and the ECM. Furthermore, expression of these receptors is associated with the expression of other developmentally important proteins affecting cell division, cell shape and cell movement.

Immunoglobulin superfamily

Expression of intercellular adhesion molecule 1 (ICAM-1), the ligand for the integrin receptor lymphocyte function-associated antigen-1 (LFA-1) found on leukocytes, has been correlated with depth of invasion and hence metastatic propensity of human malignant melanoma (Johnson *et al.*, 1989). Possible mechanisms for this effect include tumour cell binding to migratory leukocytes facilitating dissemination, heterotypic clumping in the circulation promoting arrest in capillaries and tumour cell–leukocyte interactions inducing suppression of the immune response. Release of ICAM-1 into the circulation by cells expressing the molecule could suppress the immune response by blocking the integrin receptor on cytotoxic lymphocytes. However, at the present state of knowledge it is not clear whether the observed changes in expression of ICAM-1 are the cause or an effect of increasing depth of tumour invasion.

A putative tumour suppressor gene, known as DCC (for deleted in colorectal cancer, see later), which is located on chromosome 18, and is reported to be involved in the latter stages of tumour progression in human large bowel cancer, encodes a glycoprotein which is a member of the immunoglobulin superfamily (Fearon & Vogelstein, 1990; Fearon *et al.*, 1990). It has been proposed that colorectal cancers which have lost one copy of the DCC gene have a greater propensity to metastasize (Vogelstein, 1990). Carcinoembryonic antigen (or CEA) is also a glycoprotein which may function as a CAM and play a role in metastasis. It has been hypothesized that CEA is released from large bowel cancers, taken up by Kupffer cells and hepatocytes and represented on the cell surface (Jessup & Thomas, 1989). The homophilic binding (that is, the interaction of two identical molecules) which occurs between CEA molecules expressed on diseminating cancer cells, and on cells in the liver promotes tumour cell arrest and contributes to the development of hepatic metastasis.

Integrins

There are at least three families of integrin receptor which share a common β chain, but can be distinguished by variations in the extracellular α chain. The integrins recognize a specific tripeptide amino acid sequence (Arg-Gly-Asp or RGD) in the extracellular protein. Short peptide sequences homologous to the cell-binding domain of fibronectin or laminin have been shown to reduce lung colonization when co-injected with tumour cells (Humphries *et al.*, 1986; Iwamoto *et al.*, 1987; Saiki *et al.*, 1989.

Cadherins

Cadherins represent another family of cell adhesion receptors and are probably the most important for determining binding between cells (Takeichi, 1991). These molecules are calcium-dependent and exhibit homophilic binding, that is, a cadherin molecule on one cell will only bind to an identical cadherin molecule from another cell. There are a number of subclasses, of which four have been well described: E (for epithelial), P (for placental), N (for neural) and L (liver) CAM. Cells generally express multiple classes of cadherins The cadherins are associated with cytoskeletal components of the cell, and changes in cadherin expression affect cell morphology. It has been postulated that loss or reduction of cadherin expression contributes to the release of tumour cells from the primary tumour and is associated with a more invasive phenotype (Takeichi, 1991; Hart & Saini, 1992). Although the evidence that cadherins are involved in metastasis is weak, it has been reported that E (for epithelial) cadherin acts as an 'invasion suppressor molecule' (Vleminckx *et al.*, 1991).

However, it must be emphasized that this conclusion was drawn from an *in vitro* assay measuring tumour cell invasion into fragments of chick embryonic heart and deposits of collagen type I in culture wells.

Proteolytic enzymes

Although a variety of enzymes have been reported to be associated with the invasive process, the metalloproteinase family of enzymes is probably the most extensively studied (Liotta & Stetler-Stevenson, 1991). Unfortunately, most studies of the role of enzyme activity in the metastatic process have relied on correlations between enzyme production *in vitro*, invasive capacity *in vitro*, and lung-colonizing ability *in vivo*. The discovery that there are naturally occurring inhibitors of these enzymes known as TIMPS (tissue inhibitors of metalloproteinases) has lent support to the concept of invasion suppressor proteins. Inactivation of a TIMP by whatever mechanism might be expected to result in unopposed proteolytic activity. Down-modulation of TIMP messenger RNA in Swiss 3T3 cells has been shown not only to enhance invasiveness *in vitro*, but also to cause some cells to become tumorigenic and metastatic (Khokha *et al.*, 1989). Intraperitoneal injections of recombinant human TIMP have been shown to reduce lung colonization following intravenous injection of tumour cells into mice (Schultz *et al.*, 1988). Although it has never been convincingly demonstrated that manipulation of a primary tumour at surgery contributes to the development of metastasis, it could be argued that the use of TIMPS prior to surgery might prove to be beneficial for patients shown to be free of metastasis at diagnosis.

Motility factors

Autocrine motility factor (AMF) and scatter factor have been shown to enhance cell motility, and have been implicated in tumour cell invasion and metastasis. However, evidence in support of a role for these molecules in the metastatic process is slim. Nevertheless, the concept of factors capable of stimulating motility is of great interest. AMF stimulates random movement and pseudopodial protrusion, and it has been argued that it is the binding of pseudopods to the ECM which is responsible for the initiation of directional movement of cells. AMF was identified in conditioned medium taken from cultures of the cell line which was established from a human melanoma brain metastasis. The presence of AMF was associated with an increase in the transfer of the melanoma cells across a filter *in vitro*. A similar factor has also been isolated from human colon cancer cells (Liotta *et al.*,1986). AMF appears to be a single polypeptide which is distinct from other known chemoattractants and growth factors. Experimental evidence would indicate that there is a specific cell surface receptor for this molecule.

Scatter factor (or hepatocyte growth factor), now known to be the ligand for the met receptor, is different from AMF in a number of respects. Its effects, unlike AMF, are paracrine since its production and release are limited to fibroblasts whilst response to scatter factor is seen only in epithelial cells. This molecule causes separation at epithelial junctions, increased motility and a scattering of contiguous sheets of cells (Stoker *et al.*, 1987; Gherardi *et al.*, 1989). The release of scatter factor-like molecules from fibroblasts in connective tissue could contribute to the predilection of tumour cells for certain organs.

Tumour cell dissemination/the host response

Studies of transplantable tumours indicate that, in some circumstances, thousands, perhaps millions, of cells are shed into the blood stream each day (Gullino & Liotta, 1981). The potential for interaction between disseminating tumour cells and the components of the blood stream is enormous. It has been shown that clumps of tumour cells injected into the circulation give rise to greater numbers of colonies in the lung than an equivalent inoculum of single cells (Liotta *et al.*, 1976). The presence of emboli of tumour cells and leukocytes has also been found to correlate with metastatic propensity in other experimental models (Glaves, 1983). Mechanisms by which these cellular aggregates promote colonization are not known; they might enhance arrest in the capillary beds, provide protection against attack by host defence mechanisms, act as a buffer against turbulence and shear forces, or facilitate paracrine growth stimulation.

In a light microscopic study of the sequential changes in the lung following intravenous injection of amelanotic B16 melanoma cells, tumour cell/platelet thrombi were frequently observed (Crissman *et al.*, 1985). Fibrin deposition was also seen. Electron microscopic studies showed that the platelets were degranulated, indicative of activation. The platelet/fibrin deposits appeared to cause obstruction to the vessel lumen, but within 24 h dissolution was almost complete. From these findings it was speculated that the platelet/fibrin/tumour cell thrombi contributed to the metastatic process by enhancement of trapping and adhesion to the endothelium. It was also suggested that the thrombus might protect the tumour cell from host attack and provide platelet-derived growth factors (Crissman *et al.*, 1985).

Tumour cell products, as well as normal cellular extracts, thromboplastins, have procoagulant activity. For example, a tumour cell proteinase has been identified with activation of factor X (Gasic *et al.*, 1986). Tumour cells have also been shown to have the capacity to digest fibrin *in vitro* through the action of plasminogen activator (Gasic *et al.*, 1986). Most tumour cells have the ability to activate platelets, at least *in vitro*. The mechanisms involved in inducing change in platelet shape, aggregation and secretion probably vary from tumour to tumour, but result from intimate contact. Interaction of tumour cells with platelets has the potential to induce the release of a vast array of platelet products, including serotonin, calcium, fibronectin, proteinases and platelet-derived growth factor, which could modify tumour cell behaviour in myriad ways (Gasic, 1984). The ability of tumour cells *in vitro* to produce platelet aggregation has shown good correlation with the ability of the same cells to colonize the lungs following tail vein injection. Spontaneously shed tumour cell plasma membrane vesicles have been shown to induce platelet activation, and both cathepsin B-like and thrombin enzymes have been implicated in this process (Gasic *et al.*, 1986).

The use of anticoagulants has been shown to be rather more effective in reducing organ colonization than spontaneous metastasis (Gasic *et al.*, 1986). Some of the coumarin derivatives have shown an effect even when administered 24 h after tumour cell inoculation, at a time when tumour cell-associated thrombosis would be expected to be complete. It has been postulated that a reduction in thrombin activity by the coumarins prevents the activation of tumour cell proteinases. It appears that the antimetastatic effect of warfarin may be mediated through the activation of macrophages and that functionally active NK cells are necessary for the effectiveness of anticoagulants in reducing organ colonization and metastasis; a fibrin coat could protect the tumour cells against host attack (Gasic *et al.*, 1986).

Although thousands of tumour cells probably enter the circulation each day, remarkably few survive to produce secondary tumours (Price *et al.*, 1986). This is usually attributed to the inefficiency of the metastatic process; however, looked at another way, it could indicate the operation of highly efficient host mechanisms directed against disseminating tumour cells (Pickford, 1991). A metastatic cell separated from the primary tumour mass might be considered to be more vulnerable to host attack than it is as a component of the primary tumour (Hart, 1985; Wallich *et al.*, 1985). It is known that leukocytes and tumour cells come into close proximity, but the outcome of these various interactions is yet to be determined. It is possible that T-cell responses to metastatic cells can be invoked by an association between major histocompatibility complex (MHC) class I molecules and tumour cell antigens and/or expression of novel MHC class I molecules on the surface of the tumour cell. T cells do appear to be the predominant cell type infiltrating both primary and secondary tumours, but studies have so far failed to demonstrate a clear role for T lymphocytes in the spread of tumours. If cytotoxic lymphocytes are responsible for killing tumour cells, then attentuation of class I expression might be one way by which disseminating cells avoid recognition. However, studies of class I expression by tumour cells have failed to clarify the situation: changes in class I can affect metastatic competence by mechanisms unrelated to the modulation of T-cell responses. For example, the association between these molecules and growth factor receptors may be a determinant of ligand binding (Schreiber *et al.*, 1984; Linsk & Goodenow, 1986).

NK cells have also been implicated in the eradication of disseminating tumour cells. These cells are large granular lymphocytes distinct from T and B cells. It has been hypothesized that NK selectivity is directed against cells which do not express class I molecules and so might escape attack by T cells. However, there are numerous contradictions in the data from studies of MHC class I expression in metastasis, making it difficult to draw such a conclusion. Nevertheless, there are quite persuasive data showing an inverse relationship between NK activity in peripheral blood and the incidence of metastases in experimental animals.

The idea of manipulating the host immune system to attack metastases after surgical resection of the primary tumour is clearly an attractive proposition. Unfortunately, past experience with immunotherapy has been disappointing (Early Breast Cancer Trialists' Collaborative Group, 1992). Immune therapies for cancer are currently under investigation and provide a number of different approaches to the eradication of systemic disease, including activation of macrophages, active specific immunotherapy and adoptive immunotherapy (Fidler *et al.*, 1982, 1986; Hoover *et al.*, 1985; Rosenberg *et al.*, 1985, 1986). So-called tumour-infiltrating lymphocytes or TILs expanded *in vitro* by treatment with interleukin-2 (IL2; adoptive immunotherapy) have been shown to be effective reducing lung colonies even when injected 3 days after the inoculation of tumour cells. Combination therapy of TILs, low-dose IL2 and cyclophosphamide was shown to be even more effective. This type of treatment regimen has already been introduced into clinical practice (Rosenberg, 1990). It is anticipated in some quarters that, as the molecular basis of immunity and the signalling systems involved in leukocyte activation are more clearly defined, manipulation of the host defences will become increasingly sophisticated and provide more effective immunotherapies (Guillou, 1987).

Growth and angiogenesis

Having lodged in a capillary bed and invaded a tissue, the metastatic cell must proliferate and establish its own blood supply. Cell growth is controlled by the interplay of growth-stimulatory and inhibitory factors (Zetter, 1990). The ability of disseminated tumour cells to secrete their own stimulatory factors whilst expressing the appropriate receptor might be expected to be a determinant of the metastatic phenotype. Similarly, response to locally produced stimulatory factors from either tumour cells or cells of the invaded organ would be advantageous. Organ-derived growth factors have been identified; conditioned medium from lung tissue has been shown to contain several factors with either growth-stimulatory or inhibitory activity. A lung-derived growth factor (LDGF-1) has been isolated from rat and porcine lung conditioned medium; it does not appear to be related to other known growth factors. LDGF-1 has been shown preferentially to stimulate mitogenesis in lung-colonizing tumour cells *in vitro* (Cavanaugh & Nicolson, 1989).

If a metastatic deposit is to grow beyond about 3 mm in diameter, angiogenesis is essential. Experiments in which tumour fragments were inserted into rabbit cornea showed that capillaries grew rapidly from the existing vascular bed to envelop and invade the tumour. From such experiments it was demonstrated that angiogenesis was induced by diffusible factors produced by the tumour cells. Various angiogenic factors have been identified and characterized (Evans, 1991); these include fibroblast growth factor (FGF), epidermal growth factor (EGF), angiogenin and transforming growth factor (TGF-α). Production of these angiogenic factors is not the preserve of tumour cells, but is has been shown that some cells acquire, or markedly up-regulate, angiogenic activity when they are transformed.

Clonal dominance

Studies of karyotypic markers and isoenzyme patterns have shown that human tumours are monoclonal in origin; however, they evolve during growth to comprise a heterogeneous population of cells. Nowell (1976) postulated that the increased genetic instability of tumour cells caused the production of mutants. While many of these mutants are eliminated quickly because of metabolic disadvantage or immunological destruction, others survive and some might have an additional selective advantage and so come to form a predominant clone of more aggressive cells within the tumour. Moreover, it is likely that the selective pressures vary from organ to organ, and from time to time, due to differences in abundances of growth factors, and also perhaps as a consequence of therapy. Therefore, throughout the evolution of a tumour the balance in selective pressure and genetic instability is crucial: when selective pressure is less than genetic instability there is divergence; when selective pressure is greater, there is convergence. These ideas have led to the concept of clonal dominance (Kerbel *et al.*, 1988).

The occurrence of clonal dominance in primary tumours and its relationship with the metastatic phenotype have been studied in a variety of experimental models. The method primarily used depends upon introducing into the genome of tumour cells an exogenous gene, often the *neo* gene (a bacterial gene conferring antibiotic resistance) as a selectable genetic marker. Using this method, it was shown that a mixture of two clones of the B16 melanoma gave rise to primary tumour containing both clones of cells, but that most of the metastatic deposits formed were comprised of either one or the other clone. Thus, neither of these sublines of the B16 tumour dominated the other *in vivo* and both were capable of forming metastases, probably from single cells. On the other hand, two sublines of a mouse mammary tumour were almost equally tumorigenic when injected separately into mice, but gave primary tumours composed entirely of one of them when mixtures were injected, even when the dominant subline comprised just 1% of the inoculum. This dominance occurred even in tissue culture, and proved to be due to suppression of growth of one subline by the other.

Much use has been made of the *neo* gene as a marker to investigate clonal dominance in the metastatic process. The initial series of experiments was carried out with a highly tumorigenic mouse mammary adenocarcinoma cell line which was only weakly metastatic. A mixture consisting of 50–100 individually identifiable clones of cells injected into mice produced primary tumours which predominantly comprised a single clone of cells. It was also shown that the lung metastases had arisen mainly or entirely from this dominant clone of cells. When the cells of the dominant clone were mixed with the parental tumour cells, strong selection for these cells was found *in vivo*, even when they comprised one in 10 of the inoculum. Inoculation of a mixture of a much larger number (approximately 10^4) of uniquely marked clones in the mice caused primary tumours arising from only a few (probably less than 10) clones of cells, each primary being comprised of just one or two dominant clones. Moreover, each metastasis was derived from a single clone. It would appear that during growth *in vivo* a heterogeneous mixture of tumour cells can become dominated by a single clone and it is this single clone which is the source of successful metastatic deposits.

Recently, these conclusions have been confirmed and extended to encompass the effect of organ environment on the dominating clone (Staroselsky *et al.*, 1992). Using a human renal carcinoma cell line marked with the *neo* gene it was shown that different clones became dominant in primary tumours in kidney, colon and subcutaneous sites of injection in nude mice. Moreover, it was the same clones that dominated in the kidney primaries in all mice and the clonality was retained in distant metastases. Different clones dominated in the colon, and again the clonality was retained in metastases. However, subcutaneous injection led to a random selection of dominant clones in both primary and secondary tumours. Thus, clonal dominance does occur also with this tumour, and the environment into which the cells are injected appears to have a marked effect on the clones selected.

These results notwithstanding, it has been concluded that clonal dominance as assessed by molecular markers does not mean tumour homogeneity (Bell *et al.*, 1991; Staroselsky *et al.*, 1992). Karyotypic analysis of primary tumours and metastases from both the murine adenocarcinoma and the human renal cell carcinoma cell lines showed them to be heterogeneous with respect to some marker chromosomes and homogeneous with respect to others, as well as to the exogenous genetic marker. Clearly, therefore, many of the data from experiments with *neo* marked cells require re-evaluation. A further aspect of these data has yet to be investigated: the dominance of certain *neo* clone could be due to insertional mutagenesis conferring a growth advantage on the cells and an increased propensity to complete the metastatic process.

Molecular genetics of large bowel cancer progression

Cancer is a multistep process involving initiation, promotion and progression to highly malignant and metastatic behaviour. It has long been suspected that the disturbances in cell growth and differentiation which are characteristic of malignant tumours are the result of abnormalities in the genetic material of somatic cells. Analysis of data from age incidence studies of the common malignancies predicted that carcinomas result from the accumulation within a cell of between two and seven genetic changes. Progress in molecular genetics is now providing the evidence to support this hypothesis so that we are now in a position to identify alterations in certain genes which appear to be critical for the initiation and progression of human malignancy. To date the genetic mechanisms responsible for progression to the metastatic phenotype remain elusive, although some candidate genes have been proposed.

Normal cellular genes, known as proto-oncogenes, are present in the genome of every cell. Activation of these genes via a variety of genetic events, including mutation and chromosome rearrangement, leads to the neoplastic state; proto-oncogenes are subverted to oncogenes (for review, see Pickford & Cooke, 1990). Proteins encoded by the proto-oncogenes have functions related to the control of cell proliferation and differentiation and similarities have been demonstrated between oncogene products, growth factors, growth factor receptors and activators of DNA transcription.

Although the discovery of oncogenes represented a major breakthrough in understanding cancer, the picture was incomplete. A further advance occurred with the identification of another class of cellular genes, designated tumour suppressor or anti-oncogenes (for review, see Pickford & Cooke, 1990). Loss of function of these genes appears to be a major contributory factor to the development of the malignant phenotype. Whereas the activation of one of the two cellular copies of proto-oncogene may be sufficient to override cellular control mechanisms and disrupt growth (the so-called dominant action of oncogenes), it is postulated that, as a general rule, both copies of a tumour suppressor gene must be lost or inactivated for an effect on cell behaviour to become evident. Tumour suppressor genes are said to act recessively at the cellular level. The activation of oncogenes and inactivation of tumour suppressor genes has now been demonstrated in a number of human tumours, including large bowel cancer.

Cancer results from the effects of environmental carcinogens and genetic predisposition. Many carcinogens are mutagens. Environmental factors – of which diet is probably the most important – are largely responsible for the causation of large bowel cancer (Seventh King's Fund Forum, 1990). Cancers arising from the effects of environmental agents are said to be sporadic. For patients with hereditary forms of cancer, it has been postulated that cancer susceptibility is inherited dominantly through a germ line mutation affecting one copy (or allele) of a tumour suppressor gene. Such mutations represent the first step in a recessive change leading to the malignant phenotype; the second event inactivating the normal remaining allele occurs subsequently in a somatic cell (Knudson, 1985; *Lancet*, 1984). Several hereditary causes of large bowel cancer are recognized, including familial adenomatous polyposis (FAP) and hereditary non-polyposis colorectal cancer (HNPCC; for review, see Murday & Slack, 1989). FAP is inherited in an autosomal dominant manner and is responsible for perhaps 1% of all colorectal cancers. It is characterized by multiple colorectal adenomas (the average number per patient being about 1000). Untreated, these patients will invariably go on to develop large bowel malignancy. Gardner's syndrome is a variant of FAP in which there are the extracolonic manifestations of osteomas and epidermoid cysts. HNPCC is also inherited in an autosomal dominant manner but, as the name suggests, the large bowel adenomatosis characteristic of FAP is absent in this condition. It exists in two forms, Lynch syndromes type I and type II, and probably accounts for between 4 and 13% of all large bowel cancers. The tumours in Lynch syndrome type I (also known as site-specific colon cancer) occur in the mid 40s (compared with mid 60s for sporadic colorectal cancers) and are predominantly right-sided. The affected individuals are more likely to have synchronous tumours and it is reported that 40% will develop metachronous lesions within 10 years.

The description of Lynch syndrome type II (or cancer family syndrome) is based on studies of a large family in which colorectal cancer predominates but adenocarcinomas at other sites, such as uterus and ovary, are recognized. Although hereditary cancers arguably account for less than 10–15% of all malignant tumours of the colon and rectum, the true contribution of hereditary factors is unknown. Recent evidence, based on the frequency of colorectal cancer in the first-degree relatives of patients with the disease, would suggest that inherited susceptibility is considerably greater than previous suspected (Cannon-Albright *et al.*,1988).

Genetic changes associated with the adenoma–carcinoma sequence

Colorectal cancer is now being used extensively as a model for the genetic analysis of tumour progression in humans. Large bowel tumours have proved to be particularly useful in this regard because they are characterized by a well-defined premalignant stage. Both clinical and pathological data indicate that large bowel cancers do not arise *de novo* but develop in pre-existing benign adenomatous polyps – the adenoma–carcinoma sequence.

Analysis of the genetic material from premalignant adenomatous polyps and malignant tumours has revealed a high frequency of *ras* mutations and the loss of specific chromosomal regions (allelic loss), the latter being taken as evidence that the affected regions contain tumour suppressor genes (Bos *et al.*, 1987; Vogelstein *et al.*, 1988; Fearon & Vogelstein, 1990; Cho & Vogelstein, 1992).

Vogelstein and his colleagues have constructed a genetic model for colorectal tumorigenesis based on the adenoma–carcinoma sequence (Fearon & Vogelstein, 1990). They postulate that the first genetic change in the progression, which precedes polyp formation, is mutation of a tumour suppressor gene on chromosome 5. The loss of methyl groups from DNA is deemed to be an early event and probably contributes to the derangement of mitosis, leading to the gain and loss of chromosomes by cells. Progression to increasing adenoma size and frank malignancy is associated with *ras* mutation, followed by loss of genetic material on the long arm of chromosome 18 and subsequent loss of the short arm of chromosome 17. It should be noted that, in the model described, adenomatous polyps were assigned to one of three somewhat arbitrary stages, namely early (or class I), intermediate (or class II) and late (or class III), with size, grade of dysplasia and villous component generally increasing from early to late. Such staging is clearly artificial and is not recognized as a clinicopathological classification. Although this model is presented with each of the genetic events allocated to a particular stage of tumour progression in an apparently fixed sequence, its formulators argue that it is the accumulation of changes, rather than the order of occurrence, which is important for the development of large bowel malignancy.

ras *Gene mutations*

Mutations of *ras* were found in approximately 50% of both adenomatous polyps (intermediate and late stage), and malignant tumours (Bos *et al.*, 1987). This genetic change is represented almost invariably by single-base substitution at codon 12 of the c-Ki-*ras* gene. Analysis of adenomas of less than 1 cm in size revealed that fewer than 10% contained *ras* mutations. Therefore, *ras* activation, although a relatively early event in progression, is not considered to be the first genetic alteration in the adenoma–carcinoma sequence.

The *ras* gene encodes a protein, p21, which is found bound to the inner plasma membrane. The current hypothesis regarding the function of the *ras* product is that it acts as a G-protein. The point mutation in the gene results in an amino acid substitution in p21 and appears to reduce its capacity to terminate a growth-stimulatory signal. Such an event might lead to uncontrolled growth and could represent one mechanism by which the altered protein contributes to transformation.

Allelic losses and candidate tumour suppressor genes

By comparing the genetic material from tumours with that from adjacent normal tissue, it is possible to identify regions of chromosomal losses which have occurred during tumour progression. The description of the frequency of chromosomal loss from a particular tumour type is usually called the allelotype (Vogelstein *et al.*, 1989). Generally, losses involve only one of the two parental chromosomes. Regions of chromosomes which are frequently lost (or deleted) are believed to be indicative of genetic material harbouring tumour suppressor genes. It is now recognized that the loss of specific chromosomal regions is a common occurrence during colorectal tumour progression.

Chromosome 17

The most frequent site of chromosomal loss (allelic loss) in human colorectal cancer has been found to be the short arm of chromosome 17 (greater than 75% of tumours analysed; Baker *et al.*, 1989). This event appears to occur relatively late in the progression model, occurring in the transition between late adenoma and carcinoma. However, such an event would be expected to inactivate only one of the two alternative forms (or alleles) of a tumour suppressor gene. Detailed genetic analysis has narrowed down the common region of deletion. A putative tumour suppressor gene, p53, is known to be contained within this region on chromosome 17. Since there are two copies of each gene (one maternal, one paternal), a second genetic event is required to inactivate completely tumour suppressor function. Subsequent studies have shown that the remaining p53 allele is frequently mutated, thereby inactivating this copy too. Inactivation of p53 seems to be an almost invariable component in the progression of human malignancies. The protein encoded by p53 has a DNA-binding function. A current view of the role of the normal protein is that of a 'molecular policeman', which switches off replication when DNA is damaged (Lane, 1992).

Chromosome 18

Allelic loss affecting the long arm of chromosome 18 has been demonstrated in over 70% of large bowel cancers and 47% of class III adenomas (Vogelstein *et al.*, 1988). Slightly more than 10% of class I and class II adenomas had allelic deletions affecting this chromosome arm, indicating that the genetic change usually occurs late in the progression of large bowel cancer. A gene mapping to this region on chromosome 18 has been cloned and named DCC (for deleted in colorectal cancer; Fearon *et al.*, 1990). The encoded protein of this putative candidate tumour suppressor gene shares homology with a CAM. The loss of cell–cell contacts resulting from inactivation of such a gene might well play a part in tumour progression by disrupting cellular organization and communication as well as affecting growth and differentiation.

Chromosome 5

Almost 40% of colorectal cancers have been shown to have allelic loss affecting the long arm of chromosome 5 (Vogelstein *et al.*, 1988, 1989). No evidence of allelic loss was found in class I adenomas but the frequency of loss was almost 30% in both intermediate and late polyps. In 1987 the gene responsible for FAP was mapped to the long arm of chromosome 5 (Bodmer *et al.*, 1987). However, no evidence was found of allelic loss affecting this genetic region in the DNA of adenomas from patients with FAP, indicating that the recessive change on chromosome 5 must be secondary to polyp formation (Solomon *et al.*, 1987). Bodmer and colleagues (1987) postulated that the inactivation of one copy of a tumour suppressor gene on chromosome 5 (for example, by mutation rather than by allelic loss) is sufficient to permit random fluctuations of the FAP gene product, resulting in escape from growth control and polyp formation.

Two genes have now been cloned from the region on the long arm of chromosome 5, identified by Bodmer *et al.*, as the location of the FAP gene. The first, MCC (for mutated in colorectal cancer), was shown to be mutated in sporadic large bowel cancers and was therefore proposed as a putative colorectal tumour suppressor gene (Kinzler *et al.*, 1991a). To date there is no evidence of germ line mutations of MCC in FAP patients. Therefore, MCC is unlikely to be the FAP gene. The second gene, adenomatous polyposis coli (APC), has been mapped to the same region on chromosome 5 as MCC. This gene is mutated in the germ line of patients with FAP (as well as in some sporadic tumours) and is therefore proposed as the gene responsible for FAP/Gardner's syndrome (Groden *et al.*, 1991; Kinzler *et al.*, 1991b; Cottrell *et al.*, 1992). How two closely spaced genes such as APC and MCC affect the development of sporadic colorectal carcinogenesis is, for the moment, unclear. Similarities between the protein products of the two genes have been identified, indicating involvement in the same biochemical pathways (Kinzler *et al.*, 1991b). One possibility is that the two gene products interact to form a complex.

Genetic mapping of locus predisposing to HNPCC

Recent evidence from a study of two large families suggests close linkage between a genetic locus on chromosome 2 and predisposition to HNPCC (Peltomaki *et al.*, 1993). Comparison of the genetic changes in tumours of these patients with those in 'sporadic' cancers suggests that numerous replication errors had occurred during the development of the familial tumours (Aaltonen *et al.*, 1993). No evidence for loss of heterozygosity affecting chromosome 2 has been found (in either familial or sporadic cancers), suggesting a genetic mechanism other than that expected of a tumour suppressor gene at this locus. One suggestion is that a gene generating genetic instability could represent one component of cancer predisposition (Aaltonen *et al.*, 1993; Thibodeau *et al.*, 1993).

Metastasis-associated genes

A number of approaches have been taken to identify and isolate metastasis-inducing and metastasis-suppressing genes. The transfer of genetic material between cells, known as DNA transfection, represents one of the techniques most frequently used. Another approach that has proved useful in identifying putative metastasis-associated genes is complementary DNA differential screening in which messenger RNAs from primary and secondary tumours, or metastatic variants of murine cell lines, have been compared (Elvin *et al.*, 1988; Steeg *et al.*, 1988; Ebralidze *et al.*, 1989; Hart & Easty 1991).

Oncogenes

Induction of the colonizing and/or metastatic phenotype has been achieved by transfection of cells with a number of activated oncogenes, including *ras*, *mos*, *fes*, *fms*, *src* and *myc* (Thorgeirsson *et al.*, 1985; Egan *et al.*, 1987). However, many of these studies are incomplete since they do not take into account the effect of the oncogene on tumorigenicity.

The transfer of *ras* oncogenes into a non-metastatic murine fibroblast cell line has been shown to induce highly metastatic behaviour in the recipient cells when injected into nude mice (Thorgeirsson *et al.*, 1985). Subsequent studies have shown that activated *ras* can induce colonizing or metastatic behaviour in rodent and human cells tested in experimental animals (Muschel *et al.*, 1985; Pozzatti *et al.*, 1986; Pohl *et al.*, 1988; Bonfil *et al.*, 1989). The mechanisms by which transfer of *ras* has such profound effects on metastasis remain wholly obscure. One possibility is that *ras* induces growth factor secretion (Roberts & Sporn, 1986). In one of the experimental systems the induction of the lung-colonizing phenotype in the mouse fibroblasts following transfection with the *ras* oncogene was associated with secretion of collagenase type IV (*in vitro*; Thorgeirsson *et al.*, 1985). Evidence has also been reported that the ability of murine fibroblasts transfected with *ras* to invade and metastasize is associated with the capacity to secrete and respond to AMF (Liotta *et al.*, 1986).

The profound effects of *ras* on the metastatic phenotype are not consistent with the data from Vogelstein's studies in which *ras* activation is considered to be a relatively early event in the adenoma–carcinoma sequence. Furthemore, although there was an early report that elevated levels of p21 were correlated with increasing depth of invasion for human large bowel cancers (Thor *et al.*, 1984), subsequent reports have failed to confirm this relationship (Albino *et al.*, 1984; Gallick *et al.*, 1985; Kerr *et al.*, 1986).

nm23

The gene *nm23*, identified by differential screening of variants of a murine melanoma (K-1735), has attracted a lot of attention. It is of interest because reduced *nm23* RNA levels are apparently associated with increased lung-colonizing and lung metastatic potential (Steeg *et al.*, 1988). By analogy to tumour suppressor genes, *nm23* has been labelled a metastasis suppressor gene (Leone *et al.*, 1991; Hart & Saini, 1992). The protein encoded by *nm23* has sequence homology with a developmentally regulated protein in *Drosophila*. Mutations in the *Drosophila* gene result in disordered morphology and abnormal differentiation (Rosengard *et al.*, 1989). Experiments have been reported which appear to support the claim that *nm23* is a metastasis suppressor gene (Leone *et al.*, 1991). However, careful analysis of the data reveals that the transfection of the *nm23* gene into metastatic cells not only attenuated metastatic potential, but consistently effected a loss of tumour-forming ability in the recipient cells (compared with control cells). The weight of recent evidence would, therefore, suggest that *nm23* is more likely to be a tumour suppressor gene. Furthermore, studies of *nm23* levels in human large bowel cancers failed to demonstrate a correlation with clinical stage (Steeg, 1991; Myeroff & Markowitz, 1993).

mts-1

The gene *mts-1* was identified by a modification of differential screening (Ebralidze *et al.*, 1989). It appears to be expressed specifically in metastatic cells (of a mammary carcinoma), lymphocytes and cells of lymphoid organs (Ebralidze *et al.*, 1989). The encoded protein of *mts-1* shows homology with a family of calcium-binding proteins. These proteins are found in all cells and are involved in regulating the activity of proteins, including enzymes and elements of the cytoskeletal system. The activation of the calcium-binding protein by calcium induces a change in the confirmation of the molecule, facilitating its interaction with structural protein molecules and enzymes. The role of *mts-1* in the metastatic cell has still to be elucidated. Transfection of non-metastatic tumour cells with *mts-1* complementary DNA has been shown to induce metastasis. Also of interest is the high degree of homology between the protein encoded by *mts-1* and two human proteins, MRP 14 and MRP 8 which are also calcium-binding proteins of the same subclass, and which occur at high abundance in granulocytes and macrophages in inflamed tissue. Both MRP 14 and MRP 8 are related to macrophage migration-inhibiting factor. Whether the human and mouse proteins have related functions, and how these functions might affect metastasis, are questions yet to be investigated, particularly in view of the importance of the role played by calcium ions in signal transduction pathways.

Gene encoding CD44

One further putative metastasis-related gene, encoding the lymphocyte homing receptor CD44, merits consideration. The observation that lymphocytes carry a lymph node homing receptor, and that this receptor is responsible for tissue-specific lymphocyte–endothelial cell attachment, has attracted a lot of interest (Stoolman, 1989). If metastatic tumour cells mimic lymphocytes, a similar mechanism might be responsible for the observed pattern of organ involvement in metastatic disease. The lymphocyte receptor molecule CD44 consists of a proteoglycan-like domain on the cell surface and a transmembrane domain; a large number of CD44 variants are possible, generated by alternative splicing of pre-messenger RNA (Gunthert *et al.*, 1991). Other reported functions for CD44 include anchoring of epithelium to basement membrane, attachment of fibroblasts to components of the ECM and the regulation of fibroblast motility and shape (Stoolman, 1989; Haynes *et al.*, 1991).

A CD44 variant was detected and isolated from the surface of metastatic cells of a rat pancreatic carcinoma cell line using a monoclonal antibody (Gunthert *et al.*, 1991). This particular variant was shown to have an additional 162 amino acids and was not detected on the cell surface of non-metastatic cells from the same cell line. To test the significance of this variant CD44 on metastatic propensity, DNA encoding the protein was transfected into a non-metastatic variant of the rat pancreatic cancer *in vitro*. The recipient cells were then injected into syngeneic rats and shown to be metastatic. The additional 162 amino acids, which are present in the extracellular domain of the CD44 molecule, are responsible for metastasis in this particular rat model since the non-metastatic variants were shown to express 'normal' CD44.

Moreover, it has been reported that the pattern of variant CD44 messenger RNAs distinguished between 23 tumours (breast or colon) known to have metastasized and eight that had no detectable metastases (Matsumura & Tarin, 1992).

Summary

The metastatic spread of large bowel cancer is a complex process involving the transfer of tumour cells from the primary tumour through the host tissues to the sites of secondary growth such as the liver. The mechanisms thought to contribute to this process have been reviewed. To date, metastasis research has not had a significant impact in the clinic but we are now entering a most exciting phase in molecular medicine, with the hope of major benefits for patients.

There would appear to be two groups of patients with large bowel cancer: the majority, perhaps three-quarters, die of their disease predominantly from metastasis; the remainder are cured by surgery alone. The differences between the two types of tumour or two types of patient for the moment remain elusive. Detailed molecular analysis of large bowel tumours has failed to identify genes reponsible for the metastatic process, although it would appear that loss of genetic material (sites of tumour/metastasis supressor genes?) is greater in more aggressive tumours (Kern *et al.*, 1989; Fearon & Vogelstein, 1990). Recent evidence would also suggest that new areas of genetic interest could emerge from studies of allelic losses in tumour cells of liver metastases (Ookawa *et al.*, 1993). Attempts to address differences in host responses in these two groups of patients have received little attention.

The possibility remains that metastasis is a random process and that no metastasis-specific genes will be demonstrable. Many of the cell functions discussed above may only be of secondary importance to tumour growth potential (the primary determinant of metastatic capacity?), so that variations in expression of these various phenotypes simply alter the likelihood of an individual cell completing the metastatic process.

From a clinical viewpoint the direction of much of metastasis research might be questioned. Some 40–50% of patients have established metastatic spread at diagnosis with half of the remainder suffering relapse after undergoing 'curative surgery'. Although clinical studies are under way to assess the therapeutic potential of inhibitors of signal transduction pathways to block metastatic growth following resection of the primary tumour (Kohn *et al.*, 1992), an argument can be made that a much greater emphasis should be placed on approaches aimed at controlling secondary growth (of micro- and established metastases) in organs such as the liver and lungs.

Molecular studies are beginning to impinge on clinical management of large bowel cancer. The discovery of the gene for polyposis coli will result in more effective screening. Identification of APC mutations has major implications for the patients and families afflicted with FAP. Members of FAP families can now be tested directly for mutations pre- and postnatally and such expertise will make a significant impact on genetic counselling. As more information on the mutations in the APC gene becomes available and as screening tests improve it may be possible to demonstrate that some patients with colorectal cancer (but not FAP) do indeed have inherited mutations, explaining the findings of Cannon-Albright and colleagues. It has also been reported that cells carrying genetic mutations can be detected in the stools of patients with colorectal cancers (Sidransky *et al.*, 1992). The application of such techniques might well provide a new approach to cancer screening.

As the molecular changes become better understood this will lead in turn to a clearer picture of tumour biochemistry. With clarification of the genetics of polyposis the prevention of adenoma development becomes a possibility through the identification of critical biochemical pathways. Such areas are currently being explored (Waddell *et al.*, 1989; Kinzler *et al.*, 1991b).

Finally, the surgeon performing a 'curative operation' must not contribute to tumour dissemination either locally or distally. Adjuvant therapy with TIMPs or synthetic peptides (to block interaction with the ECM) could prove to be beneficial.

References

Aaltonen LA, Peltomaki P, Leach FS *et al.* (1993) Clues to the pathogenesis of familial colorectal cancer. *Science* **260**, 812–816.

Alberts B, Bray D, Lewis J, Raff M, Roberts K & Watson JD (eds) (1983) *Molecular Biology of the Cell.* New York: Garland.

Albino AP, Le Strange R, Oliff AI, Furth ME & Old LJ (1984) Transforming *ras* genes from human melanoma: a manifestation of tumour heterogeneity? *Nature* **308**, 69–72.

Alexander P (1983) Dormant metastases – studies in experimental animals. *J. Pathol.* **141**, 379–383.

Baker SJ, Fearon ER, Nigro JM *et al.* (1989) Chromosome 17 deletions and p53 gene mutations in colorectal carcinomas. *Science* **244**, 217–221.

Bell C, Frost P & Keber RS (1991) Cytogenetic heterogeneity of genetically marked and metastatically competent 'dominant' tumour cell clones. *Cancer Genet. Cytogenet.* **54**, 153–161.

Bodmer WF, Bailey CJ, Bodmer J *et al.* (1987) Localisation of the gene for familial adenomatous polyposis on chromosome 5. *Nature* **328**, 614–616.

Bonfil RD, Reddel RR, Ura H *et al.* (1989) Invasive and metastatic potential of a V-Ha-*ras* transformed human bronchial epithelial cell line. *J. Natl Cancer Inst.* **81**, 587–594.

Bos JL, Fearon ER, Hamilton SR, de Vries MV, van Boom JH, van der Eb AJ and Vogelstein B (1987) Prevalence of *ras* gene mutations in human colorectal cancers. *Nature* **327**, 293–303.

Cannon-Albright LA, Skolnick MH, Bishop DT, Lee RG & Burt RW (1988) Common inheritance of susceptibility to colonic adenomatous polyps and associated colorectal cancers. *N. Engl. J. Med.* **319**, 533–537.

Carlsen SA, Ramshaw IA & Warrington RC (1984) Involvement of plasminogen activator production with tumour metastases in a rat model. *Cancer Res.* **44**, 3012–3016.

Carter RL (1982) Some aspects of the metastatic process. *J. Clin. Pathol.* **35**, 1041–1049.

Cavanaugh PG & Nicolson GL (1989) Purification and some properties of a lung-derived growth factor that differentially stimulates the growth of tumour cells metastatic to the lung. *Cancer Res.* **49**, 3928–3933.

Chambers AF & Ling V (1984) Selection of experimental metastatic ability of heterologous tumour cells in the chick embryo after DNA-mediated transfer. *Cancer Res.* **44**, 3970–3975.

Cho KR & Vogelstein B (1992) Genetic alterations in the adenoma–carcinoma sequence. *Cancer* **70**, 1727–1731.

Cottrell S, Bicknell D, Kaklamanis L & Bodmer WF (1992) Molecular analysis of APC mutations in familial adenomatous polyposis and sporadic colon carcinomas. *Lancet* **340**, 626–630.

Crissman JD, Hatfield J, Schaldenbrand M, Sloane BF & Honn KV (1985). Arrest and extravasation of the B16 amelanotic melanoma in murine lungs. *Lab. Invest.* **53**, 470–478.

Early Breast Cancer Trialists' Collaborative Group (1992) Systemic treatment of early breast cancer by hormonal, cytotoxic or immune therapy. *Lancet* **339**, 71–85.

Ebralidze A, Tulchinsky E, Grigorian M *et al.* (1989) Isolation and characterisation of a gene specifically expressed in different metastatic cells and whose deduced gene product has a high degree of homology to a Ca^{2+}-binding protein family. *Genes Dev.* **3**, 1086–1093.

Egan SE, Wright JA, Jarolim L, Yanagihara K, Bassin RH & Greenberg AH (1987) Transformation by oncogenes encoding protein kinases induces the metastatic phenotype. *Science* **238**, 202–205.

Elvin P, Kerr IB, McArdle CS & Birnie GD (1988) Isolation and preliminary characterisation of cDNA clones representing mRNAs associated with tumour progression and metastasis in colorectal cancer. *Br. J. Cancer* **57**, 36–42.

Evans CW (1991) *The Metastatic Cell*, pp. 104–107. London: Chapman & Hall.

Fearon ER & Vogelstein B (1990) A genetic model for colorectal tumorigenesis. *Cell* **61**, 759–767.

Fearon ER, Cho KR, Nigro JM *et al.* (1990) Identification of a chromosome 18q gene that is altered in colorectal cancers. *Science* **247**, 49–56.

Fidler IJ (1973) Selection of successive tumour lines for metastasis. *Nature New Biol.* **242**, 148–149.

Fidler IJ (1986) Rationale and methods for the use of nude mice to study the biology and therapy of human cancer metastasis. *Cancer Metastasis Rev.* **5**, 29–49.

Fidler IJ (1991) Orthotopic implantation of human colon carcinomas into nude mice provides a valuable model for the biology and therapy of metastasis. *Cancer Metastasis Rev.* **10**, 229–243.

Fidler IJ & Kripke ML (1977) Metastasis results from preexisting variant cells within a malignant tumour. *Science* **197**, 893–895.

Fidler IJ, Barnes Z, Fogler WE, Kirsh R, Bugelski P & Poste G (1982) Involvement of macrophages in the eradication of established metastases following IV injection of liposomes containing macrophage activators. *Cancer Res.* **42**, 496.

Fidler IJ, Jessup JM, Fogler WE, Staerkel R & Mazunder A (1986) Activation of tumoricidal properties in peripheral blood monocytes of patients with colorectal carcinoma. *Cancer Res.* **45**, 994–998.

Gallick GE, Kurzrock R, Kloetzer WS, Arlinghaus RB & Gutterman JU (1985) Expression of p21 *ras* in fresh primary and metastatic human colorectal tumours. *Proc. Natl Acad. Sci. USA* **82**, 1795–1799.

Gasic GJ (1984) Role of plasma, platelets and endothelial cells in tumour metastasis. *Cancer Metastasis Rev.* **3**, 99–116.

Gasic GJ, Tuszynski GP & Gorelik E (1986) Interaction of the haemostatic and immune systems in the metastatic spread of tumour cells. In: Richter GW (ed), *International Review of Experimental Pathology*, pp. 173–212. London: Academic Press.

Gherardi E, Gray J, Stoker M, Perryman M & Furlong R (1980) Purification of scatter factor, a fibroblast-derived basic protein that modulates epithelial interactions and movement. *Proc. Natl Acad. Sci. USA* **86**, 5844–58.

Giavazzi R, Alessandri G, Spreafico F, Garattini S & Mantovani A (1980) Metastasizing capacity of tumour cells from spontaneous metastases of transplanted murine tumours. *Br. J. Cancer* **42**, 462–472.

Glaves D (1983) Correlation between circulating cancer cells and incidence of metastases. *Br. J. Cancer* **48**, 665–673.

Groden J, Thliveris A, Samowitz W *et al.* (1991) Identification and characterisation of the familial adenomatous polyposis coli gene. *Cell* **66**, 589–600.

Guillou PJ (1987) Potential impact of immunobiotechnology on cancer therapy. *Br. J. Surg.* **74**, 705–710.

Gullino PM & Liotta LA (1981) Cell shedding by tumours. In: Weiss L & Gilber HA (eds) *Bone Metastasis*, pp. 11–20. Boston, MA: GI Hall.

Gunthert U, Hofmann M & Rudy W (1991) A new variant of glycoprotein CD44 confers metastatic potential to rat carcinoma cells. *Cell* **65**, 13–24.

Hanna N (1982) Role of natural killer cell in control of cancer metastasis. *Cancer Metastasis Rev.* **1**, 45–65.

Hart IR (1985) Molecular basis of tumour spread. *Nature* **315**, 274–275.

Hart IR & Easty D (1991) Identification of genes controlling metastatic behaviour. *Br. J. Cancer* **63**, 9–12.

Hart IR & Fidler IJ (1980) Cancer invasion and metastasis. *Q. Rev. Biol.* **55**, 121–142.

Hart IR & Saini A (1992) Biology of tumour metastases. *Lancet* **339**, 1453–1457.

Haynes BF, Liao H-X & Patton KL (1991) The transmembrane hyaluronate receptor (CD44): multiple functions, multiple forms. *Cancer Cells* **3**, 347–350.

Heald RJ (1988) The 'holy plane' of rectal surgery. *J. R. Soc. Med.* **81**, 503–508.

Hoover HC, Surdyke MG, Dangel RB, Peters LC & Hanna MG (1985) Prospectively randomized trial of adjuvant active-specific immunotherapy for human colorectal cancer. *Cancer* **55**, 1236–1243.

Humphries MJ, Olden K & Yamada KM (1986) A synthetic peptide from fibronectin inhibits experimental metastasis of murine melanoma cells. *Science* **233**, 467–470.

Iwamoto Y, Robey FA & Graf J (1987) YIGSR, a synthetic laminin pentapeptide, inhibits experimental metastasis formation. *Science* **238**, 1132–1134.

Jessup JM & Thomas P (1989) Carcinoembryonic antigen: function in metastasis by human colorectal carcinoma. *Cancer Metastasis Rev.* **8**, 263–280.

Johnson JP, Stade BG, Holzmann B, Schwable W & Rietmuller G (1989) *De novo* expression of intercellular-adhesion molecule in melanoma correlates with increased risk of metastasis. *Proc. Natl Acad. Sci. USA* **86**, 641-644.

Kerbel RS, Waghorne C, Korczak B, Lagarde A & Breikman ML (1988) Clonal dominance of primary tumours by metastatic cells: genetic analysis and biological implications. *Cancer Surv.* **7**, 597–629.

Kern SE, Fearonf ER, Tersmette KWF *et al.* (1989) Allelic loss in colorectal carcinoma. *J.A.M.A.* **261**, 3099–3103.

Kerr IB, Spandidos DA, Finlay IG, Lee FD & McArdle CS (1986) The relation of *ras* family oncogene expression to conventional staging criteria and clinical outcome in colorectal carcinoma. *Br. J. Cancer* **53**, 231–235.

Khokha R, Waterhouse P & Yagel S (1989) Antisense RNA-induced reduction in murine TIMP levels confers oncogenicity on Swiss 3T3 cells. *Science* **243**, 947–950.

Kinzler KW, Nilbert MC, Vogelstein B *et al.* (1991a) Identification of a gene located at chromosome 5q21 that is mutated in colorectal cancers. *Science* **251**, 1366–1370.

Kinzler KW, Nilbert MC, Su L-K *et al.* (1991b) Identification of FAP locus genes from chromosome 5q21. *Science* **253**, 661–669.

Kleinman HK, McGarvey ML & Hassell JR (1986) Basement membrane complexes with biological activity. *Biochemistry* **25**, 312–318.

Knudson AG (1985) Hereditary cancer, oncogenes and antioncogenes. *Cancer Res.* **45**, 1437–1443.

Kohn EC, Holmes K & Liotta LA (1992) Signal transduction therapy of metastasis. *Clin. Exp. Metastasis* **10** (suppl. 1), 66.

Kozlowski JM, Fidler JJ, Campbell D, Xu Z-I, Kaighn ME & Hart IR (1984) Metastatic behaviour of human tumour cell lines grown in the nude mouse. *Cancer Res.* **44**, 3522–3529.

Lancet (1984) Clues from familial cancer. *Lancet* 1219–1220.

Lane DP (1992) p53, Guardian of the genome. *Nature* **358**, 15–16.

Leone A, Flatow U & Richter-King C (1991) Reduced tumour incidence, metastatic potential and cytokine responsiveness of nm 23-transfected melanoma cells. *Cell* **65**, 25–35.

Ling V, Chambers F, Harris JF & Hill RP (1985) Quantitative genetic analysis of tumour progression. *Cancer Metastasis Rev.* **4**, 173–192.

Linsk RL & Goodenow RS (1986) Immunological and non-immunological roles of the major histocompatibility complex in tumorigenesis. *Cancer Rev.* **6**, 40–62.

Liotta LA & Stetler-Stevenson WG (1991) Tumour invasion and metastasis: an imbalance of positive and negative regulation. *Cancer Res.* **51**, 5054–5059.

Liotta LA, Kleinerman J & Saider GM (1976) The significance of hematogenous tumour cell clumps in the metastatic process. *Cancer Res.* **36**, 889–894.

Liotta LA, Rao CN & Barsky SH (1983) Tumour invasion and the extracellular matrix. *Lab. Invest.* **49**, 636–649.

Liotta LA, Mandler R, Murano G *et al.* (1986) Tumour cell autocrine motility factor. *Proc. Natl Acad. Sci. USA* **83**, 3302–3306.

McArdle CS, Hole D, Hansell D, Blumgart LH & Wood CB (1990) Prospective study of colorectal cancer in the west of Scotland: 10 year follow up. *Br. J. Surg.* **77**, 280–282.

Matsumura Y & Tarin D (1992) Significance of CD44 gene products for cancer diagnosis and disease evaluation. *Lancet* **340**, 1053–1058.

Murday V & Slack J (1989) Inherited disorders associated with colorectal cancer. *Cancer Surv.* **8**, 139–157.

Muschel RJ, Williams JE, Lowy DR & Liotta LA (1985) Harvey *ras* induction of metastatic potential depends upon oncogene activation and the type of recipient cell. *Am. J. Pathol.* **121**, 1–8.

Myeroff LL & Markowitz SD (1993) Increased nm23-H1 and nm 23-H2 messenger RNA expression and absence of mutations in colon carcinomas of low and high metastatic potential. *J. Natl Cancer Inst.* **85**, 147–152.

Nowell PC (1976) The clonal evolution of tumour cell populations. *Science* **194**, 23–28.

Ookawa K, Sakamoto M, Hirohashi S *et al.* (1993) Concordant p53 and DCC alterations and allelic losses on chromosomes 13q and 14q associated with liver metastases of colorectal carcinoma *Int. J. Cancer* **53**, 382–387.

Paget S (1889) The distribution of secondary growths in cancer of the breast. *Lancet* **1**, 571–573.

Peltomaki P, Aaltonen LA, Sistonen P, Pylkkanen L, Mecklin J-P & Jarvinen H (1993) Genetic mapping of a locus predisposing to human colorectal cancer. *Science* **260**, 810–812.

Pickford IR (1991) Immunity and tumour metastasis. In: Pollock AV (ed). *Immunology in Surgical Practice* pp. 150–175. London: Edward Arnold.

Pickford IR & Cooke TG (1990) Oncogenes. *Curr. Pract. Surg.* **2**, 195–201.

Pohl J, Radler-Pohl A, Franks LM & Schirrmacher V (1988) Analysis of metastatic competence of mouse bladder carcinoma cells after transfection with activated Ha-*ras* or N-*ras* oncogenes. *J. Cancer Res. Clin. Oncol.* **114**, 373–379.

Pozzatti R, Muschel R, Williams J *et al.* (1986) Primary rat embryo cells transformed by one or two oncogenes show different metastatic potentials. *Science* **232**, 223–227.

Price JE, Ankerman SL & Fidler IJ (1986) Evidence that the process of murine melanoma metastasis is sequential and selective and contains stochastic elements. *Cancer Res.* **46**, 5172–5178.

Roberts AB & Sporn MB (1986) Growth factors and transformation. *Cancer Surv.* **5**, 405–412.

Rosenberg SA (1990) Immunotherapy with recombinant cytokines and activated lymphocytes in patients with advanced cancer. *Clin. Exp. Metastasis* **8** (suppl. 1), 13.

Rosenberg SA, Lotze MT & Muul LM (1985) Observations of the systemic administration of autologous lymphokine-activated killer cells and recombinant interleukin-2 patients with metastatic cancer. *N. Engl. J. Med.* **313**, 1485–1492.

Rosenberg SA, Spiess P & Lafreniere R (1986) A new approach to the adoptive immunotherapy of cancer with tumour-infiltrating lymphocytes. *Science* **223**, 1318–1321.

Rosengard AM, Krutzsch HC & Shearn A (1989) Reduced Nm 23/Awd protein in tumour metastasis and aberrant *Drosophila* development. *Nature* **342**, 177–180.

Saiki I, Murata J & Iida J (1989) Antimetastatic effects of synthetic polypeptides containing repeated structures of the cell adhesive Arg-Gly-Asp (RGD) and Tyr-Ile-Gly-Ser-Arg (YIGSR) sequences. *Br. J. Cancer* **60**, 722–728.

Schreiber AB, Schlessinger J & Edidin M (1984) Interaction betwen major histocompatibility complex antigens and epidermal growth factor receptors on human cells. *J. Cell Biol.* **98**, 725–731.

Schultz RM, Silberman S, Persky B, Bajkowski AS & Carmichael DF (1988) Inhibition by human recombinant tissue inhibitor of metalloproteinases of human amnion invasion and lung colonisation by murine B16-F10 melanoma cells. *Cancer Res.* **48**, 5539–5545.

Seventh King's Fund Forum Consensus Statement (1990) Cancer of the Colon and Rectum. *BMJ* **300**, 1675.

Sharkey FE & Fogh J (1979) Metastasis of human tumours in athymic nude mice. *Int. J. Cancer* **24**, 733–738.

Sidransky D, Tokino T, Hamilton SAR *et al.* (1992) Identification of *ras* oncogene mutations in the stool of patients with curable colorectal tumours. *Science* **256**, 102–105.

Solomon E, Voss R, Hall V *et al.* (1987) Chromosome 5 allele loss in human colorectal carcinomas. *Nature* **328**, 616–691.

Stackpole CW (1981) Distinct lung-colonising and lung-metastasising cell populations in B16 mouse melanoma. *Nature* **289**, 798–800.

Stackpole CW (1983) Generation of phenotypic diversity in the B16 mouse melanoma relative to spontaneous metastasis. *Cancer Res.* **43**, 573–580.

Staroselsky AN, Radinsky R, Fidler IJ, Pathak S, Chernajovsky Y & Frost P (1992) The use of molecular genetic markers to demonstrate the effect of organ environment on clonal dominance in a human renal-cell carcinoma grown in nude mice. *Int. J. Cancer* **51**, 130–138.

Steeg PS (1991) Genetic control of the metastatic phenotype. *Cancer Biol.* **2**, 105–110.

Steeg PS, Bevilacqua G, Kopper L *et al.* (1988) Evidence for a novel gene associated with low tumour metastatic potential. *J. Natl Cancer Inst.* **80**, 200–204.

Stoker M, Gherardi E, Perryman M & Gray J (1987) Scatter factor is a fibroblast-derived modulator of epithelial cell mobility. *Nature* **327**, 239–242.

Stoolman LM (1989) Adhesions molecules controlling lymphocyte migration. *Cell* **56**, 907–910.

Sugarbaker EV (1981) Patterns of metastasis in human malignancies. In: Marchalonis J, Hanna MG & Fidler IJ (eds) *Cancer Biology Reviews*, Vol. 2, pp. 235–278. New York: Marcel Dekker.

Takeichi M (1991) Cadherin cell adhesion receptors as a morphogenetic regulator. *Science* **251**, 1451–1455.

Terranova VP, Hujanen ES, Loeb DM, Martin GR, Thornburg & Glushko V (1986) Use of reconstituted basement membrane to measure cell invasiveness and select for highly invasive tumour cells. *Proc. Natl Acad. Sci USA* **83**, 465–469.

Thibodeau SN, Bren G & Schaid D (1993) Microsatellite instability in cancer of the proximal colon. *Science* **260**, 816–819.

Thor A, Horan Hand P, Wunderlich D, Caruso A, Muraro R & Schlom J. (1984) Monoclonal antibodies define differential *ras* gene expression in malignant benign colonic diseases. *Nature* **311**, 562–565.

Thorgeirsson UP, Turpeenniemi-Hujanen T, Williams JE *et al.* (1985) NIH/3T3 cells transfected with human tumour DNA containing activated *ras* oncogenes express the metastatic phenotype in nude mice. *Mol. Cell. Biol.* **5**, 259–262.

Vleminckx K, Vakaet L, Mareel M, Fiers W & Van Roy F (1991) Genetic manipulation of E-cadherin expression by epithelial tumour cells reveals an invasion suppressor role. *Cell* **66**, 107–119

Vlodavsky I, Korner G, Ishai-Michaeli R, Bashkin P, Bar-Shavit R & Fuks Z (1990) Extracellular matrix-resident growth factors and enzymes: possible involvement in tumour metastasis and angiogenesis. *Cancer Metastasis Rev.* **9**, 203–226.

Vogelstein B (1990) Genetic alterations underlying colorectal tumorigenesis. *Clin. Exp. Metastasis* **8** (suppl. 1), 3.

Vogelstein B, Fearon ER, Hamilton SR *et al.* (1988) Genetic alterations during colorectal tumour development. *N. Engl. J. Med.* **319**, 525–532.

Vogelstein B, Fearon ER, Kern SE *et al.* (1989) Allelotype of colorectal carcinomas. *Science* **244**, 207–211.

Waddell WR, Gansen GF, Cerige EJ & Loughry RW (1989) Sulindac for polyposis of the colon. *Am. J. Surg.* **157**, 175–179.

Wallich R, Bulbuc N, Hammerling GJ, Katzov S, Segal S & Feldman M (1985) Abrogation of metastatic properties of tumour cells by *de novo* expression of H-2K antigens following H-2 gene transfection. *Nature* **315**, 301–305.

Wang BS, McLoughlin GA, Ritchie JP & Mannick JA (1980) Correlation of the production of plasminogen activator with tumour metastasis in B16 mouse melanoma cell lines. *Cancer Res.* **40**, 288–292.

Weiss L (1986) Metastatic inefficiency: causes and consequences. *Cancer Rev.* **3**, 1–24.
Weiss L, Holmes JC & Ward PM (1983) Do metastases arise from pre-existing subpopulations of cancer cells? *Br. J. Cancer* **47**, 81–89.
Weiss L, Grundmann E & Torhorst J (1986) Haematogenous metastatic patterns in colonic carcinoma: an analysis of 1541 necropsies. *J. Pathol.* **150**, 195–203.
Zeidman I (1965) The fate of circulating tumour cells. *Acta Cytol.* **9**, 136–140.
Zetter BR (1990) The cellular basis of site-specific tumour metastasis. *N. Engl. J. Med.* **322**, 605–612.

2

Imaging hepatic metastases

Derek Glenn

Patients with limited hepatic metastases due to colorectal cancer have a low 2-year survival rate. The 5-year survival rate after attempted cure by resection is around 30% (Morrow *et al.*, 1981; Scheele *et al.*, 1991).

The role of the radiology department is to:

1. Identify as accurately as possible all sites of metastatic disease in the liver.
2. Identify extrahepatic disease.
3. Demonstrate vascular anatomy.

The aim of radiological activity is to select those patients who will benefit from surgical resection and to prevent unnecessary laparotomies. Resection is useful only in the absence of extrahepatic disease and with fewer than four metastases restricted to an area that is resectable (Sugarbaker, 1990).

The modalities available are computed tomography (CT), magnetic resonance imaging (MRI) and ultrasound, combined with angiography.

Computed tomography

Dynamic CT

There are various formulae for the conduct of CT examinations for hepatic metastases. The major differences lie in the rate of infusion of intravenous contrast agent. The problem faced in judging the rate of infusion of contrast is the optimization of the differential contrast behaviour between normal hepatic parenchyma and metastatic disease.

The role of intravenous contrast is to opacify vascular structures, making them easier to identify, and to exploit the differential rate of opacification between normal hepatic parenchyma and primary or metastatic tumours.

Most hepatic tumours do not increase in density with the administration of intravenous contrast as quickly as normal hepatic parenchyma. The key to successful scanning is to time the peak opacification of normal hepatic parenchyma with the time of scanning through the liver, before liver tumours have significantly opacified.

If the injection of contrast is completed too early, tumours have time to opacify and the contrast differential between tumour and normal liver is lost. If the injection is too slow, hepatic parenchyma will not be opacified, and the differential between tumour and normal liver will not be established. Unfortunately, the contrast behaviour of tumours is not constant, as it depends upon the rate of blood supply of tumour compared to normal parenchyma. Vascular tumours, such as metastatic melanoma, some thyroid metastases and some hepatocellular carcinomas will enhance at a rate similar to or greater than normal parenchyma, with a resultant loss of conspicuity.

Colorectal metastatic disease is, however, almost invariably less vascular than normal hepatic parenchyma and achieving a satisfactory contrast bolus technique is relatively easy.

Scanning protocols

The simplest method is dynamic scanning with a bolus of intravenous contrast, providing up to about 40 g of intravenous iodine. There have been a wide range of injection rates and scanning delays proposed. Peak opacification of hepatic parenchyma depends upon the rate of infusion of contrast, the rate of flow in the portal vein and the hepatic artery, the volume of the liver and the total amount of iodine infused. The rate of flow in the portal vein and hepatic artery is in turn influenced by the cardiac output, and the resistance of the hepatic vascular bed.

Optimizing hepatic enhancement is futile unless the CT scanner is capable of scanning the liver entirely during the period of optimum enhancement. At this point protocols have to be modified to take into account the capacity of the available equipment to scan the liver – usually about 17 10 mm slices – in the time span required. The most recent slip-ring-equipped scanners can scan a liver from top to bottom in 40 s. A more usual time for older equipment is 150 s. The timing and rate of injection of contrast must be adjusted locally to accommodate the available equipment.

The rationale of all these techniques is to provide time and sufficient contrast to opacify the hepatic veins and normal hepatic parenchyma but to allow the minimum time for enhancement of hepatic metastatic disease.

Angio-CT/CT portography

CT arterial portography is the most sensitive preoperative imaging modality available to detect and localize hepatic colorectal metastases (Heiken *et al.*, 1989; Nelson *et al.*, 1989). Precise and rational preoperative planning depends upon knowledge of the number and location of metastases.

There is debate about the wisdom of performing conventional angiography before CT angio-portography (CTAP). Any infusion of contrast prior to conduct of CTAP must increase the overall density of the liver and metastatic disease, and theoretically can reduce lesion/liver contrast. No study has yet been performed that demonstrates improved diagnostic certainty with omission of angiography. The advantage of angiography in practical terms is that the splanchnic vasculature is demonstrated preoperatively. Splanchnic arteries are subject to considerable normal variation with, for example, replacement of the right hepatic artery by a vessel arising from the superior mesenteric artery being present in 12.5% of the normal population (Fig. 2.1). If placement of a hepatic arterial catheter is considered, either primarily or if resection is shown to be unfeasible at laparotomy, knowledge of

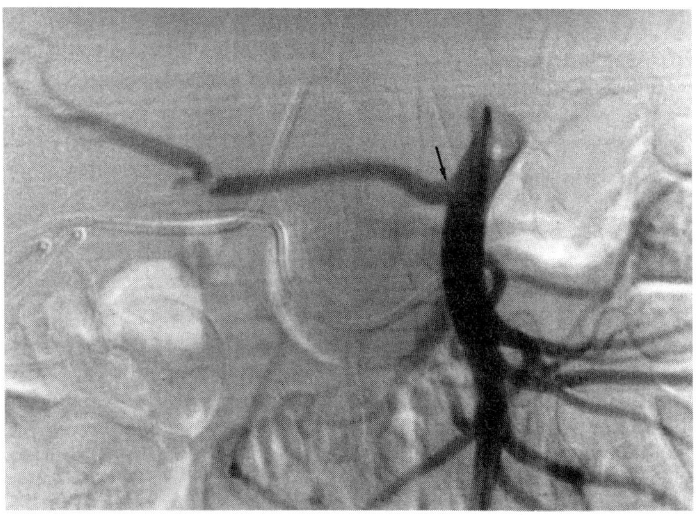

Figure 2.1 Right hepatic artery arising from the superior mesenteric artery (arrow). This case also illustrates the use of two separate hepatic artery catheters for infusion of chemotherapeutic agents.

the vascular variations may be of value, although surgeons at our hospital routinely use intraoperative methylene blue to assess adequacy of perfusion and maintain that the aberrant vessels are relatively constantly placed.

Technique

After conventional superior mesenteric and coeliac axis angiography, the catheter is placed into the superior mesenteric artery and secured at the groin. The patient is transferred to the CT scanner whilst a slow infusion of heparinized saline runs, keeping the catheter patent. The scans are performed in the dynamic mode, at the maximum possible rate, during an infusion of 200 ml 50% solution intra-arterial contrast. Scans are performed from the diaphragm to the inferior margin of the liver. The scanning sequence is repeated at the end of the first set, yielding an examination resembling a standard CT with intravenous contrast. The timing of the injection is set to provide opacification of the hepatic veins, which corresponds to commencement of scanning at 50 s after the start of the injection. Some centres administer 40 mg papaverine hydrochloride immediately prior to administration of intra-arterial contrast to increase portal vein flow.

The rationale of CT portography is to obtain dense opacification of the portal vein during scanning. Hepatic metastatic disease receives supply preferentially from the hepatic artery, and the dense opacification of the portal vein by this technique provides the greatest possible conspicuity of metastatic lesions by exploiting this effect. Normal hepatic parenchyma is much more vividly enhanced than metastatic disease. The disadvantage of the technique is that the mixing of densely opacified blood draining the area perfused by the superior mesenteric artery catheter and non-opacified blood can be incomplete. The result is large areas of non-perfusion on the initial scan which do not correspond to areas of metastatic disease. This problem is partially ameliorated by the second scan, which does not demonstrate this artefact (Figs 2.2, and 2.3). Analysis of the images is then conducted with reference to both sets, and segmental areas of non-perfusion can usually be eliminated as areas of metastatic disease. If there is remaining ambiguity, a delayed scan at 6 h can be performed to employ the capacity of normal hepatic parenchyma to excrete contrast into biliary radicals as a means of differentiating metastatic disease from normal liver (Fig. 2.4).

The common sites of flow-related perfusion defects are adjacent to the porta hepatis and adjacent to the fissure for ligamentum teres.

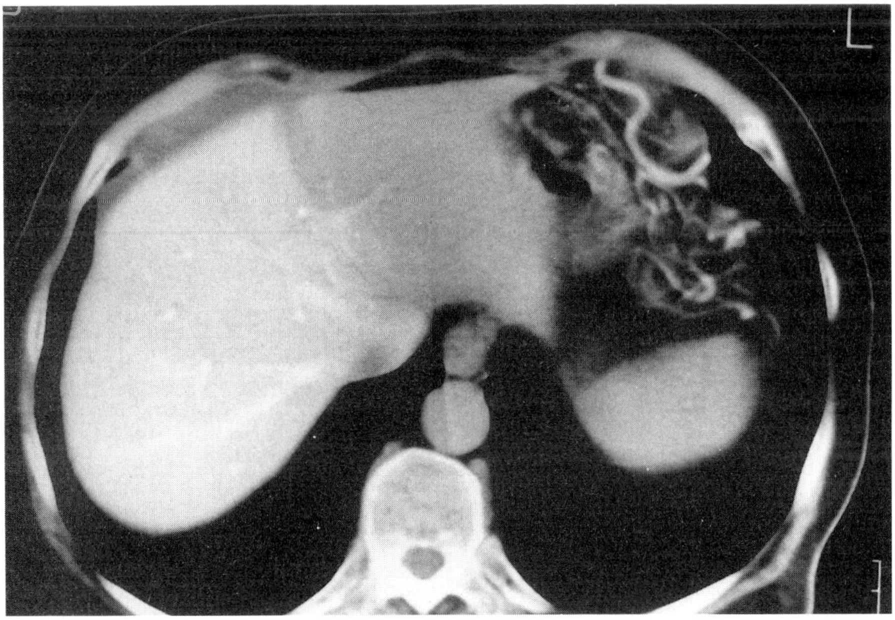

Figure 2.2 The lateral segment of the left lobe is poorly opacified in the angio-CT.

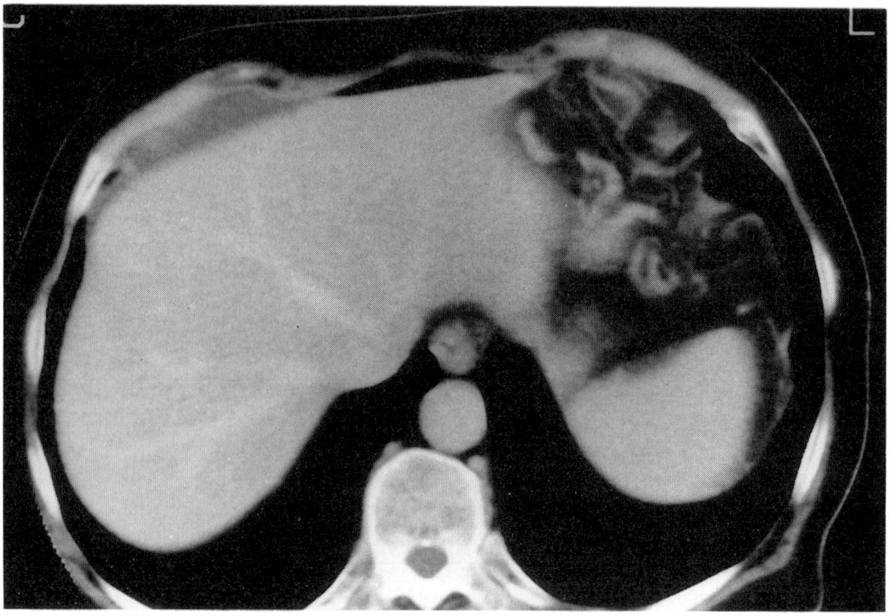

Figure 2.3 The second set of images, obtained immediately upon completion of the first set, eliminates the artefact shown in Figure 2.2

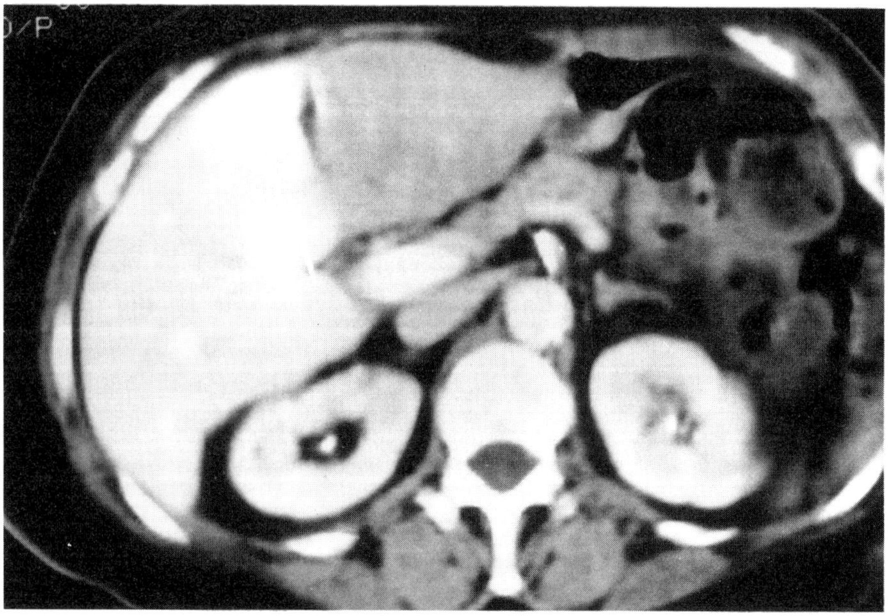

a

Figure 2.4 Three images obtained (a) during angio-CT; (b) immediately after angio-CT; (c) 6 h after angio-CT illustrate the return of lesion contact in the delayed images. This can be used to resolve ambiguity due to perfusion defects.

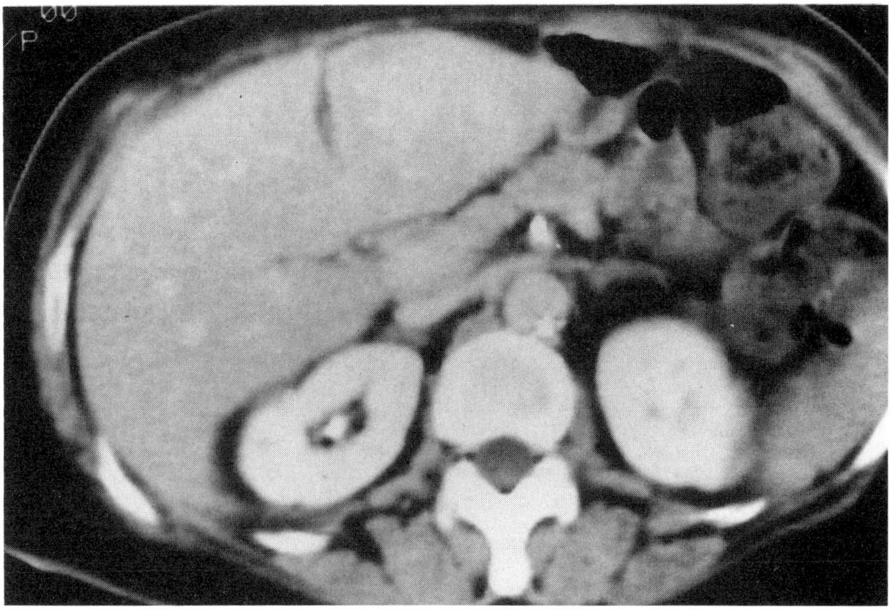

b

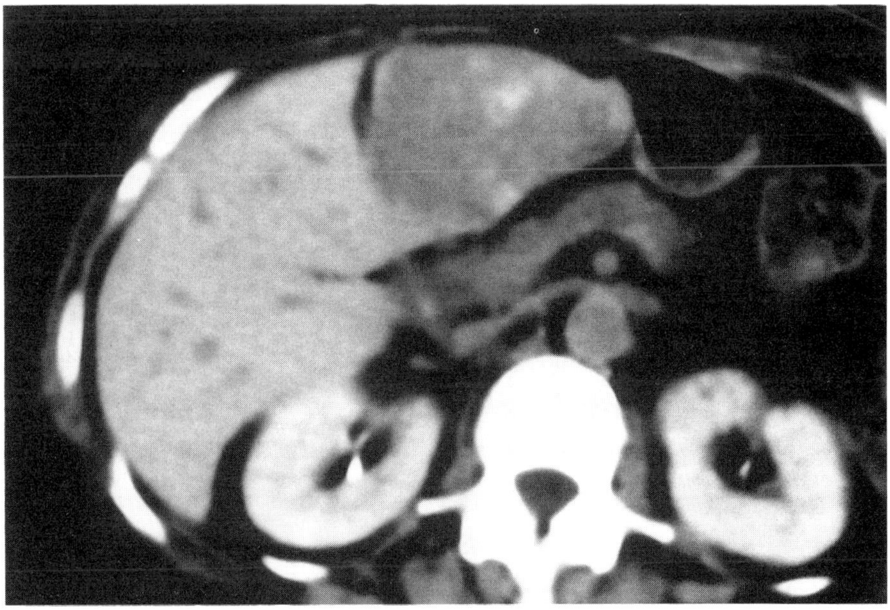

c

Both of these sites give rise to rounded defects, which may cause diagnostic difficulty, even with a delayed scan (Fig. 2.5).

In addition to these perfusion anomalies, central lesions disrupt portal flow, producing characteristic wedge-shaped perfusion defects. These can usually be differentiated from real lesions by their typical broad base on the liver capsule, as they correspond to a portal branch. the second scan is useful to resolve ambiguity in this area.

Advantages

The advantages of CT portography are:

1. It maximizes lesion/normal liver contrast.
2. It is relatively operator-independent.

Disadvantages

The disadvantages of CT portography are:

1. It requires angiography.
2. It is susceptible to artefacts.
3. It administers approximately 250 ml of contrast.
4. It is insensitive to micro-metastases.

Delayed CT

A repeat conventional CT of the liver may be performed at 6 h post CTAP. The aim of this delayed examination is to exploit the capacity of normal hepatocytes to excrete contrast. This renders intact hepatic tissue dense, and in a similar fashion to angio-CT, leaves the metastases unopacified. This technique has the advantage over angio-CT that there no flow artefacts – the principal cause of false-positive results with CT-angiography – but it is less sensitive. Delayed CT may be used where the angio-CT result remains ambiguous despite the second sequence, principally to determine the nature of perfusion defects at the porta hepatis.

Extrahepatic disease

CT has an important role in the demonstration of extrahepatic disease. In colonic carcinoma extrahepatic disease has been reported in a wide variety of sites, including retroperitoneal lymph nodes, lungs, pancreas, bone or brain. Of these, retroperitoneal lymphadenopathy is the commonest site of metastatic disease.

Careful inspection of the retroperitoneum, particularly the para-aortic region, is essential. Comparison with previous examinations is desirable, as even nodes less than 1 cm in diameter may be significant if they are new, or if there are more than a few present. The coeliac axis nodes are often difficult to appreciate, the area is subject to the cupping artefact, and anatomical ambiguity in the region of the cardio-oesophageal junction is common (Fig. 2.6). Careful inspection of the lesser curve is necessary in all cases of colonic malignancy.

There are two sites where lymphadenopathy may be unexpectedly encountered in the angio-CT phase of work-up. There is an inconstant node at the inferior margin of the caudate lobe, variously described as the caudate node or, more commonly, as the portacaval node (Fig. 2.7). This node may be up to 1.5 cm in diameter in normal adults. It is occasionally the sole site of metastatic disease and can be seen to enlarge with serial scans. The second site is in the pericardiac lymph nodes, where central anterior nodes are occasionally involved. Disease at either of these sites is unresectable (Fig. 2.8).

CT interpretation

Artefacts

In conventional CT the common artefacts that mimic metastases are:

Cupping

At the point of a rapid transition between two densities, a streak of low density may appear in line with the transition layer. In practical terms this means an ill-defined lucent wedge in the lateral aspect of the left lobe adjacent to the stomach, at the level of the gastric air bubble (Fig. 2.9).

Beam hardening

Selective attenuation of the X-ray beam by bone changes the physical characteristics of the beam, producing a wedge of lucency subtending the bone. This is evident as lucent areas adjacent to the ribs in the right lobe of the liver.

Movement

Particularly with long scan times on older equipment, the movement of the liver with

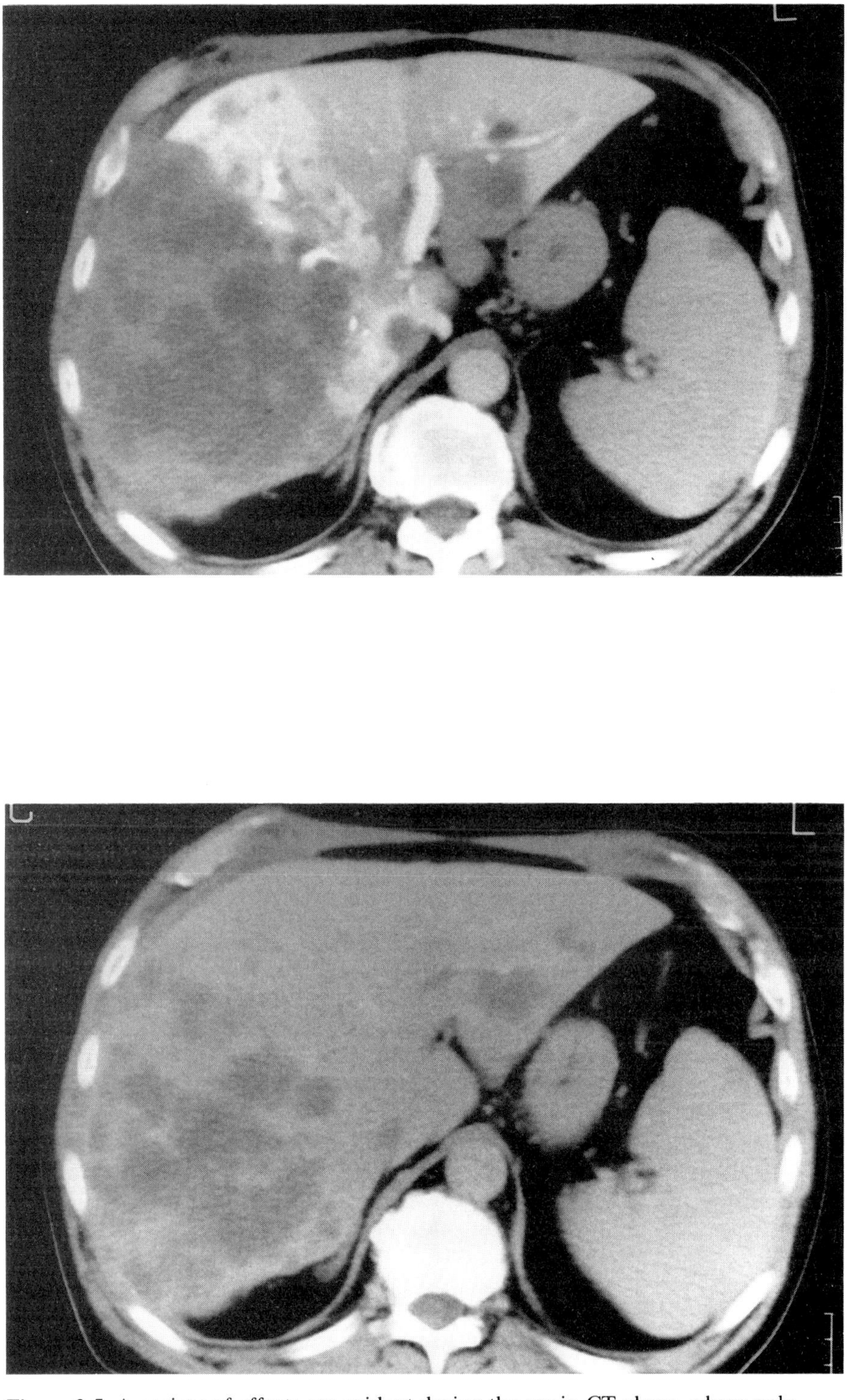

a

b

Figure 2.5 A variety of effects are evident during the angio-CT phase, where only segment 4 is well-perfused due to centrally placed metastases disrupting portal flow. There is a small perfusion defect adjacent to the left portal vein (a). These artefacts are abolished on the second set of images (b).

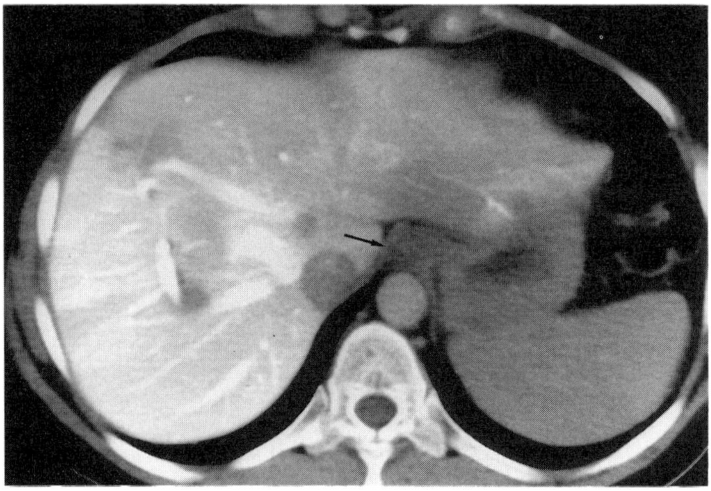

Figure 2.6 The cardio-oesophageal junction can mimic coeliac axis nodes (arrow), and careful inspection of the images above and below the ambiguity is necessary.

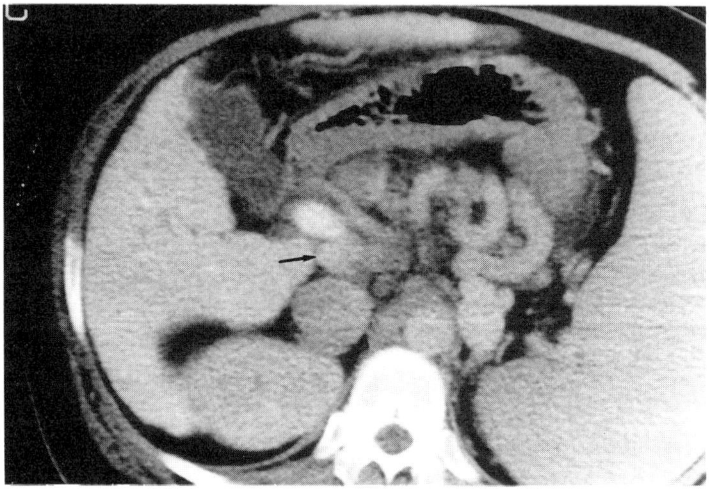

Figure 2.7 The portacaval node, illustrated here (arrow) in a case of portal hypertension.

respiration in uncooperative or distressed patients produces a cusp of lower density parallel to the liver margin, usually most conspicuous anteriorly.

Surgical decision-making with the angio-CT

Hepatic veins

The proximity of lesions to the hepatic veins is important in judging resectability. Contrast administration during CT should reflect this requirement.

Portal veins

Proximity to either of the main portal veins raises the possibility of unresectability, and should be checked carefully.

Inferior vena cava

Lesions may abut the inferior vena cava, but still be dissectible from the vein. CT is not a reliable indicator of caval invasion.

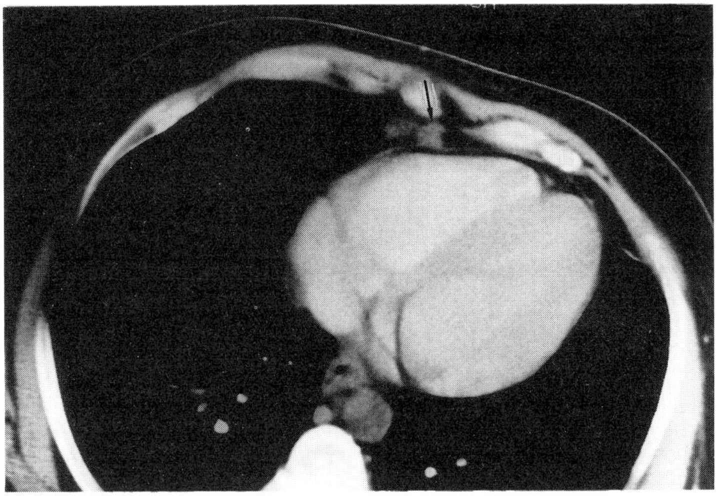

Figure 2.8 A pericardial node, in the pericardial chain.

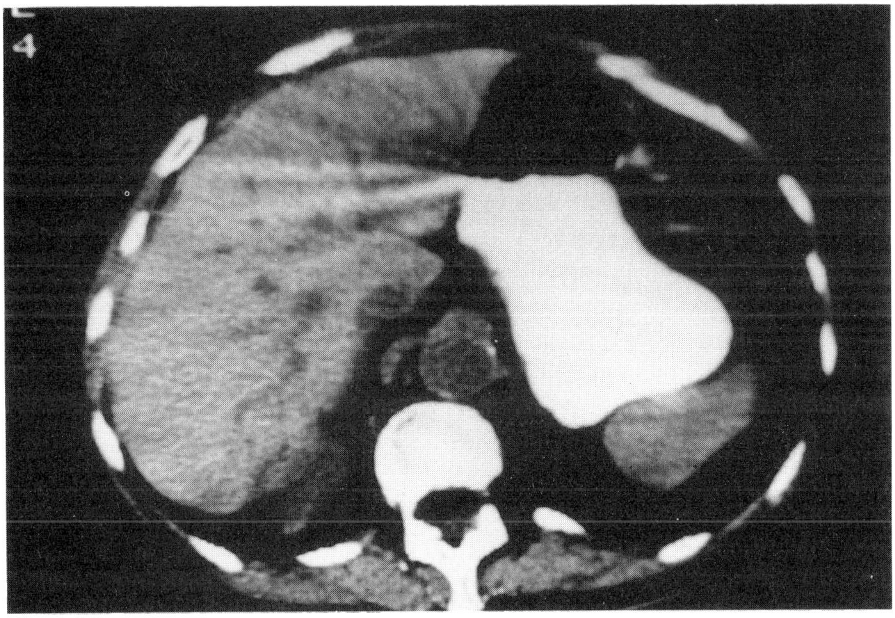

Figure 2.9 The cupping artefact, evident as dark horizontal streaks on this image, occurs where there are rapid transitions between densities, and is particularly troublesome at the lateral margin of the left lobe.

Number of lesions

If there are more than four lesions present, resection is not advised in colorectal cancer. The usual basis of failure is manifestation of metastases previously undetected, either at operation or evident soon after resection.

Diaphragmatic involvement

The shape of the diaphragm, nearly parallel to the plane of section of CT, renders CT unreliable in assessing diaphragmatic involvement. Clear manifestations such as masses on both sides of the diaphragm should not be ignored,

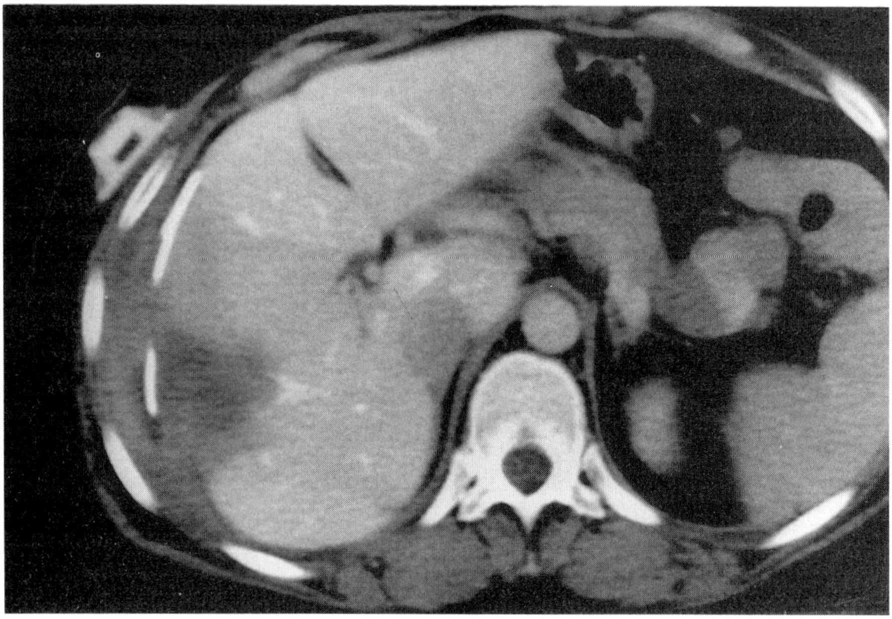

Figure 2.10 Apparent diaphragmatic involvement, not confirmed surgically.

but these are rare. More common is a lesion abutting the diaphragm, where diaphragmatic involvement is uncertain. Most of these cases are resectable (Fig. 2.10).

Volume remaining postresection

The residual volume after resection should be considered. If there will be less than 35% of the original functioning liver remaining, resection should not be undertaken. This situation is most likely to arise with an extended right resection, leaving the Couinaud segments 1, 2 and 3.

Differential diagnosis of colorectal metastases on CT

Hepatocellular carcinoma

Assuming the diagnosis is not apparent from markers or the clinical context, there are some morphological characteristics of hepatocellular carcinoma on CT that are very unusual in colorectal metastatic disease. Vascular invasion, particularly growth in to the portal vein, is unusual. The presence of a large mass with satellite lesions is suggestive of hepatocellular carcinoma. Colorectal metastases, when numerous, tend to be within one or two orders of magnitude of size to each other. The contrast enhancement characteristics are not reliable.

Haemangioma

Lesions larger than 5 cm do not usually cause difficulty. They have a characteristic enhancement pattern on dynamic CT, with opacification of 1–2 cm lobules at the periphery of the lesion. Lesions of this size can also be accurately diagnosed with a labelled red cell scan. Smaller lesions are more difficult. There are no reliable CT, ultrasound or angiographic criteria that can be used to differentiate small haemangiomata (<2 cm) from enhancing metastases. MRI may become useful, but has not yet gained widespread clinical application. Depending upon circumstances, biopsy or direct evaluation at surgery will be necessary.

Focal nodular hyperplasia and adenomata

There is substantial overlap in the radiographic appearance of these lesions, and between them and colorectal metastases. Outside a suggestive clinical context and without suitable evidence from markers, biopsy will be necessary. Occasionally large adenomata and focal nodular hyperplastic lesions have characteristic angiographic appearances that enable the diagnosis to be made with certainty. This is not however the norm.

Ultrasound

The role of ultrasound can be divided into preoperative assessment and intraoperative assessment/localization.

Preoperative assessment

The value of ultrasound in preoperative assessment of the liver prior to resection is controversial. A formal analysis of the entire liver based upon segmental anatomy is the ideal standard which is not achievable in some patients. Even in ideal candidates, the sensitivity of ultrasound is less than CT (Nelson *et al.*, 1989). Ultrasound is also more operator-dependent than CT, with a higher false-negative rate for detection of hepatic metastases.

The main disadvantage of ultrasound is in the detection of extrahepatic disease. The ability of ultrasound to image beyond solid organs is compromised by bowel gas. The detection rate for retroperitoneal lymphadenopathy and local recurrence is poor. Imaging of other important structures such as lungs and bones is not possible. Ultrasound therefore must be supplemented by other modalities, and is of little value as a screening examination.

Intraoperative assessment

During resection surgery, intraoperative ultrasound permits the operator to identify metastatic deposits in the non-resected segment for other management, such as cryotherapy. Dubious findings on the preoperative studies may be subject to further evaluation.

Perfusion defects, common at the porta hepatis and adjacent to the fissure for ligamentum teres, can be evaluated by intraoperative ultrasound, determining the feasibility of resection. The sensitivity of intraoperative ultrasound is comparable to CT portography (Soyer *et al.*, 1992).

Technical aspects

The technical advantage of intraoperative ultrasound over conventional ultrasound is due to two factors. Intraoperatively the probe is placed directly on to the surface of the liver. This permits use of higher-frequency probes with improved resolution. Comparatively inaccessible areas can be imaged directly using intraoperative probes with adequate liver mobilization.

Various different shapes of probes are available – long-handled, short-handled, T-piece. One manufacturer offers a transducer which fits inside the surgeon's glove. All probes must be presented within some form of sterile envelope or adequately sterilized. Autoclaving destroys ultrasound transducer elements.

The use of intraoperative ultrasound in relation to liver resection and cryotherapy is covered in later chapters of this book.

Magnetic resonance imaging

Introduction

Curent MRI technology remains unsuitable for routine work-up and assessment of hepatic metastatic disease. Examination times remain too long, and although excellent images are obtained in cooperative volunteers, image quality in routine work remains variable. New pulse sequences may resolve this problem.

There is persistent debate about the merits of high field strength (1.5 T) versus mid-field strength (0.5 T). Motion artefact is a more severe problem at higher field strengths, but signal-to-noise ratio and the availability of fast pulse sequence are better with high-field strength machines. There is a trend towards high-field strength in neurological applications.

There is marked variation in image quality and contrast relationships between different pulse sequences. The spleen has similar signal characteristics to hepatic metastases, where the spleen itself is normal. This permits assessment of the results of an unfamiliar pulse sequence on the basis of spleen/liver contrast, as opposed to lesion/liver contrast with CT.

In general, tumours have relatively more free water than normal liver. This results in prolongation of T1 and T2 times, resulting in relatively dark lesions on T1-weighted images, and bright lesions on T2-weighted images. This parallels the behaviour of tumours elsewhere in the body.

MRI in colorectal metastatic disease

Early experience with low and mid-field MRI was hampered by technical limitations in the conduct of T1-weighted images, and as a consequence T2-weighted imaging was emphasized. This introduced long imaging times, with inevitable motion artefact degradation. Recently, technical advances in high-field-strength MRI have made T1-weighted imaging possible within a single breath-hold (Semelka *et al.*, 1990). Experience with conventional pulse sequences at high field strengths indicated that T2-weighted spin echo was the most sensitive for lesion detection (Foley *et al.*, 1987). Later technical advances demonstrated T2-weighted fat-suppressed spin echo imaging to be more sensitive (Semelka *et al.*, 1990). Currently there are a wide range of pulse sequences proposed for both lesion detection and characterization. Studies are now being published comparing dynamic contrast-enhanced CT and MRI for imaging hepatic metastatic disease (Semelka *et al.*, 1990). The conclusions so far are that a statistically significant difference cannot yet be demonstrated, despite a trend towards superiority with MRI. MRI can however be demonstrated to be statistically superior to non-enhanced CT and delayed CT alone.

References

Foley WD, Kneeland JB, Cates JD *et al.* (1987) Contrast optimisation for the detection of focal hepatic lesions by MR imaging at 1.5 T. *Am. J. Radiol.* **149**, 1155–1160.

Heiken JP, Weyman PJ, Lee JKT *et al.* (1989) Detection of focal hepatic masses: prospective evaluation with CT, delayed CT, CT during arterial portography and MR imaging. *Radiology* **171**, 47–51.

Morrow CE, Grage TV, Suthaland DER & Najarian JS (1982) Hepatic resection of secondary neoplasms. *Surgery* **92**, 610–614.

Nelson RC, Chezmar JL, Sugarbaker PH & Bernadino ME (1989) Hepatic tumours: comparison of CT during arterial portography, delayed CT, and MR imaging for preoperative evaluation. *Radiology* **172**, 27–34.

Scheele J, Stangl R, Altendorf-Hofmann A & Gall FP (1991) Indicators of prognosis after hepatic resection for colorectal secondaries. *Surgery* **110**, 13–29.

Semelka RC, Shoenut JP, Kroeker MA *et al.* (19??) (1a) Focal liver disease: comparison of dynamic contrast-enhanced CT and T2-weighted fat-suppressed, FLASH, and dynamic gadolinium-enhanced MR imaging at 1.5 T.

Semelka RC, Chew W, Hricak H, Tomei E & Higgins CB (1990) Fat saturation MR imaging of the upper abdomen. *Am. J. Radiol.* **155**, 1111–1116.

Soyer P, Levesque M, Elias D *et al.* (1992) Detection of liver metastases from colorectal cancer: comparison of intraoperative US and CT during arterial portography. *Radiology* **183**, 541–544.

Sugarbaker PH (1990) Surgical decision making for large bowel cancer metastatic to the liver. *Radiology* **174**, 621–626.

3

The detection of occult liver metastases: use of alternative techniques

E. Leen and Colin S. McArdle

The presence of occult liver metastases in patients with colorectal cancer was first described by Finlay and colleagues using meticulously performed ultrasound (US) and the first generation of computed tomography (CT) (1982). It has since been shown that the presence or absence of these occult liver metastases at the time of surgery determines the likelihood of death from disseminated disease following an apparently curative resection (Finlay & McArdle, 1986).

Conventional imaging techniques such as US, CT and magnetic resonance imaging (MRI) are limited in the diagnosis of small liver metastases because there is a threshold size and contrast, below which discrimination between normal and abnormal tissue is impossible. Recent technical advances in liver imaging techniques, including contrast-enhanced MRI, intraoperative US, CT during arterial portography and high-resolution CT, have resulted in an increase in the detection rate of small (less than 1.0 cm) hepatic lesions (Ferrucci, 1990). However these lesions are often too small to have any characteristic morphology that would be of diagnostic value. Follow-up with repeated radiological examinations is required to determine the true nature of these lesions, as biopsy may be technically difficult. Furthermore, whilst it is justified to use these advanced techniques to stage the liver for the purpose of resection, these methods are altogether far too expensive or invasive to be used as a screening method for liver metastases detection. Alternative non-invasive technique are therefore required.

It has long been known that the presence of even small liver tumours is associated with subtle changes in the liver blood flow. Whereas the normal liver receives approximately 25% of its blood supply via the hepatic artery and about 75% via the portal vein, liver metastases derive a much greater proportion of their blood supply from the hepatic arterial flow and a lesser proportion from the portal venous flow. Breedis and Young (1954) and subsequently Healey (1965) demonstrated the paradox by injecting dyes and plastic into the blood vessels of a postmortem liver specimen. More recently, this was confirmed by Ridge and colleagues (1987) using dynamic scintigraphy following hepatic arterial and portal venous perfusion with radiolabelled amino acids and ammonia. Measurement of the relative hepatic arterial contribution to total liver blood flow might therefore provide an alternative method for the detection of liver tumours.

Dynamic scintigraphy: hepatic perfusion index

In the past these subtle changes in liver blood flow have been measured indirectly using dynamic scintigraphy (Sarper *et al.*, 1981). By measuring the first pass of an intravenous bolus injection of a radioactive colloid through the

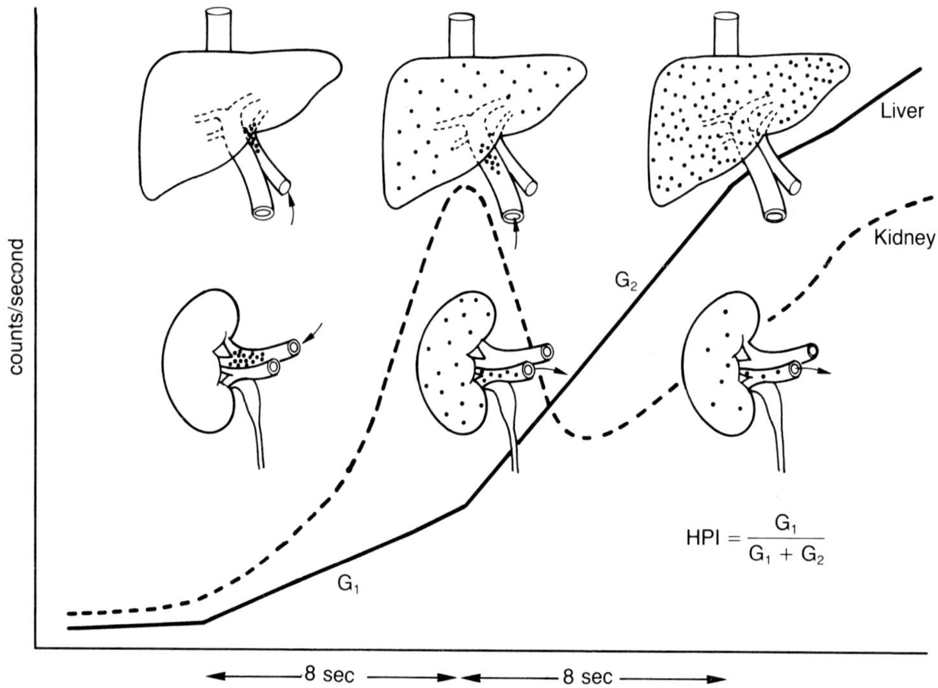

Figure 3.1 The initial increase in the time–activity curve of the liver is due to the arrival of the radionuclide to the liver via the hepatic artery. However, the second rise in the time–activity curve results from radionuclide reaching the liver via the portal vein, which is delayed relative to the hepatic arterial inflow. Thus the time–activity curve can be divided into the hepatic arterial inflow and portal venous inflow.

The hepatic arterial contribution to total liver blood flow can be calculated as the ratio of G_1 to $G_1 + G_2$, whereby G_1 represents the hepatic arterial inflow and G2 represents the portal venous inflow. This ratio was termed the hepatic perfusion index (HPI). Modified from Leveson *et al.* (1985).

liver and kidney, and using the peak activity over the right kidney to define the hepatic arterial and portal venous phases, it is possible to measure the ratio of hepatic arterial to total liver blood flow or hepatic perfusion index (HPI) from the activity–time curve of the liver (Fig. 3.1).

In a preliminary study of 100 patients with primary gastrointestinal malignancy, the Leeds group showed that the HPI measurements might be of clinical value in improving the detection of hepatic metastases (Leveson *et al.*, 1983; Parkin *et al.*, 1983). The surgical findings were correlated with the preoperative HPI measurements, and almost all patients with overt liver metastases were found to have abnormally elevated HPI values. However, about 50% of patients with no evidence of liver metastases on the basis of laparotomy findings also had abnormally elevated HPI values. Whether these patients were harbouring occult liver metastases would be determined by the results of long-term follow-up.

The 1-year follow-up results in 150 patients with gastrointestinal cancer were subsequently reported by the same group of workers in 1985 (Leveson *et al.*, 1985). Forty-seven of 50 patients with overt liver metastases were found to have an abnormal HPI value. One year after presentation, a total of 50 patients who had an apparently disease-free liver on the basis of laparotomy finding had been reviewed. Eighteen of the 29 patients with an elevated HPI value prior to laparotomy had developed liver metastases. All 21 patients with a normal HPI remained disease-free.

More recently, from the same centre, the outcome of the same cohort of patients with gastrointestinal cancer with a longer follow-up period was reported by Cooke *et al.* (1987). Overt hepatic metastases were found in 50 patients at initial laparotomy. On follow-up, liver secondaries developed in 18 in the first year, 12 in the second year and 1 in the third year. Overall, 31 patients had subsequently developed liver metastases, 27 of whom had an abnormal HPI value. Of the 81 patients with occult and overt liver metastases, HPI was abnormal in 74 patients, giving an overall sensitivity of 91%. The sensitivity of HPI for overt metastases was 94% (47/50), whilst for occult metastases it was 87% (27/31). Of the whole group of 150 patients, 90 had elevated HPI. Of the 60 patients with a normal preoperative HPI value, 7 were found to have liver metastases either at laparotomy (3 patients) or during follow-up (4 patients).

However, this technique is well-recognized to be susceptible to numerous errors in the derivation of the index. The separation of the hepatic arterial and portal venous phases is dependent on the activity being given as a fast bolus; otherwise there would be too much overlap of the phases to derive accurate gradients from the time–activity curve. The presence of intrahepatic portosystemic shunting is likely to reduce the HPI value and result in false-negative results. Although portosystemic shunting had been shown not to be significant in the presence of colorectal liver metastases, it is occasionally associated with large tumours and following multiple biopsy attempts. Furthermore, factors such as choice of region of interest, the inadvertent inclusion of lung bases and kidneys, and variations in the time period over which the gradient of the slopes are calculated will affect the quality of the time–activity curves.

It is therefore not surprising that other centres had been unable to reproduce the high sensitivity and specificity of the HPI technique as described by the Leeds group. In a study of 109 patients with colorectal cancer using a minor modification of the method of Parkin *et al.* (1983), Ballantyne and colleagues (1990) reported that only 68% of patients with liver metastases had abnormal HPI values. In a study of 180 patients referred for any reason, Laird *et al.* (1987) also reported that a proportion of patients with liver metastases had HPI values within the normal range and that HPI was raised in some cases of cholestasis and cirrhosis.

More recently, the reproducibility and accuracy of the HPI measured in two different centres were assessed (Maughan *et al.*, 1992). *In vitro* validation tests using a flow model showed that variations occurred at different centres. Following repeated HPI measurements on the same volunteers in the two centres, the correlation between two observers at one centre was high, but considerably less between the two centres. Of the 40 patients recruited, 12 cases were rejected because of technical or other factors (e.g. poor renal function, poor injection or prolonged circulation time). The authors suggested that direct comparison or extrapolation of HPI values obtained at different centres must be viewed with caution and that each centre should generate its own normal range of HPI values.

Numerous attempts had been made to refine the technique in order to improve its accuracy in the clinical setting. Perkins and co-workers (1987) had proposed the use of the time–activity curve of the left kidney to define the demarcation of the arterial and venous portal venous phases of the liver blood flow, because it was associated with fewer unevaluable studies. However, in a recent study using the modified technique, no significant improvement in the accuracy was achieved in the clinical setting – the sensitivity of HPI in detecting liver metastases was actually lower (Ballantyne *et al.*, 1990).

Furthermore, the dose of radionuclide commonly used (80–111 MBq) to measure HPI produces relatively low counts in the region of interest which can reduce the statistical reliability in the curve analysis. When the regions of interest are made artificially small to reduce the counts, the interobserver variation can be high (Leng *et al.*, 1987). In an attempt to improve the reproducibility of the technique, Hemingway and colleagues (1991) increased the dose of radionuclide to 400 MBq. The authors concluded that there were indications of a reduction in the variability in reprocessing through using the higher activity.

A major deficiency of the HPI technique is the fact that benign parenchymal liver diseases such as cholestasis and cirrhosis are also associated with abnormally elevated HPI values. In an attempt to increase the specificity of the method, an intravenous infusion of a vasoactive agent, angiotensin II, had been used to increase further the HPI value in patients with hepatic metastases (McGregor *et al.*, 1987). However, in a study of a small group of patients with hepatic metastases as well as a control group of patients with benign parenchymal liver disease, the use of the angiotensin II infusion did not increase the diagnostic power of the technique, as the increase in HPI occurred to a similar degree and frequency in both groups of patients (Goldberg *et al.*, 1989).

Despite all the attempts to refine the technique, there has been little or no improvement in the accuracy obtained from other centres to match the clinical results of the Leeds group. Dynamic scintigraphy may be too indirect a method of flow measurement to achieve the accuracy required clinically.

Duplex/colour Doppler sonography: Doppler perfusion index

Recent technical advances in duplex/colour Doppler sonography (DCDS) have made it possible to measure blood flow directly. Its accuracy has been demonstrated in studies of animal and patients (Sato *et al.*, 1987; Nakamura *et al.*, 1989; Robertson *et al.*, 1992; Leen *et al.*, 1991a). In contrast to dynamic scintigraphy, DCDS is a more direct method of flow measurement and is therefore likely to be more accurate. It also has the advantage of being non-invasive, independent of hepatic function and more readily standardized.

Over the last 2 years, we developed and employed a new technique using DCDS to measure hepatic arterial and portal venous blood flows in control subjects with no evidence of any liver disease, and patients with gastrointestinal carcinoma. Blood flow in each vessel was calculated as the product of the time-averaged velocity (TAV) and time-averaged cross-sectional area (TACSA) of the vessel. The Doppler perfusion index (DPI), termed as an analogy to the HPI, was calculated as the ratio of the hepatic arterial to the sum of the hepatic arterial and portal venous blood flow. The Doppler flow ratio (DFR), defined as the ratio of the hepatic arterial to portal venous blood flow, was also calculated. In addition to being able to measure blood flow directly, DCDS can assess the hepatic arterial vascular impedance, thus giving a pathophysiological insight into hepatic haemodynamics.

Technique of DPI measurement

A Diasonics Spectra scanner (Diasonics Sonotron, Bedford, UK), which consists of duplex and colour Doppler facilities, was used with a 3.5 MHz convex, phased linear array probe. In the Doppler mode, ultrasound waves were emitted and received by a single 3.5 MHz probe at a frequency of 3 MHz with a repetition frequency of 3.7 kHz. It was possible to steer the Doppler beam to any location and the angle between the axis of the Doppler beam to that of the vessel examined could be measured from the monitor. An angle range of 50–68° was used for velocity measurement. Special analysis was performed using fast Fourier transformation and the Doppler shift signal was displayed on the monitor. The system was equipped with software to compute the TAV from the velocity spectral display automatically following placement of the callipers at the start and end of one or more cardiac cycles. The cross-sectional area of the vessel was measured by mapping the perimeter of the vessel lumen with the tracker ball.

A transverse scan was made at the epigastrium to locate the common hepatic artery in its longitudinal axis (Plate 1). The Doppler cursor was placed over the lumen of the artery segment as near to the origin as possible, at the point where it first became horizontally straight. The Doppler sample volume and beam angle were adjusted and the TAV was calculated over four cardiac cycles (Plate 2). The cross-sectional area of the artery was measured at the same point at right angles to the vessel (Plate 3). The TACSA was calculated by taking the mean of the areas measured separately over four different cardiac cycles. The same parameters were obtained for the portal vein in a similar manner at the mid-level of the vein (Plates 4 and 5). All measurements were performed under respiratory suspension in expiration to allow optimal visualization of the portal vein and enabled a more acute angle to be achieved for Doppler purposes. Each measurement was performed repeatedly until the most satisfactory spectral patterns were obtained – no spectral broadening or aliasing. The duration of all these measurements lasted between 15 and 45 min.

The hepatic arterial vascular impedance was assessed through the measurement of the hepatic arterial resistive index (HARI), defined as the ratio of the peak systolic velocity (PSV) minus the end-diastolic velocity (EDV) to the PSV. The HARI was measured in all subjects from the velocity spectral display obtained while carrying out the TAV measurement. HARI was calculated automatically by the computer software, simply by placing the callipers at the PSV and at the end of the EDV of a cardiac cycle. A mean value for HARI was obtained from four separate cardiac cycles.

The splanchnic vascular impedance was also assessed by measuring the superior mesenteric arterial resistive index (SMARI). From a sagittal scan at the epigastrium, the superior mesenteric artery can be identified lying anterior to the aorta and inferior to the origin of the coeliac axis. The Doppler cursor was placed over the lumen of the vessel and, following angle and sample volume correction, the velocity spectral display could be obtained. From the velocity waveform the SMARI can be calculated automatically by placing the callipers at the PSV and at the EDV in the same way as HARI was calculated.

The whole examination was carried out by an independent ultrasonologist without knowledge of the preoperative CT and ultrasound findings. No sonographic assessment of the liver parenchyma was made while performing the DPI measurement.

Percentage hepatic replacement measurement

The percentage hepatic replacement (PHR) was measured in all patients with histologically proven liver metastases using an IGE 9800 CT scanner. Non-enhanced scans of the liver were first performed with contiguous 10 mm-thick slices and 2 s scan time. Enhanced CT scans were then obtained following a bolus intravenous injection of 100 ml of Ultravist 370 (Iopromide) via an injector (Angiomat CT, Digital Injector System) with contiguous 10 mm-thick slices and 2 s scan time. Scanning began about 45 s after the bolus injection, and the entire liver was scanned within an average of 4 min.

The cross-sectional areas of all the metastatic lesions in each slice and that of the liver in each slice were measured automatically using the scanner software. This was done by mapping the perimeter of the region of interest with the help of the tracker ball, after which the area of the region was determined. The PHR by metastases was calculated from the ratio of the sum of the areas of all lesions in all slices to the sum of the areas of the liver in all slices multiplied by 100.

In vitro, in vivo and reproducibility tests

The value of the qualitative data provided by DCDS is widely recognized clinically, but there is still some doubt as regards the value of the quantitative measurements. Whilst the accuracy and reproducibility of flow measurements have been well documented *in vitro* and *in vivo* at research level, there is still some scepticism regarding its application in clinical practice. The wide variety of commercially available duplex Doppler systems which have not been properly calibrated has led to inconsistency of quantitative data. Kimme-Smith and colleagues (1990) have compared measurements of peak velocities obtained using 17 different Doppler ultrasound machines, with values obtained from calibrated phantoms. The variation among the various systems averaged 23% under identical conditions. Some units gave peak velocities which were over 100% too high when compared with calibrated peak velocities. The authors advised that quantitative measurements obtained using Doppler sonography should be reported with information on the calibration of the equipment.

We have previously demonstrated the accuracy of duplex/colour Doppler flowmetry *in vitro* and the reproducibility of the hepatic arterial and portal venous blood flow measurements *in vivo* (Leen *et al.*, 1991 a, b; Robertson *et al.*, 1992). *In vitro* validation tests using a flow circuit model of tissue-equivalent material had been performed in order to calibrate the DCDS against an electromagnetic flowmeter. These had shown that only a single multiplicative correction factor of 0.819 was required to obtain accurate flow measurements in absolute units in vessels of a wide range of diameters for both pulsatile and continuous flow.

Reproducibility tests were carried out in 12 subjects (7 control subjects and 5 patients with colorectal cancer, of whom 3 had hepatic metastases and 2 had disease-free livers) for measurement of HARI, DPI and DFR repeated on a subsequent occasion within a period of 2 weeks. In the control group, the mean changes for the DPI, DFR and HARI were 0.004, –0.010 and –0.010 respectively. The root mean square changes for the DPI, DFR

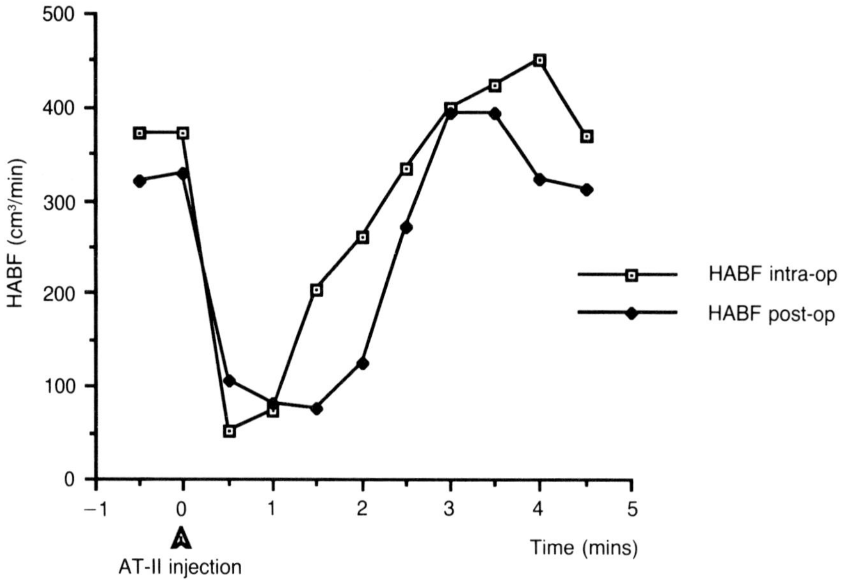

Figure 3.2 Concordance in blood flow measurements between duplex/colour Doppler sonography and another flowmeter during intra-arterial infusion of angiotensin II(AT-II). HABF = Hepatic arterial blood flow.

and HARI were 0.04, 0.08 and 0.02, respectively. In the group of patients with colorectal cancer, the mean changes for the DPI, DFR and HARI were 0.02, 0.15 and 0.01, respectively, and the root mean square changes were 0.05, 0.35 and 0.02, respectively. The DPI, DFR and HARI values of controls measured on the second occasion were within normal range, and those for patients with overt liver metastases remained in the abnormal range.

Following repeated measurements of the flow parameters in each vessel for 5 healthy volunteers, the mean coefficients of variation for TAV, cross-sectional area and blood flow were 4.5, 6.1 and 7.6% respectively. More recently, using another calibrated Doppler flowmeter, we carried out continuous measurements of hepatic arterial blood flow intraoperatively during an infusion of angiotensin II via a hepatic arterial catheter in 6 patients. Within 2 weeks of the operation, hepatic arterial blood flow was measured in the same group of patients using DCDS, during a similar infusion of angiotensin II via the hepatic arterial catheter. There was high concordance in the blood flow measurements between the two flowmeters, with the postoperative temporal flow changes paralleling those measured intraoperatively (Leen *et al.*, 1993b; Fig. 3.2).

Anatomical variations were present in 30% (20 of 67) of our patients with liver metastases as confirmed by hepatic arteriography, and 24% (16 of 68) of patients with an apparently clear liver on the basis of DCDS scan only. Control subjects with anatomical variations were excluded from the study. The variation easily identified on DCDS in this study was that the left hepatic artery arose from the coeliac axis and the right hepatic artery from the superior mesenteric artery. When hepatic arterial anatomical variations occurred, the total hepatic arterial blood flow was taken as the sum of the blood flows from the individual hepatic arteries.

Although we took account of anatomical variations when detected, underestimation of hepatic arterial blood flow would occur, particularly when the left hepatic artery and/or an accessory left hepatic artery arises from the left gastric artery, as they would not have been identified on DCDS. If that were the case in patients with an abnormal DPI, the true DPI value would be even higher. Underestimation of hepatic arterial flow, could, in theory, lead to

Table 3.1 Clinical results

	CONTROLS N = 50 mean +/- sd	LIVER METASTASES N = 70 mean +/– sd	CLEAR LIVER N = 130 mean +/– sd
HA/AREA mm²	17.0 +/– 5.0	33.0 +/– 14.5#	21.8 +/– 7.9
HA/TAV cm/s	19.0 +/– 10.0	33.1 +/– 12.4#	27.6 +/– 11.0
HABF ml/min	194 +/– 125	635 +/– 333#	346 +/– 173
PV/AREA mm²	129.0 +/– 36.0	99.3 +/– 26.6*	97.2 +/– 25.1
PV/TAV cm/s	15.0 +/– 6.0	11.1 +/– 4.0*	12.8 +/– 3.9
PVBF ml/min	1200 +/– 570	675 +/– 342#	727 +/– 268
TLBF ml/min	1390 +/– 640	1350 +/– 580	1053 +/– 315
DPI	0.14 +/– 0.06	0.50 +/– 0.12#	0.33 +/– 0.12

HA/AREA: Cross-sectional area of the hepatic artery; HA/TAV: Time average velocity of blood in the hepatic artery; HABF: Hepatic arterial blood flow; PV/AREA: Cross-sectional area of the portal vein; PV/TAV: Time average velocity of blood in the portal vein; PVBF: Portal venous blood flow; TLBF: Total liver blood flow; DPI: Doppler perfusion index; *$P<0.001$ & #$P<0.0001$

false-negative results, but no patient with a normal DPI has as yet developed liver metastases.

We are aware of further potential sources of error involved in flow measurements using DCDS, namely:

1. Non-uniform insonation of the vessel.
2. Spectral broadening.
3. Angle correction.
4. Area estimation.
5. Errors in the processing facilities of the system.

However, some of these can be minimized by standardizing the technique used to make each measurement. We also found that the addition of the colour Doppler facility to the conventional duplex Doppler ultrasound was of great advantage, with ease of precise assessment of vessel geometry, accurate identification of vessels of interest and showing anatomical variations, and with significant reduction in the duration of scanning. This technique is, however, operator-dependent and a dedicated ultrasonologist is essential for meticulous standardized examinations to be performed. Following the HPI experience, we recommend that each centre should derive its own normal range of DPI values.

Clinical results

To date we have investigated a cohort of 50 control subjects without evidence of neoplastic or liver disease and 200 patients with colorectal cancer. On the basis of laparotomy findings and preoperative CT scan findings, 70 patients with colorectal cancer had proven liver metastases and 130 patients had an apparently disease-free liver. The results are summarized in Table 3.1. There was a significant increase in the TAV and TACSA of the hepatic artery in patients with liver metastases compared with controls ($P<0.0001$). The hepatic arterial blood flow was therefore significantly elevated in the metastases group ($P<0.0001$; Table 3.1). However, there was a significant reduction in the TAV and TACSA of the portal vein in patients with hepatic metastases compared with the control group ($P<0.001$, $P<0.0001$ respectively). The portal venous blood flow was significantly lower in patients with liver metastases ($P<0.0001$ Table 3.1). No significant difference was demonstrated in the total liver blood flow among the two groups.

The upper limit of the normal range of DPI values was 0.25. The DPI values were significantly higher in females compared with males in the control group ($P<0.01$) but no correlation was demonstrated between DPI and body weight or age.

The range of DPI values for patients with hepatic metastases was 0.30–0.77. Clear separation of the DPI and DFR values was observed between controls and patients with overt liver metastases ($P<0.0001$; Fig. 3.3). When the sex difference was taken into account, the separation of DPI values between the control group

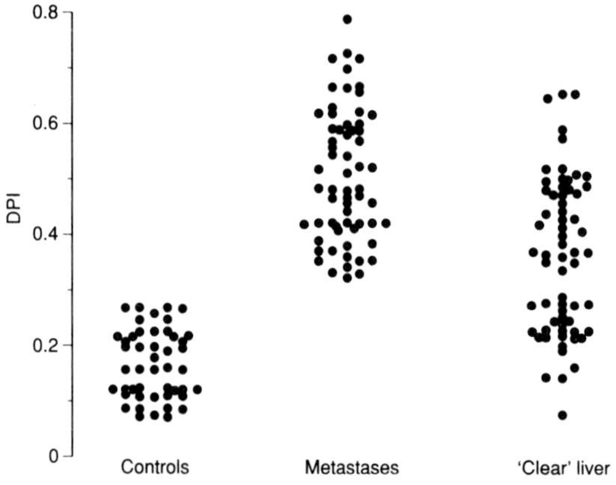

Figure 3.3 Doppler perfusion index (DPI) values of control subjects, patients with overt liver metastases and patients with an apparently 'clear' liver.

and patients with established metastases was even greater. As one would expect, there was an even wider gap between those two groups when DFR was considered compared with DPI.

The PHR by metastases as measured by CT scans showed no correlation with the DPI values (Fig. 3.4). This again suggests that the

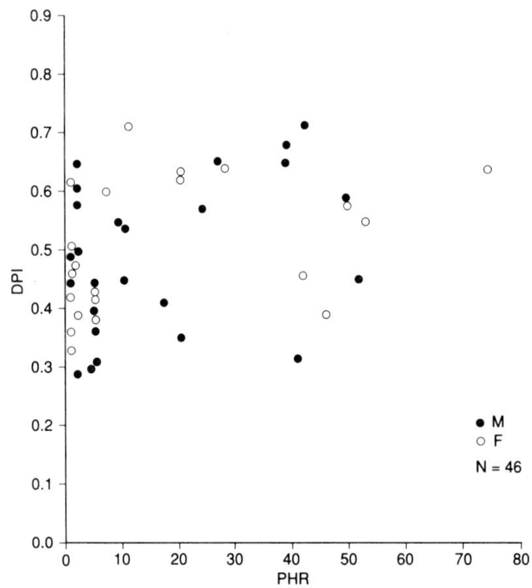

Figure 3.4 Relationship between Doppler perfusion index (DPI) and percentage hepatic replacement by metastases (PHR). No correlation was demonstrated for the number of patients studied.

mere presence of small liver tumours in itself is enough to cause measurable alterations in liver blood flow. It also casts some doubts on the initial belief that the changes in liver blood flow are primarily due to an increase in hepatic arterial blood flow to supply the liver metastases. More recently, numerous studies based on the liver metastasis model in the rat have confirmed the changes in liver blood flow with the development of overt liver tumours and, more importantly, the changes occurred before the appearance of macroscopic metastasis (Notts *et al.*, 1989; Hemingway *et al.*, 1991). The alteration in the liver blood flow was reported to be due to a reduction in the portal venous inflow, as opposed to a rise in the hepatic arterial blood inflow. Studies carried out by the same group of investigators suggested that the alteration in the portal venous flow might be mediated by an unknown vasoactive humoral agent which would increase the splanchnic vascular resistance, thereby reducing the splanchnic blood flow.

Although in this study we have shown an increase in the hepatic arterial blood flow in the presence of liver tumours, the portal venous blood flow reduction is probably the primary change. The rise in hepatic arterial blood flow may be a secondary component, as a result of the reciprocal relationship between hepatic arterial and portal venous flow to maintain homeostasis, demonstrated in non-tumour-bearing animal models and humans. However, it is also possible that some contribution to the increase in the hepatic arterial supply may be a result of an increase in functional demand by the normal liver tissue.

The HARI was significantly reduced in patients with overt liver metastases when compared with controls ($P<0.0001$) and correlates with the significant increase in hepatic arterial blood flow in the presence of liver tumours. In contrast, there was a significant reduction in the SMARI ($P<0.001$), correlating with the reduction in portal venous blood flow.

Malignant neoplastic growth is known to be correlated with increased blood supply by the host (Eddy & Casarett, 1973). Neovascularization takes place around and/or within the lesions (Folkman *et al.*, 1989). These tumour vessels are primitive and it has been suggested that there may be associated arteriovenous shunting. One would expect that, with increasing size of metastases, there would be an increase in arteriovenous shunting and a corresponding decrease in HARI. However, no correlation was found between HARI and PHR in patients with overt liver metastases. This supports previous observations that arteriovenous shunting in hepatic metastases is not significant (Goldberg *et al.*, 1987).

Follow-up results

The DPI result of patients in the third group (those with an apparently disease-free liver, $n = 130$) is of more interest, overlapping with those of controls and patients with overt liver metastases. Of these patients, 55% had an abnormally elevated DPI (Fig. 3.5). Clearly, the question is whether these patients with an abnormal DPI at the time of primary resection will subsequently develop overt liver metastases.

At 1-year follow-up, 68 patients with an apparently disease-free liver on the basis of laparotomy and preoperative CT scan findings had been reviewed. The outcome is illustrated in Figure 3.5. Twenty-one of the 38 (55%) patients had developed liver metastases and 9 had died. Two additional patients had died with local recurrence of the primary tumour but hepatic metastases could not be excluded at the time of death. Another 2 patients died at home of unrelated causes and no postmortem was carried out. Thirteen patients with abnormal DPI have not as yet shown evidence of hepatic metastases, but 5 of these have evidence of local dissemination; further follow-up is continuing. The remaining 30 patients with normal DPI are still alive and remain disease-free on the basis of clinical examination, biochemical indices, ultrasound and CT scans. At 1-year follow-up (excluding the 4 patients in whom the liver status was unknown), the sensitivity and negative predictive value of the DPI technique were both 100%.

Of the 30 patients who had an apparently curative resection of the primary tumour with a normal DPI value, 10 (33%) patients had a Dukes stage C disease, 19 (63%) had a Dukes stage B disease and 1 (3%) had a Dukes stage A disease. Of the 21 patients who subsequently developed overt liver metastases within 1 year of follow-up, 18 (86%) patients had a Dukes stage C disease and 3 (14%) had a Dukes stage B disease; vascular invasion by the primary tumour was present in 6 (29%) cases.

In the same group of 68 patients with an apparently clear liver at the time of initial presentation, intraoperative US was also performed at the time of laparotomy. Metastatic lesions were detected in only 2 of the 21 patients who subsequently developed liver metastases, whilst DPI had diagnosed all 21 cases. The intraoperative US scan was normal in all 30 patients who as yet show no evidence of hepatic metastasis.

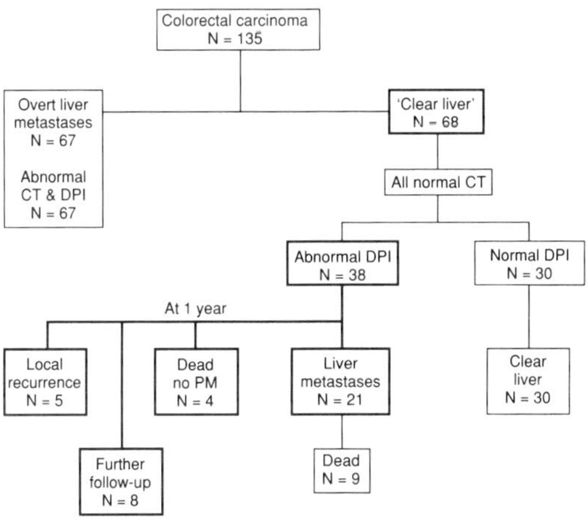

Figure 3.5 One-year follow-up: outcome of patients who had an apparently 'clear' liver at initial presentation. CT = Computed tomography; DPI = Doppler perfusion index; PM = postmortem.

Specificity of DPI

In a study of 72 patients with gastric (35), oesophageal (10), carcinoid (7) and breast carcinomas (20), all those with proven liver metastases (21) were also associated with abnormally elevated DPI values, resulting in 100% sensitivity; the negative predictive value as yet remains 100%. However, compared with patients with colorectal carcinoma, a smaller proportion (25%) of patients with gastric carcinoma with an apparently clear liver on the basis of laparotomy or CT scan findings at initial presentation had an elevated DPI value (Leen *et al.*, 1993c). Three of these patients have subsequently developed liver metastases over a period of 6 months. Follow-up is continuing for the remaining patients.

A well-recognized deficiency of dynamic scintigraphy is that HPI is elevated not only in the presence of liver metastases but also by

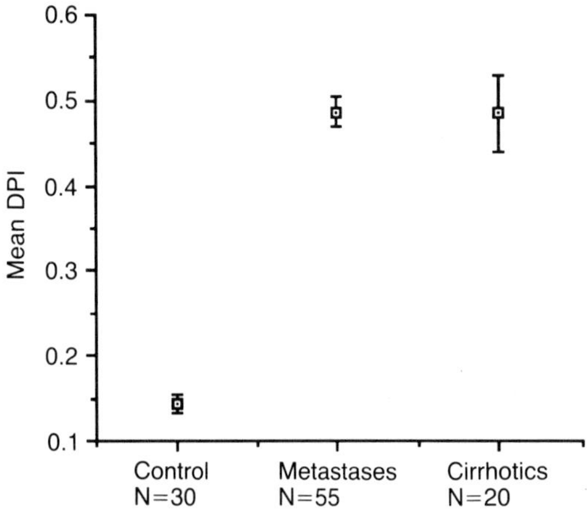

Figure 3.6 Doppler perfusion index (DPI) values of control subjects, patients with overt liver metastases and patients with cirrhosis.

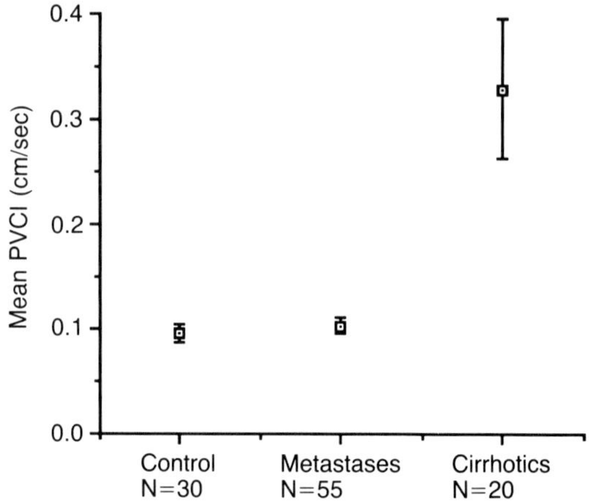

Figure 3.7 Portal venous congestive index (PVCI) values of control subjects, patients with overt liver metastases and patients with cirrhosis.

hepatic cirrhosis. The cause in the case of cirrhosis, in contrast to metastases, is an increased intrahepatic portal resistance; however, the subtly different haemodynamic effects cannot be distinguished by the scintigraphic technique. The greater information provided by DCDS allowed the haemodynamic effects of benign and malignant liver disease to be clearly differentiated. Hepatic arterial and portal venous blood flows were measured in 30 controls, 20 patients with cirrhosis (mean Child Pugh score 7.1) and 55 patients with overt liver metastases. DPI and the congestive index (ratio of cross-sectional area of the vessel to TAV of blood flow in the vessel) of the hepatic artery (HACI) and portal vein (PVCI) were calculated. The hepatic arterial blood flows of the cirrhotic and metastatic groups were significantly elevated compared with that of controls and the portal venous blood flows of the former groups were reduced ($P<0.0001$). The DPIs of the cirrhotic and metastatic groups were therefore significantly elevated compared with those of controls ($P<0.0001$; Fig. 3.6). No significant difference was noted in HACI values among the three groups. However, the PVCI values of the cirrhotic group were significantly elevated compared with those of controls and patients with metastases ($P<0.0001$; Fig. 3.7). The data suggest that DCDS measurement of PVCI may be of value in differentiating the hepatic perfusion changes due to cirrhosis from those as a result of hepatic metastases, thereby increasing the diagnostic power of the technique (Leen *et al.*, 1993a). The limits of this technique in distinguishing cases of early benign and malignant disease remain to be explored.

In conclusion, the data suggest that DCDS measurement of DPI can reliably detect overt liver metastases and confirm its ability to detect occult liver metastases at an earlier stage. This technique is also more sensitive than intraoperative US and conventional CT scan in the global detection of liver metastases in patients with colorectal cancer.

Implications

Despite more than 6000 randomized patients having been reported in published trials, the effect of adjuvant systemic chemotherapy upon mortality remains unclear. An overview suggests that 5-fluorouracil-containing regimens administered systemically over an extended period of time may reduce the odds of death by about 17%, resulting in an increase in 5-year survival of approximately 3% (Buyse *et al.*, 1988). However, these regimes may be associated with varying degrees of toxicity.

An alternative approach was adopted by Taylor and his colleagues (1985); they developed the concept of portal vein perfusion chemotherapy. Based on the premises that metastases, which are released by handling of the primary tumour, reached the liver via the portal vein and that these micrometastases subsequently develop into overt liver metastases, Taylor *et al.* infused 5-fluorouracil into the portal vein during the immediate postoperative period. After a median follow-up of 4 years, 22% in the group receiving cytotoxic liver perfusion and 43% in the control group had died. The benefit appeared to be limited to patients with Dukes B colon cancer.

Subsequent studies undertaken by Metzger *et al.* (1987), Gray *et al.* (1987), Wereldsma *et al.* (1990) and Wolmark and colleagues (1990) using 5-fluorouracil alone or in combination with mitomycin failed to confirm the magnitude of mortality reduction reported by Taylor *et al.* An overview suggests that portal vein infusion chemotherapy may confer a survival benefit similar to that of systemic chemotherapy.

More recently the combination of 5-fluorouracil and levamisole has been evaluated in patients following apparently curative resection of Dukes B and C colonic tumour (Moertel *et al.*, 1990). There was a 41% reduction in recurrence risk in the group receiving levamisole plus 5-fluorouracil. The overall mortality was reduced by 33%. However, 30% of patients discontinued therapy prematurely because of toxicity.

Following these encouraging results, the National Cancer Institute suggested that adjuvant chemotherapy should be regarded as standard practice in stage C carcinoma of the colon and that 'no treatment' controls are no longer justifiable. If so, we would expect that about 75 000 patients in western Europe (including 8100 in UK) and 45 000 in the USA would receive adjuvant therapy each year. Most regimes of systemic adjuvant chemotherapy are associated with varying degrees of toxicity and about 36 000 patients would be expected to discontinue therapy prematurely because of toxicity (Moertel *et al.*, 1990). However, half of the patients undergoing a curative resection do not require adjuvant therapy; therefore, if patients at high risk could be identified reliably, adjuvant chemotherapy could be administered on a selective basis. This would prevent inappropriate therapy and avoid unnecessary morbidity. The results of the follow-up studies suggest that DCDS has an important role to play in this respect.

Whilst the 1-year follow-up results clearly demonstrated that DCDS measurement of DPI can detect both occult as well as overt colorectal liver metastases, a longer follow-up period is still required and it is important for other centres to reproduce our results with the same degree of accuracy.

References

Ballantyne KC, Charnley RM, Perkins AC *et al.* (1990) Hepatic perfusion index in the diagnosis of overt metastatic colorectal cancer. *Nucl. Med. Commun.* **11**, 23–28.

Breedis C & Young G (1954) The blood supply of neoplasms in the liver. *Am. J. Pathol.* **30**, 969–985.

Buyse M, Zeleniuch-Jacquotte A & Chalmers TC (1988) Adjuvant therapy of colorectal cancer. Why we still don't know. *J.A.M.A.* **259**, 3571–3578.

Cooke DA, Parkin A, Wiggins P *et al.* (1987) Hepatic perfusion index and the evolution of liver metastases. *Nucl. Med. Commun.* **8**, 970–974.

Eddy HA & Casarett GW (1973) Development of the vascular system in the hamster malignant neurilemmoma. *Microvasc. Res.* **6**, 63–82.

Ferrucci JT (1990) Liver tumour imaging: current concepts. *AJR* **150**, 473–484.

Finlay IG & McArdle CS (1986) Occult hepatic metastases in colorectal carcinoma. *Br. J. Surg.* **73**, 732–735.

Finlay IG, Meek DR, Gray HW *et al.* (1982) Incidence and detection of occult hepatic metastases in colorectal carcinoma. *Br. Med. J.* **284**, 803–805.

Folkman J, Watson K, Ingber D *et al.* (1989) Induction of angiogenesis during the transition from hyperplasia to neoplasia. *Nature* **339**, 58–61.

Goldberg JA, Bradnam MS, Kevv DJ *et al.* (1987) Arteriovenous shunting of microspheres in patients with colorectal liver metastases: errors in assessment due to free pertechnetate and the effect of angiotensin II. *Nucl. Med. Commun.* **8**, 1033–1046.

Gray BN, deZwart J, Fisher R *et al.* (1987) The Australian and New Zealand trial of adjuvant chemotherapy in colon cancer. In: Salmon SE (ed) *Adjuvant Therapy of Cancer* V, pp. 357–456. New York: Grune & Stratton.

Healey J (1965) Vasular pattern in human metastatic liver tumours. *Surg. Gynecol. Obstet.* **120**, 1187–1193.

Hemingway DM, Cooke TG, Grime SJ *et al.* (1991) Changes in hepatic haemodynamics and the hepatic perfusion index during the growth and development of hypovascular HSN sarcoma in rats. *Br. J. Surg.* **78**, 326–330.

Kimme-Smith C, Hussain R, Duerinckz A, Tessler F & Grant E (1990) Assurance of consistent peak-velocity measurements with a variey of duplex Doppler instruments. *Radiology* **177**, 265–272.

Laird EE, Williams D, Williams ED *et al.* (1987) Can the hepatic perfusion index improve routine diagnosis of liver disease? *Nucl. Med. Commun.* **8**, 959.

Leen E, Goldberg JA, Robertson J *et al.* (1991a) Detection of hepatic metastases using duplex colour Doppler sonography. *Ann. Surg.* **214**, 599–604.

Leen E, Goldberg JA, Robertson, Sutherland GR & McArdle CS (1991b) The use of duplex sonography in the detection of colorectal liver metastases. *Br. J. Cancer* **63**, 323–325.

Leen E, Goldbert JA, Anderson JR, Moule B, Cooke TG & McArdle CS (1993a) Hepatic perfusion changes in patients with hepatic metastases: comparison with those in patients with cirrhosis. *Gut* **34**, 554–557.

Leen E, Angerson WJ, Warren H *et al.* (1993b) Hepatic arterial haemodynamics changes following intra-arterial angiotensin II infusion: duplex /colour Doppler sonography. *Clin. Radiol.* **47**, 321–324.

Leen E, Anderson JR, Robertson J, Wotherspoon H, Cooke TG & McArdle CS (1993c) Detection of hepatic metastases secondary to gastric carcinoma: an alternative method. *Gastroenterology* **104(4)**, A420.

Leng B, O'Driscoll MP, Majeed FA *et al.* (1987) Hepatic perfusion index in cirrhotic livers: investigation of imaging and analytical procedures. *Nucl. Med. Commun.* **8**, 1001–1010.

Leveson SH, Wiggins PA, Nasiru TA *et al.* (1983) Improving the detection of hepatic metastases by the use of dynamic scintigraphy. *Br. J. Cancer* **47**, 719–721.

Leveson SH, Wiggins PA, Giles GR *et al.* (1985) Deranged liver blood flow in the detection of liver metastases. *Br. J. Surg.* **72**, 128–130.

McGregor JR, Galloway DJ, Hilditch TE *et al.* (1987) Enhanced perfusion scintigraphy in metastatic liver disease. *Br. J. Surg.* **74**, 1148–1149.

Maughan J, Parkin A, Smith AH *et al.* (1992) Hepatic perfusion index: a multicentre trial. *Nucl. Med. Commun.* **13**, 161–167.

Metzger U, Mermillod B, Aeberhard P *et al.* (1987) Intraportal chemotherapy in colorectal carcinoma as an adjuvant modality. *World J. Surg.* **ii**, 452.

Moertel CG, Fleming TR, MacDonald JS *et al.* (1990) Levamisole and fluorouracil for adjuvant therapy of resected colon carcinoma. *N. Engl. J. Med.* **322**, 352–358.

Nakamura T, Moriyasu F, Ban N *et al.* (1989) Quantitative measurement of abdominal arterial blood flow using image directed Doppler US: superior mesenteric, splenic and common hepatic arterial blood flow in normal adults. *J. Clin. Ultrasound* **17**, 261–268.

Notts DM, Grime SJ, Yates J *et al.* (1989) Changes in the hepatic perfusion index during the development of experimental liver tumours. *Br. J. Surg.* **76**, 259–263.

Parkin A, Robinson PJ, Baxter P *et al.* (1983) Liver perfusion scintigraphy – method, normal range and laparotomy correlation in 100 patients. *Nucl. Med. Commun.* **4**, 395–402.

Perkins AC, Whalley DR, Ballantyne KC *et al.* (1987) Reliability of the hepatic perfusion index for the detection of liver metastases. *Nucl. Med. Commun.* **8**, 982–989.

Ridge JA, Bading JR, Gelbard AS *et al.* (1987) Perfusion of colorectal hepatic metastases. *Cancer* **59**, 1547–1553.

Robertson J, Leen E, Goldberg JA *et al.* (1992) Flow measurement using duplex Doppler ultrasound: haemodynamic changes in patients with colorectal liver metastases. *Clin. Phys. Physiol. Meas.* **13**, 709–921.

Sarper R, Fajman WA, Rypins EB *et al.* (1981) A non-invasive method for measuring portal venous/total hepatic blood flow by hepatosplenic radionuclide angiography. *Radiology* **141**, 179–184.

Sato S, Ohnishi K, Sugita S *et al.* (1987) Splenic artery and superior mesenteric artery blood flow: non-surgical Doppler ultrasouind measurement in healthy subjects and patients with chronic liver disease. *Radiology* **164**, 347–352.

Taylor I, Machin D, Mullee M *et al.* (1985) Randomised controlled trial of adjuvant portal vein cytotoxic perfusion in colorectal cancer. *Br. J. Surg.* **74**, 455–459.

Wereldsma JCJ, Bruggink EDM, Meijer WS *et al.* (1990) Adjuvant portal liver infusion in colorectal cancer with 5-fluorouracil/heparin versus urokinase versus control. *Cancer* **65**, 425.

Wolmark N, Rockette H, Wickerham DL *et al.* (1990) Adjuvant therapy of Duke A, B and C adenocarcinoma of the colon with portal vein 5-fluorouracil hepatic infusion: preliminary results of NSABP protocol C-02. *J. Clin. Oncol.* **8**, 146.

4

Resection: how to do it

Russell W. Strong

Hepatic resection for colorectal metastases is the standard treatment for resectable disease. However, from the large group of patients with colorectal cancer who develop metastatic disease, only a small number will be found suitable to undergo resection of their liver metastases and only a small subset will be cured by such surgery. It is a prerequisite that any surgeon who is contemplating resective surgery for colorectal liver metastases should select those patients who are likely to benefit from the procedure. The necessity to perform liver resection with almost zero mortality is mandatory or the perceived benefits will be negated.

Patients referred with hepatic metastases from colorectal cancer either have synchronous disease, identified during the primary resection, or metachronous disease, diagnosed at a variable interval after operation. The course of management will depend on whether the patient has synchronous or metachronous disease. With synchronous disease, baseline imaging of the liver is performed using ultrasound. If the metastatic disease is small in volume, this author advocates leaving the patient for 6 months before undertaking more extensive investigations. This allows time for the patient to recover from the resective surgery and, in some cases, reveals more widespread disease which would negate hepatic resection conferring any benefit to the patient. The author has not seen any patient who was disadvantaged by this delay but has observed a number of patients who revealed more widespread intrahepatic or extrahepatic disease that was present but not manifest at the time of the original surgery. If the metastasis is large in volume, the waiting period is not necessary, as the metastatic disease has been present for a period of time that would allow the manifestation of other intrahepatic or extrahepatic disease. In this situation, hepatic resection is performed once the patient has recovered from the colonic resection – about 4–6 weeks.

Patients referred with metachronous metastases to the liver usually have the disease identified by follow-up with protocol serial blood tests for carcinoembryonic antigen (CEA) or CA 19.9 and from liver imaging. Occasionally, investigations are prompted by the presence of some mild right upper quadrant pain or a palpable liver.

The preoperative investigations are directed towards the exclusion of extrahepatic disease, the identification of resectable disease with an adequate clear margin (1 cm or greater) and an assessment of the patient's ability to be able to tolerate major liver surgery. Clinical examination of the abdomen, including rectal examination, is aimed at identifying any evidence of abdominal recurrence outside the liver. Local recurrence following the primary resection usually occurs within 2 years. Metachronous liver metastases diagnosed after this period are less likely to be complicated by local recurrent disease.

If the chest X-ray is clear, computer tomography (CT) of the chest and abdomen is performed. This endeavours to identify the presence or absence of pulmonary metastases or intra-abdominal disease outside the liver, as well as the extent of liver involvement. The author has found ultrasonography of the liver a much more reliable modality than CT scan for the detection of non-resectable metastases as well as the relationship of the tumour masses to important vascular structures.

Preoperative preparation

Hepatic angiography is necessary for preoperative assessment in cases of gallbladder and high bile duct cancer but is not required prior to resection for metastatic disease. Inexperienced hepatic surgeons may find it a useful 'road map' in the early period of their experience. Perhaps a better reason for arteriography is to allow CT portography, which is currently the most sensitive preoperative imaging modality. Whilst CT portography is certainly sensitive, it relatively frequently produces false-positive results in certain parts of the liver (see Chapter 2).

The preoperative assessment is aimed at assessing the patient's ability to tolerate the procedure, to aid in assessing potential problems in the postoperative period and to predict the need for ventilatory support. They also form a baseline for reference, subsequent to resection. Clinical assessment of cardiorespiratory function should include an electrocardiogram and spirometry. Preoperative chest physiotherapy and breathing exercises are given to all patients. This period of therapy may need to be prolonged and accompanied by the use of bronchodilators in patients with chronic airways disease.

The blood tests will include full blood count, multiple biochemical analysis and a coagulation profile. The patient's blood group is determined. The quantity of blood to be cross-matched will be dependent on the preoperative haemoglobin, the type of resection and the experience of the surgeon. A coagulation profile in the normal range is a prerequisite for the insertion of an epidural catheter, which has become a routine for postoperative analgesia.

The anticipation of an open abdomen and rib retraction for a prolonged period of time, in addition to extensive handling of a portion of liver with probable necrotic tumour, necessitates the use of prophylactic antibiotics to cover the operative and immediate postoperative period. The author's preference has been amoxycillin and an aminoglycoside.

Thromboembolism is an important complication of liver resection and heparin 5000 units subcutaneously twice daily is used routinely.

Operative procedures

An epidural catheter is inserted by the anaesthetist prior to the commencement of a general anaesthetic. Intravenous and intra-arterial lines will be necessary for adequate infusions and monitoring but some of these are delayed until the laparotomy confirms that resection will proceed. The patient should be placed supine on the operating table with a warming blanket to maintain normothermia. The operating table should allow cholangiography to be performed. The right arm of the patient should be suitably retained by the side, thereby avoiding ulnar nerve damage from forced abduction by the second assistant during the procedure.

The major portion of the liver is high under the right costal margin and is not easy to access. Retraction of the costal margins is essential and can be achieved by the use of a solid, self-retaining retractor, fixed to the operating table. The abdomen is opened via an oblique right subcostal incision. This allows preliminary assessment of whether the patient has resectable disease and can then be extended as necessary. The incision most commonly employed is a bilateral subcostal incision with a xiphisternal midline extension (Fig. 4.1). On occasions, the right subcostal incision extended vertically to the xiphisternum is adequate. A thoracoabdominal incision is never used by the author. On only three occasions in 585 liver

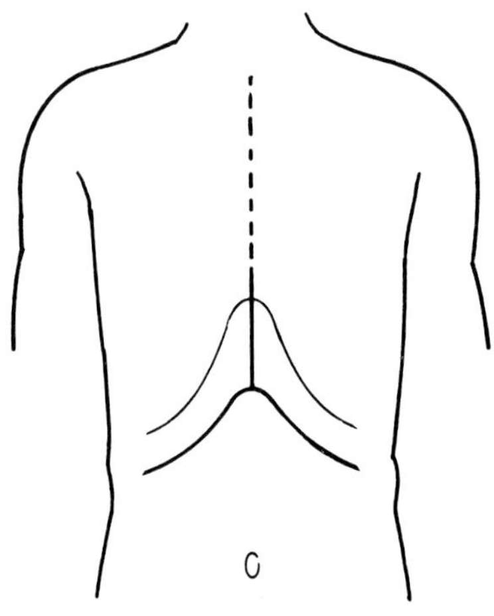

Figure 4.1 Abdominal incision.

resections for all causes did the size and position of the lesion to be resected necessitate a median sternotomy extension.

Abdominal exploration is directed towards the exclusion of extrahepatic disease and the demonstration of resectable disease in the liver. Adhesions from previous colorectal surgery may make a general laparotomy difficult. As best as possible, the surgeon needs to define if there is any evidence of local recurrence, peritoneal or omental tumour or enlarged lymph nodes in the area of drainage of the primary tumour. Attention is then directed to the presence or absence of enlarged lymph nodes in the hepatoduodenal ligament, peripancreatic and coeliac regions. A suspicious node should be sent for frozen section. If there is no evidence of extrahepatic disease, a thorough examination of the liver is performed. If preliminary palpation indicates resectable disease, the abdominal incision is extended. The ligamentum teres is ligated and divided and, with the assistant retracting the liver posteriorly, the falciform ligament is divided with electrocautery up to the suprahepatic inferior vena cava. Thorough bimanual palpation is performed. It may be necesary to mobilize the right lobe in order to carry out a complete examination.

Intraoperative ultrasound

Intraoperative ultrasound has become an important adjunct in the management of hepatic metastases. Combined with palpation, it offers greater sensitivity in the detection of small nodules not delineated by preoperative imaging modalities. It is valuable in localizing the lesion to a particular anatomical segment and where appropriate permits the performance of a segment-oriented resection. The learning curve to attain proficiency is prolonged and it is advised that the surgeon seek the assistance of an experienced radiologist during the early phase of its use. Once proficiency is attained, it becomes an indispensable tool in the armamentarium of the hepatic surgeon.

Anatomy

The liver has a complex vasculature but little in the way of surface landmarks to indicate the location of either the inflow portal elements or the outflow hepatic veins. The morphological anatomy of the liver bears little relationship to the more recently described and accepted functional anatomy which is based on the distribution of the portal pedicles and location of the hepatic veins (Bismuth, 1982). Confusion has resulted from the different nomenclature based on either the morphological or functional anatomy of the liver. In this chapter, the segmental content of each resection will be enumerated. The liver is divided functionally into two hemilivers, each independent with regard to arterial and portal venous inflow and biliary drainage. There is no surface marking to indicate the division. The principal plane between the right and left hemilivers (Cantlie's line) runs from the gallbladder fossa to the inferior vena cava and contains the middle hepatic vein. With the liver in its normal position, the plane is inclined 30–60° to the right (Fig. 4.2). It will be shown later that this has important implications in positioning the liver during resection.

Further subdivision of the liver into sectors and segments is made on the basis of the distribution of the portal triad. The portal vein and hepatic artery divide into right and left branches outside the liver. The portal pedicles to the right side of the liver divide into anterior and posterior branches which, after a further 2 cm inside the liver, divide into cranial and caudal branches. The biliary drainage, with some aberrations, generally follows the same pattern. The right hemiliver is composed of an anterior sector comprising caudal segment V

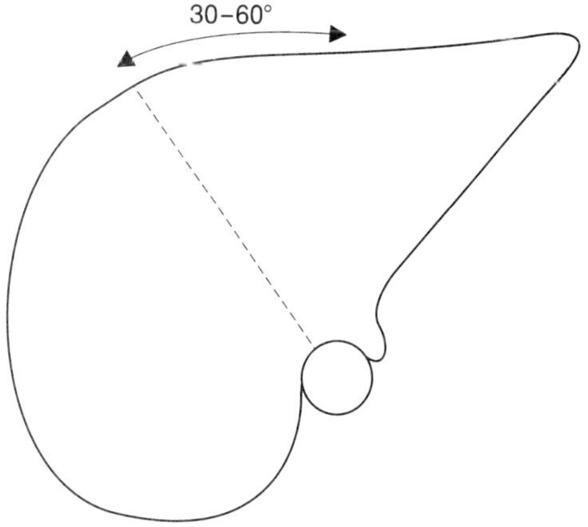

Figure 4.2 Transverse section through the liver as seen on computed tomography scan. The principal plane is inclined between 30–60° to the right.

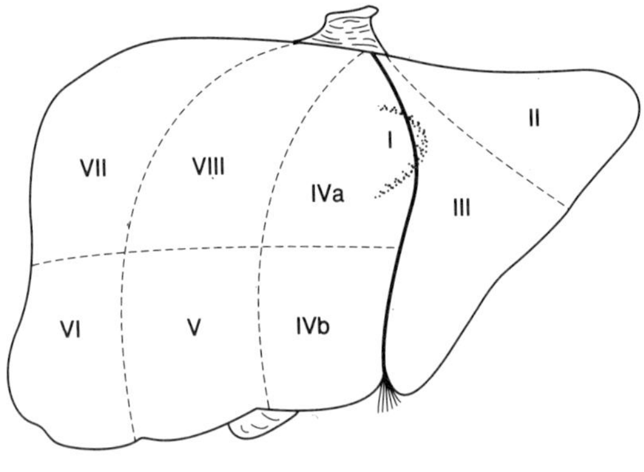

Figure 4.3 Segmental anatomy of the liver.

and cranial segment VIII and a posterior sector comprising caudal segment VI and cranial segment VII Fig 4.3).

For the left hemiliver, the portal vein curves anteriorly at the posterior end of the umbilical fissure, passing forwards to insert at the ligamentum teres. The branch to segment II is given off at the curve. The branches to segments III and IV are given off near the insertion into the ligamentum teres. The hepatic artery and bile duct give off the segment IV branches prior to division into cranial and caudal branches (II and III respectively) in a similar fashion to the right side. Scheele (1989) has proposed that segment IV is divided into a smaller apical portion as segment IV(a) and the larger caudal portion as segment IV(b), both on an anatomical and surgically useful basis. This gives an almost symmetrical structure to both halves of the liver (Fig. 4.3). Segmental borders are delineated on the longitudinal axis by the path of the hepatic veins and on the transverse axis by the portal pedicle branching. The caudate lobe (segment I), including the caudate process, is somewhat separate and autonomous. It is situated posteriorly on the left side of the inferior vena cava with the caudate process extending to the right, behind the portal structures, in front of the inferior vena cava. It receives arterial and portal supply from both the left and right branches and the main trunks and its biliary drainage is usually to the confluence of the right and left hepatic ducts. The hepatic veins drain directly into the inferior vena cava via a number of short branches.

With the exception of resection of segments II and III (the left lateral segment), all liver resections require full mobilization of the right lobe. As outlined previously, the plane of resection through Cantlie's line is approximately 30–60° to the right, from the vertical. When the right lobe has been mobilized and the position maintained with packs behind the liver, the plane of resection between the right and left hemilivers is vertical. It is considerably easier to perform and maintain the plane of resection when it is vertical rather than oblique. The vertical plane can be achieved in all resections except between the anterior (segments V and VIII) and posterior (segments VI and VII) sectors of the right lobe, where a horizontal plane is present with the liver in its normal position, and an oblique plane (60°) with the liver mobilized and retained with packs.

The right lobe is mobilized by division of the peritoneal reflections to the bare area. This is most conveniently achieved by lifting the liver anteriorly and commencing the division of the posterior coronary ligament (Fig. 4.4). Passing laterally, the division continues with the right triangular ligament and, with retraction of the right lobe to the left, continues medially with division of the anterior coronary ligament towards the inferior vena cava. The entire bare area is exposed up to the inferior vena cava. At times, the right adrenal gland is firmly adherent to the liver and may require a ligature on the adrenal gland side prior to separation. The inferior vena cava is obscured by a sheath of fibrous tissue in its superior part, the so-called inferior vena caval ligament. Division of this ligament displays the posterior aspect of the

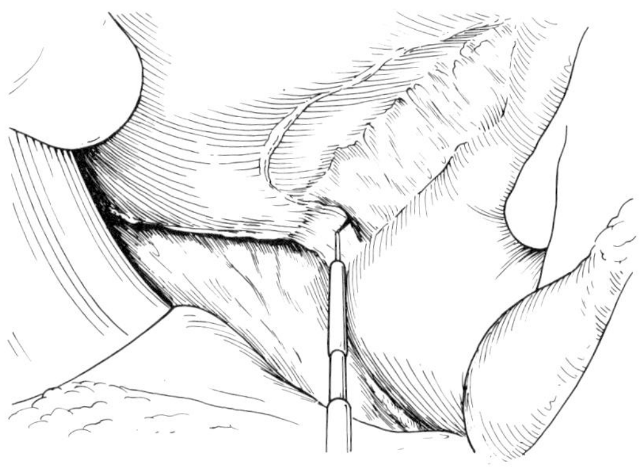

Figure 4.4 Division of peritoneal reflection over bare area. This is the commencement of mobilization of the right lobe.

junction of the right hepatic vein with the inferior vena cava. When fully mobilized, the right lobe of the liver can be rotated completely into the wound.

Metastatic colorectal cancers may be found attached to the diaphragm. It may be possible to dissect the tumour free from the diaphragm but, if this is not possible, resection of a portion of the diaphragm, with the tumour, is necessary. The diaphragmatic defect is repaired with non-absorbable suture. Histology usually indicates inflammatory adhesion between the tumour and the diaphragm, rather than malignant invasion.

Right hemihepatectomy (segments V–VIII)

Retraction of the inferior surface of the liver displays the gallbladder and portal structures. Calot's triangle is dissected and the cystic artery is ligated and divided. The cystic duct is dissected, ligated and divided, leaving a long cystic duct stump (see later; Fig. 4.5). Cholecystectomy is performed. The peritoneum overlying the structures in the hepatoduodenal ligament is incised. The right hepatic artery (sometimes two) is dissected and encircled with a rubber vessel loop. Rotation of the right lobe anteriorly aids in the dissection of the right portal vein (Fig. 4.6), which sometimes divides outside the liver into its anterior and posterior branches. The portal vein or veins are encircled with a rubber vessel loop. In dissecting the vein, care must be taken to avoid tearing the short branch to the caudate process. Vascular clamps

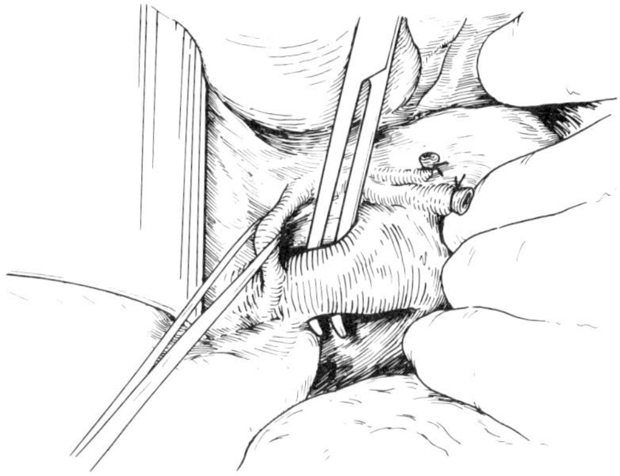

Figure 4.6 Dissection of the hilum of the liver, to identify and sling the right hepatic artery and right portal vein.

are applied to the right hepatic artery and right portal vein. A clear line of demarcation will appear on the liver surface, indicating the line of transection between the right and left hemilivers. The right hepatic artery is ligated and divided. The right portal vein is doubly clamped with angle vascular clamps. The portal vein is partially divided between the clamps and a 4/0 or 5/0 vascular suture commenced on the proximal stump. The sequence of division and suture continues until the full width of the portal vein is secured. The clamp can then be safely removed. The distal stump is transfixed with the vascular suture and the clamp removed (Fig. 4.7). Dissection of the confluence of the hepatic ducts and division of the right hepatic duct are not performed at this stage. Division of the right hepatic duct is carried out after transection of the liver in the principal plane,

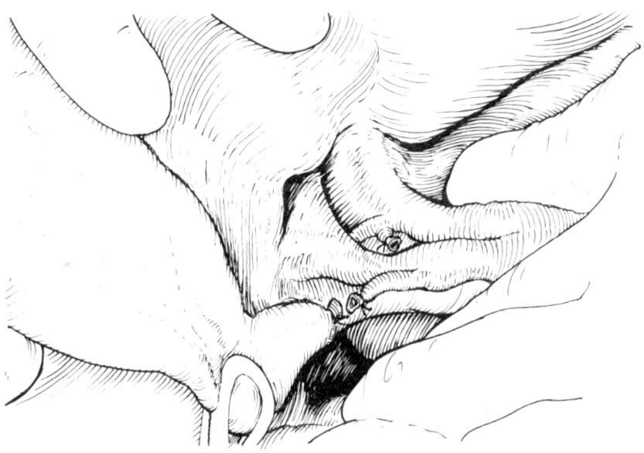

Figure 4.5 Dissection of Calot's triangle with ligation and division of the cystic artery and duct.

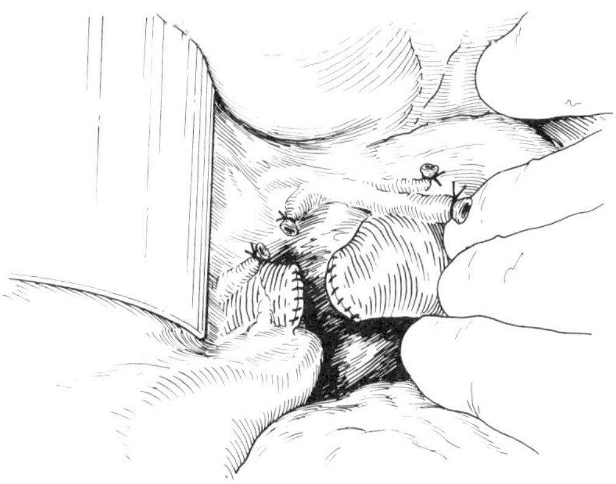

Figure 4.7 Division and ligation of the right hepatic artery and division and suture of the right portal vein.

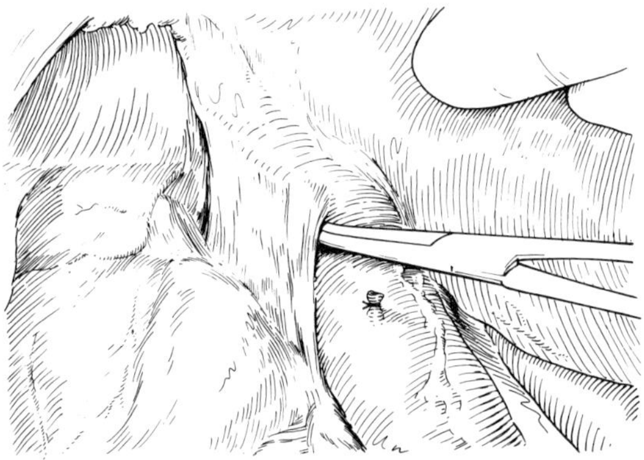

Figure 4.8 After division and ligation of the short hepatic veins, the inferior vena caval ligament is displayed.

thereby avoiding potential damage to the left hepatic duct or the confluence.

Rotation of the mobilized right lobe of the liver to the left and upwards displays the inferior vena cava and the inferior short hepatic veins. Commencing behind the caudate process, these veins are ligated and divided in sequence, from caudad to craniad. Any vein of substance should be sutured rather than ligated. The inferior vena caval ligament is a sheath of fibrous tissue overlying the inferior vena cava in its superior portion (Fig. 4.8). This ligament requires division to display the inferior vena cava, where it is joined by the right hepatic vein (Fig. 4.9). When this junction is extrahepatic and easily encircled, the application of clamps, division and suture with 3/0 or 4/0 vascular suture is performed (Fig. 4.10). When the junction is buried in liver tissue and difficult to dissect or encircle or when a tumour bulges or abuts this area, extrahepatic dissection should not be attempted. Abdominal packs are placed behind the right lobe to bring the transection plane to the vertical position (Fig. 4.11). Electrocautery is used to divide the liver capsule at the line of demarcation produced by clamping the inflow vessels. The divided capsule extends from the inferior vena cava superiorly, across the anterior surface of the liver to the gallbladder fossa and then across the

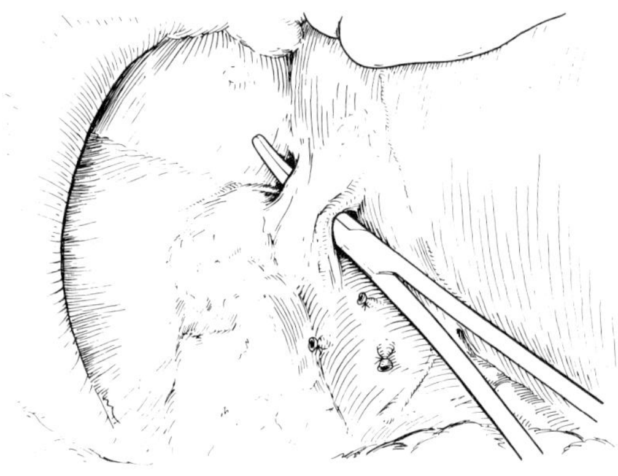

Figure 4.9 Right hepatic vein dissected.

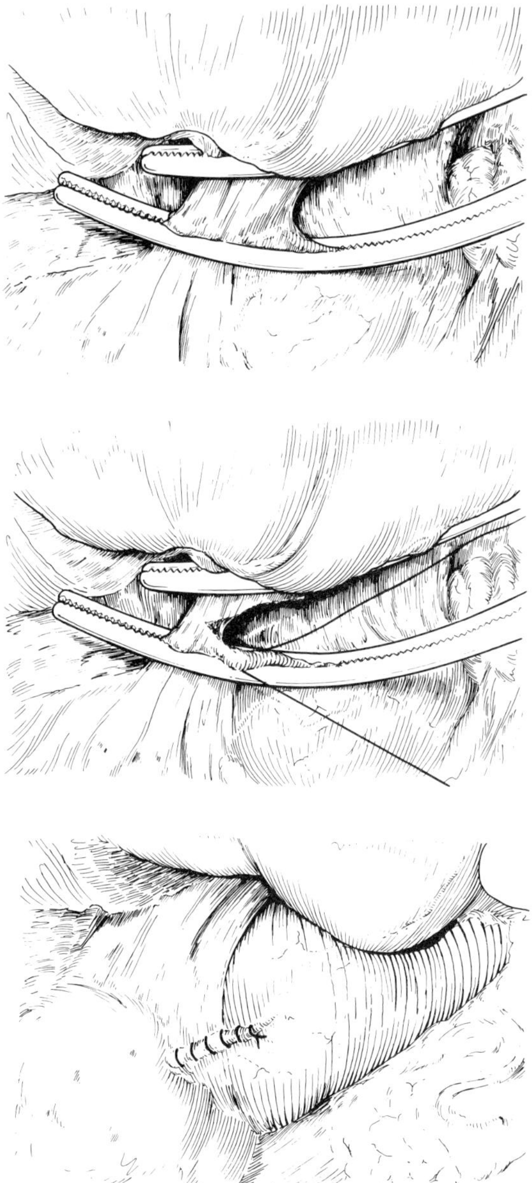

a

b

c

Figure 4.10 (a–c) Stages of division and suturing of right hepatic vein.

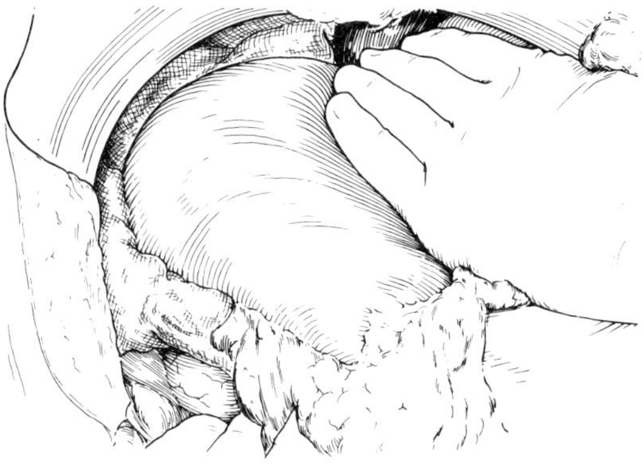

Figure 4.11 Packs behind the right lobe, bringing the resection plane to the vertical position.

gallbladder bed and caudate process at the right side of the inferior vena cava.

The parenchymal transection can be performed by a number of methods, such as finger fracture, Kelly clamp crush, dissection with a fine metal sucker or the use of more sophisticated and expensive devices such as the ultrasonic dissector or waterjet dissector. The author prefers the ultrasonic dissector. The transection commences at the liver edge and progresses posteriorly and superiorly. The small vessels and ducts crossing the plane of transection are divided after ligating the left side with fine silk and applying metal clips to the right side, which is to be removed. Large structures are sutured with a 4/0 or 5/0 vascular suture. At the hilum, the right hepatic duct, ensheathed in Glisson's capsule, is safely encircled away from the confluence, ligated and divided (Fig. 4.12).

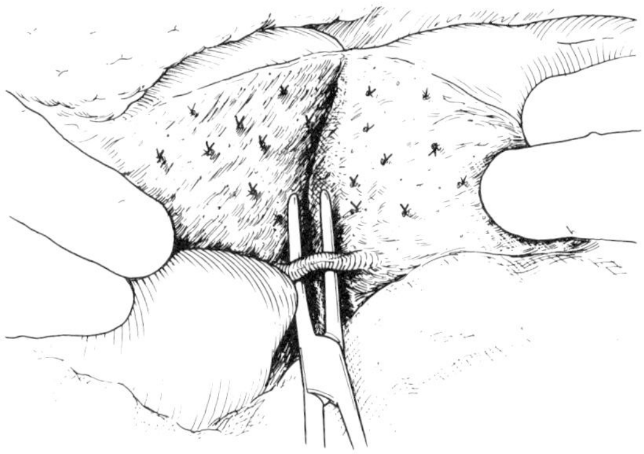

Figure 4.12 Right hepatic duct dissected and divided away from the confluence.

Once the transection extends deep into the liver, the posterior packs are removed in sequence, commensurate with the increasing depth of resection, to allow the field to open out like a book. The plane of transection extends along the right side of the middle hepatic vein which is visible along its length at the completion of the resection. Inferiorly, the caudate process is transected at the right margin of the inferior vena cava. The resection continues superiorly, removing the right liver from the inferior vena cava. The short hepatic veins have already been ligated and divided. The right hemiliver is gradually retracted to the right as the resection proceeds superiorly. The left hand is placed above and behind the liver with the forefinger placed along the groove between the liver and the inferior vena cava and the thumb along the resected surface of the right hemiliver.

Forward lifting with the forefinger and retraction laterally with the thumb allow the final portion of the liver to be transected with safety and relative ease (Fig. 4.13a). In cases where a large tumour in segments VII and VIII prevents this manoeuvre the surgeon can place his left hand from below with the forefinger in the same position and the thumb pushing the resected surface of the left hemiliver to the left. Alternatively, this can be carried out by the assistant using his left hand (Fig. 4.13b).

In those cases where the right hepatic vein has not been divided and sutured from behind it is dissected to allow application of a curved vascular clamp to the vena caval side and a long haemostat to the side to be removed. The vein is partially divided and a 3/0 vascular suture commenced, thereby avoiding any catastrophe should the vein slip out of the clamp before the vein is secured (Fig. 4.14). The sequence of division and suture continues until the vein is secure and the specimen is removed (Fig. 4.15).

The surface of resection should be dry at the completion of the procedure. However, if there is any ooze, it can be controlled by compression, diathermy or suture. An umbilical catheter is inserted into the long cystic duct, retained at cholecystectomy. The injection of saline together with finger compression of the lower common bile duct will indicate any site of biliary leak which can be secured with a fine suture. After removal of the catheter, the cystic duct is ligated.

a

b

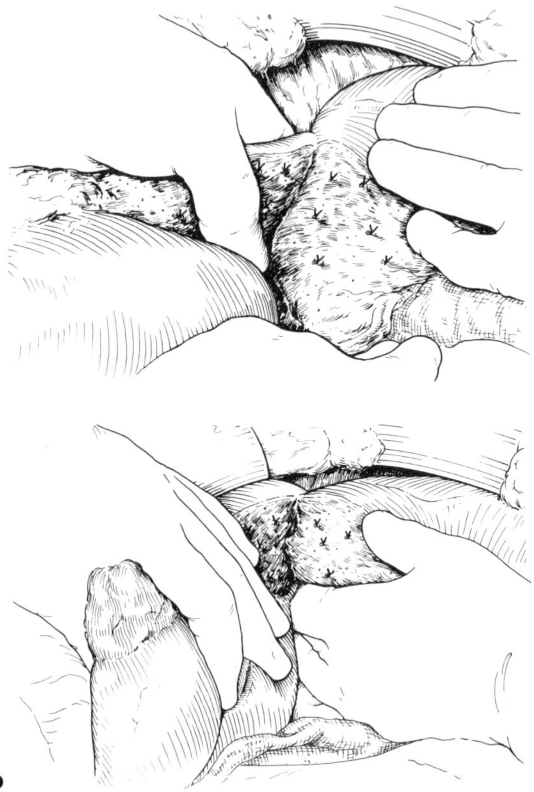

Figure 4.13 In the final portion of the resection, the left hand of the surgeon is used to lift the liver forward, either from above (a) or by the assistant from below (b).

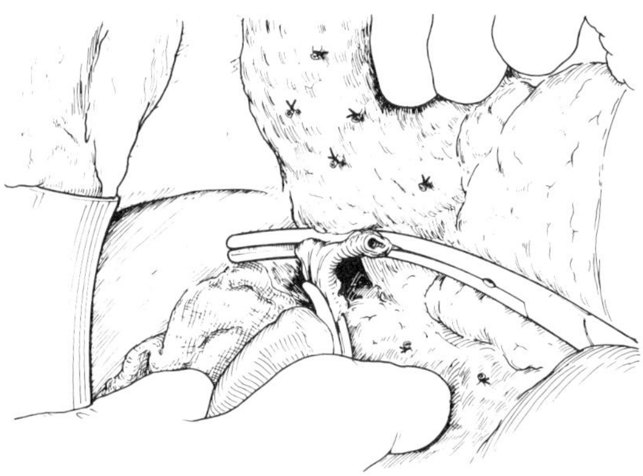

Figure 4.14 When extrahepatic division and suture of the right hepatic vein is not possible, the procedure is performed from within the liver, as the final step in the resection.

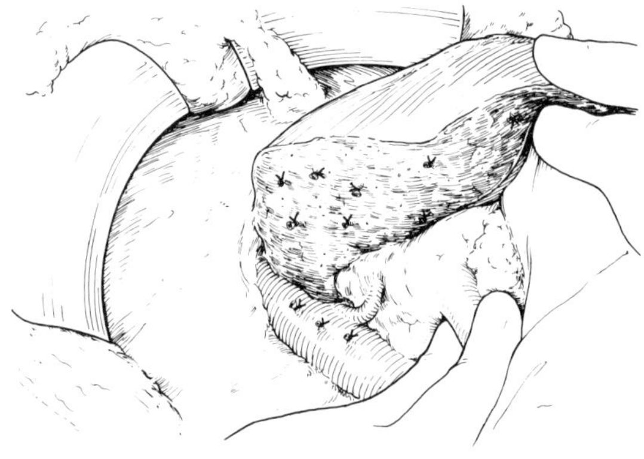

Figure 4.15 The completed resection.

Extended right hepatectomy (segments IV–VIII)

The preliminary steps in performing an extended right hepatectomy are the same as for the right hemihepatectomy. The hepatic mass in segments II and III must be of sufficient size to sustain adequate hepatic function. Compensatory hypertrophy of this liver tissue will have occurred when a large tumour mass has replaced a major portion of the liver to be removed. The consequences of resection on hepatic reserve are minimal. However, there would be a high risk of fatal liver failure with resection of an equivalent amount of liver, for small, unfavourably placed tumours, which would not be accompanied by compensatory hypertrophy. Under these circumstances, a segment-oriented resection may be advantageous.

The cystic duct and artery are ligated and divided as with a right hemihepatectomy but the gallbladder does not need to be removed. The right hepatic artery and right portal vein are managed in the same way as described for a right hemihepatectomy. The base of the quadrate lobe (segment IV) requires dissection to free the confluence of the hepatic ducts. This requires division of the hilar plate – the fusion of the Glisson's capsule with the connective tissue enclosing the portal triad (Fig. 4.16) (Bismuth *et al.*, 1982). When the hilar plate has been divided, the base of segment IV can be elevated, allowing the right hepatic duct or ducts to be encircled, ligated and divided (Fig. 4.17). Further dissection posteriorly frees the left portal structures from the base of segment IV.

The line of transection is to the right of the

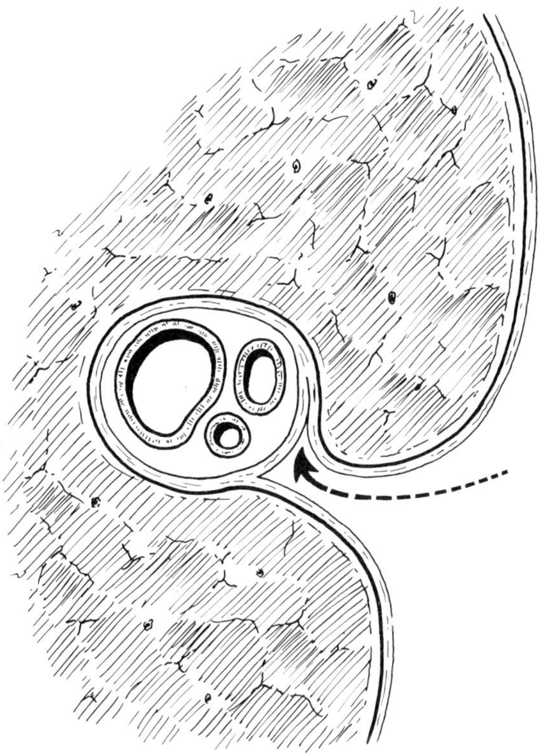

Figure 4.16 Access to the bile duct by incision of the Glisson's capsule at the base of the quadrate lobe. (Reproduced with permission, Surgery of the Liver and Biliary Tract. L. Blumgart (Ed). Churchill Livingstone).

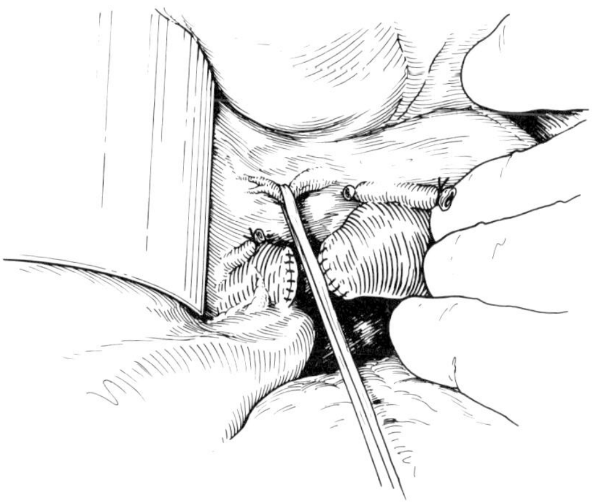

Figure 4.17 Ligation and division of the right hepatic artery and division and suture of the right portal vein as in right hemihepatectomy. Following division of the hilar plate, the right hepatic duct is encircled, retracted, ligated and divided.

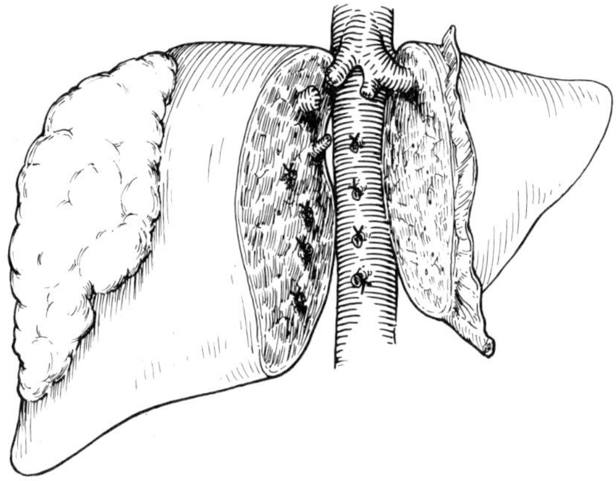

Figure 4.18 The near completed extended right hepatectomy exposing the inferior vena cava with ligated short hepatic veins and divided and sutured middle and right hepatic veins.

falciform ligament and umbilical fissure, where the feedback structures pass to segment IV, and can be secured without damage to the main structures supplying the left liver. The capsule of the liver is incised with electrocautery, extending from the middle of the inferior vena cava superiorly, along the right side of the falciform ligament and umbilical fissure. The presence of a bridge of liver tissue over the ligamentum teres between segments III and IV is variable. If present, it can be divided with electrocautery.

Parenchymal transection, using the ultrasonic dissector, commences at the anterior edge and proceeds superiorly and posteriorly. The feedback structures are isolated, ligated and divided. The resection continues posteriorly towards the inferior vena cava. Superiorly, the resection crosses the middle hepatic vein, close to its site of insertion into the left hepatic vein or inferior vena cava. It is dissected, divided and ligated or sutured. The resection then continues from caudad to craniad, dissecting the liver off the inferior vena cava, in a similar fashion to that described for right hemihepatectomy. The short hepatic veins will have already been ligated and divided, and the right hepatic vein will be treated in a similar fashion to that previously described (Fig. 4.18).

Left hemihepatectomy (segments II–IV)

Left hemihepatectomy involves much the same dissection as for right hemihepatectomy, but

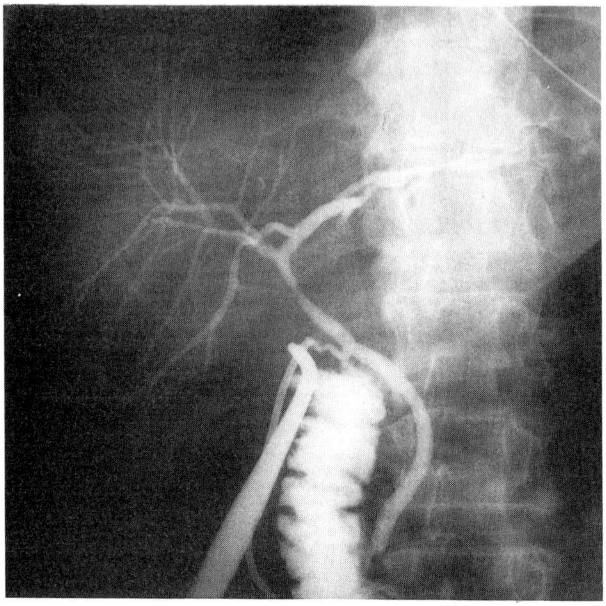

Figure 4.19 Operative cholangiogram demonstrating a right segmental duct entering the left hepatic duct above the apparent confluence of the hepatic ducts.

with some very important differences. The right lobe is mobilized as previously described. However, the inferior vena caval ligament and the short hepatic veins are left intact. The left lobe of the liver is mobilized by dividing the left triangular ligament. The placement of an abdominal pack high up under the left lobe, protecting the underlying stomach and spleen, allows the ligament to be divided with ease and safety using electrocautery. Care must be taken not to damage the left hepatic vein as the division approaches the inferior vena cava. When the mobilized left lateral segment is lifted forwards, the thin gastrohepatic omentum is displayed and can be divided close to the liver. If a left hepatic artery arises from the left gastric artery, it is easily visible in the gastrohepatic omentum where it is ligated and divided.

When performing left hemihepatectomy it is important to perform a cholangiogram. It is not infrequent for one of the right sectoral or segmental ducts to join with left hepatic duct well to the left side (Fig. 4.19). Delineation of this anatomical situation will avoid inadvertent ligation and division. Access to the left hepatic duct is obtained by dividing the hilar plate as previously described, lifting the base at segment IV upwards and encircling the left hepatic duct which can then be ligated and divided. The left hepatic artery is ligated and divided. The caudate lobe is not usually resected in this operation and the left portal vein should be divided distal to the origin of the caudate branches and sutured with 4/0 or 5/0 vascular suture (Fig. 4.20). The line of demarcation, as with the right hemihepatectomy, is from the gallbladder fossa to the inferior vena cava. The plane of resection needs to be brought to the vertical, in the same way as for the right-sided resection by the placement of packs behind the

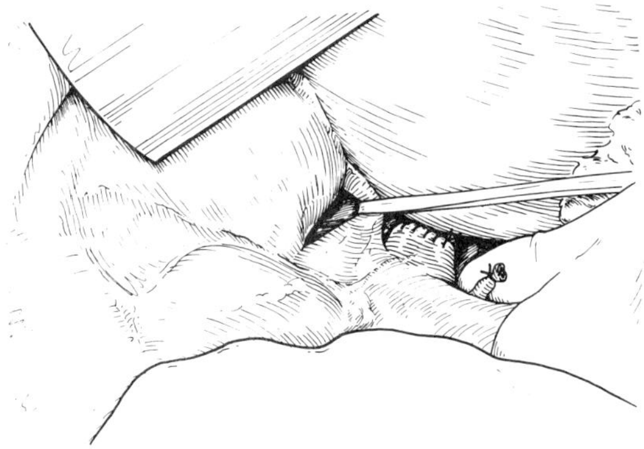

Figure 4.20 The ligated and divided left hepatic artery, divided and sutured left portal vein and dissected and slung left hepatic duct, in preparation for left hemicolectomy.

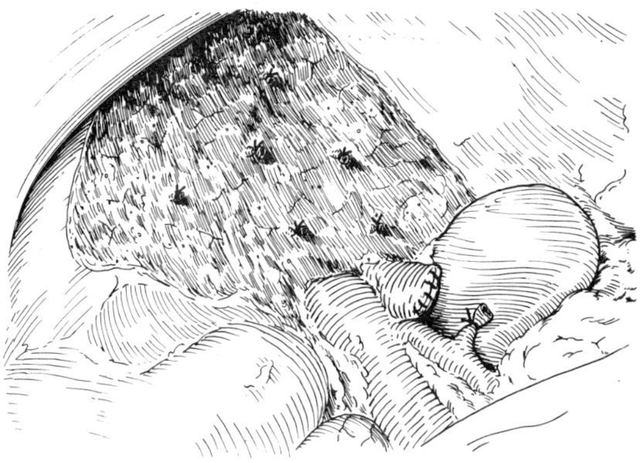

Figure 4.21 The completed left hemihepatectomy. The right hemiliver is in the normal anatomical position, demonstrating the oblique principal plane.

right lobe. The resection proceeds in a similar fashion, along the left side of the middle hepatic vein. The final structure to be dealt with is the left hepatic vein, which is clamped and sutured in a similar fashion to the right hepatic vein, as previously described. The middle hepatic vein most commonly enters the left hepatic vein near the inferior vena cava and it is usually preserved unless the proximity of tumour necessitates a wider resection. When the packs are removed from behind the right lobe and the right lobe settles back in its normal postion, the oblique principal plane is clearly seen (Fig. 4.21).

Resection of segments II and III (left lateral segmentectomy)

This is the simplest of the more commonly performed hepatic resections. Control of the inflow vessels at the hilum is not required. The left lobe of the liver is mobilized by dividing the left triangular ligament and gastrohepatic omentum as previously described. The presence of a bridge of the liver tissue over the ligamentum teres between segments III and IV is variable. If present, it can be divided with electrocautery. The resection line is just to the left of the ligamentum teres and falciform ligament to avoid damage to the segment IV vessels and duct. The liver capsule is divided in the line of resection using electrocautery. The parenchymal division is performed using the ultrasonic dissector, commencing at the anterior edge and progressing superiorly and posteriorly. The major inflow structures that will be encountered are at the base of the umbilical fissure where they will be isolated, ligated and divided. The transection continues superiorly towards the left hepatic vein which is dissected, clamped and sutured as previously described.

These four standard operations are the most commonly performed hepatic resections. Some variation may be necessary when a tumour is large or in an awkward position in relationship to important intrahepatic structures, such as the middle hepatic vein. In these circumstances, the resection line will need to be redirected into a neighbouring area of liver to gain adequate clearance of the tumour. This may be performed without the necessity to remove all the adjoining segment. For example, a large tumour in segments V and VIII, pushing the middle hepatic vein towards the left side, could be adequately resected by a right hemihepatectomy plus resection of the right portion of segment IV which would include the middle hepatic vein. This would preserve a portion of segment IV which would be lost if an extended right hepatectomy was performed. This type of resection would be termed a right hemihepatectomy extended into segment IV.

Extended left hepatectomy (segments II–V, VIII and ± I)

This is technically one of the most demanding of hepatic resections. It is usually performed for large tumours, centrally placed, but which cannot be accomplished with either a left hemihepatectomy or extended right hepatectomy. Although the necessity to perform this operation is relatively uncommon, the author has employed the operation on 17 patients, mainly for primary malignancy but also for metastatic disease. A detailed description is beyond the capacity of this book. However, readers are referred to the excellent description of the technique by Blumgart (1988).

Segmental resections

Although segmental resections are regarded as somewhere between a local excision and a major resection, this is a misconception. Certainly with regard to volume of liver removed, they are in the middle of the spectrum. However, with regard to technical difficulty, they generally exceed that required for the standard liver resections. In the right hemiliver, the use of segmental resection permits adequate resection without unnecessary removal of a large amount of normal liver tissue.

Segment-oriented resections can be numerous in their design, which will be specifically related to the number, size, position and extent of the disease and the necessity to leave the patient with an adequate hepatic mass to prevent postoperative liver failure. Segment-oriented resections can be classified as follows (after Scheele, 1989):

1. Monosegmentectomy – the removal of a single anatomical unit as previously defined.
2. Multiple segmentectomies – simultaneous segmentectomies performed on different parts of the liver e.g. VII, IVb.
3. Bi- and polysegmentectomies – removal of interconnected individual segments e.g. V, VIII and IV, V and VIII.
4. Segment-oriented modifications of classical resections – a subgroup of polysegmentectomies e.g. left hemihepatectomy (II–IV) plus VII.

Detailed descriptions of the various types of segmental resection are beyond the scope of this book. Readers are referred to more detailed descriptions by Bismuth, Houssin and Castaing (1982) and Scheele (1989).

Local excision, often described as a wedge excision, still has a limited place in the treatment of metastatic tumour. The tumour should be not greater than 3 cm in size, subcapsular in position and well clear of portal structures and hepatic veins. The ideal position for such local excision is a lesion at the outer edge of the left lateral segment. It must be remembered that the lesion is somewhat like an iceberg in that the intrahepatic extent of the tumour is always greater than is obvious from the surface. The resection needs to be in the form of a large arch and must gain a clearance of at least 1 cm.

Before wound closure, the cut surface should be dry. This will have been achieved during the transection procedure, so that little in the way of diathermy or suture ligation is necessary after the resection is completed. Haemostatic agents, such as fibrin glue, are rarely required and it is unnecessary to attempt to cover the cut surface with peritoneum or omentum.

The remaining liver is allowed to settle into its most natural position which causes no problems when performing any left-sided resection. When a large tumour has been resected on the right side, there is a tendency for the left-sided remnant to rotate over into the large fossa created by the resection. There is a danger that the left hepatic vein and/or the inferior vena cava may become kinked. This can be prevented by suturing the falciform ligament to the peritoneum of the anterior abdominal wall. The space created will be obliterated by the downwards movement of the diaphragm and the upwards displacement of the right colon. The insertion of two or three closed suction drainage tubes (3 mm) is adequate to drain the relatively minimal serosanguineous fluid which occurs over the few days after operation. The wound is closed with nylon.

Postoperative management

A major advance in the postoperative management has been the introduction of epidural analgesia which is continued for 3 days after operation. The improved ability to perform deep-breathing exercises and to cough has reduced respiratory complications. Patients commence mobilization on the first postoperative day. The closed-suction drains are usually removed by the third day. The vast majority of patients will be discharged from hospital within 10 days.

References

Bismuth H (1982) Surgical anatomy and anatomical surgery of the liver. *World J. Surg.* **6**, 3–9.

Bismuth H, Houssin D & Castaing D (1982) Major and minor segmentectomies 'réglées' in liver surgery. *World J. Surg.* **6**, 10–24.

Blumgart L (ed) (1988) Liver resection – liver and biliary tumours. In *Surgery of the Liver and Biliary Tract*, vol 1, pp. 13–14; vol 2, 1268–1270. Churchill Livingstone.

Scheele J (1989) Segment-orientated resection of the liver: rationale and technique. In: Lygidakis N & Tytgart G (eds) *Hepato-biliary and Pancreatic Malignancies*, pp. 219–247. New York: Thieme.

5

Hepatic metastasis resection: results

Glenn Steele, Jr

Colon cancer is a highly prevalent disease throughout the world, particularly in North America where 152 000 new cases occurred in 1993 (Boring *et al.*, 1993). Although the death rate has decreased over the last few years, particularly in patients who have rectal carcinoma, at least 58 000 patients will die each year and the predominant pattern of failure will include liver as either the first or major site of distant disease spread (Steele, 1994a). For the purposes of this chapter, we will be concerned mainly with liver as the only site of metastatic failure. In this extraordinarily biologically select subset, it is estimated that approximately 18 000 patients will be diagnosed each year in North America (Steele, 1994b).

Before examining the outcome of resection of hepatic metastases from colorectal carcinoma or, in fact, any regional treatment approach, one must first understand the degree of selection involved in defining a group of patients with isolated, potentially resectable liver metastases. Pestana *et al.* (1964) reported that liver was involved in 75–80% of all patients who died from disseminated colon and rectum carcinoma. Numerous studies of the natural history of colorectal carcinoma, including our own (Goslin *et al.*, 1982), have shown that liver metastasis, although the primary determinant of patient survival, is most often only one site in a diffuse picture of disseminated disease. Obviously, disseminated disease will be irrelevant to the surgeon. For effective regional therapy, there must be no extraregional disease. And, as shown in a number of relatively recent prospective adjuvant trials, the liver is the first or only site of failure in fewer than 20% of patients who experience recurrence after primary colon or rectum cancer resection (Gastrointestinal Tumour Study Group, 1984, 1985). Naturally, some of these patients will show rapid proliferation of disease outside the liver, obviating any significant regional therapy with curative intent. In addition, over one-third of the patients who have liver-only or predominantly liver colorectal cancer metastases staged by any of the presently available non-invasive diagnostic tests will be found at surgery to have extrahepatic disease or metastases to the liver too diffuse to allow surgical resection (Steele *et al.*, 1991). Newer staging techniques, such as intraoperative ultrasound applied either laparoscopically or at the time of surgical exploration before any hepatic metastasis resection is peformed, will exclude even more patients found to have additional liver metastases deep within the parenchyma of the right or left lobes, sometimes as small as 2–4 mm in diameter (Forse *et al.*, 1993). For the astute reader of this review, it will become apparent that, as the surgeon becomes stricter in excluding patients with multiple liver lesions or with disease outside the liver, results from metastasis resection will, of course, seem better. Furthermore, as the surgeon selects patients with more indolent disease (in other words, metastasis isolated to liver or lung that grow more slowly), results

Grant support: National Institute of Health, PO1CA44704 and T32 CA09580 from resection will also seem better, even though what one might be dealing with is lead time or length time bias. These varying and often unknown selection biases may explain differences in outcome among the many single-institution hepatic metastasis resection series already published (Steele and Ravikumar, 1989). Composite series should offer a more realistic survival estimate but are just as difficult to analyse because they are equally subject to selection processes and are compromised by retrospective analysis (Hughes *et al.*, 1986, 1988a, 1988b).

In an earlier review, Steele and Ravikumar (1989) analysed most available single-institution experiences with liver metastasis resection and also included the Hughes *et al.* (1986, 1988a, 1988b) retrospective hepatic metastasis registry data. It was obvious that Adson (1983, 1987) and Foster and Berman (1977) perhaps best estimated the maximum potential therapeutic benefit. They assumed in the 1980s that if 50% of approximately 150 000 patients who at that time were incident cases with colon and rectum carcinoma would fail within 5 years, approximately 70 000 patients would be at risk for liver metastases as part of their recurrence pattern. Eventually, 60–70% of these patients would, of course, have liver as one of the involved organs, as stated above. However, only 20%, or 9000 at most, would be considered for liver resection since the liver would be the first or predominant site only in this subset. If one assumes some probability of comorbid disease excluding any major operation, then perhaps another 1000–1500 patients would be excluded from surgery. At the time of surgery, one-third, at the very least, of the 7500 patients would be found ineligible for resection because of the increased staging capacity of laparotomy itself. Thus, only 5000 patients would be potential candidates for resection each year. If one accepts the cumulative operative mortality of approximately 5%, 250 patients would die in the immediate postoperative period. Thus, with the theoretical 4750 patients operated on alive after their operation and with a 20–25% 5–10-year disease-free survival, perhaps no more than 1000 patients per year could be cured by surgical resection. This put the clinical discussion into proper context until the most recent prospective trial in which, as we will show below, there may be very little chance that even 1000 patients are cured with appropriate surgery even after the most rigorous selection of the 'best biology' disease.

Our original investment in patients with liver metastases from colon and rectum carcinoma came from a rebirth of interest in hepatic arterial chemoperfusion. This was essentially the same conceptual approach as defined by Cady and colleagues from the Lahey Clinic in 1970. The rationale for the rebirth came from the technical advances that led to the design and application of the Infusaid (Metal Bellows Corp., Sharon, MA) pump. Unfortunately, our own (Weiss *et al.*, 1983) and subsequent multi-institutional studies showed that, by and large, although patients with predominantly liver or liver-only metastatic colon and rectum carcinoma had a higher chance of liver tumour response when 5-fluorouracil or FUdR was given persistently through the hepatic artery, survival was mitigated because of increased prevalence of extrahepatic disease occurrence. In addition, toxicity from the hepatic arterial approach was consequential (Steele, 1987).

Prior to taking the next step, which was leading us to an inevitable increase in our indications for liver resection in patients who presented with isolated, potentially resectable liver metastases, we chose to review the available natural history series and we defined our own natural history series since it became apparent that the use of historical controls in defining outcome might, in fact, be artificially biasing in favour of whatever the presumed regional approach might be. In other words, we felt that perhaps the patients coming to us with isolated liver metastases were an extraordinarily biologically privileged group with relatively indolent tumour growth. Would they do well regardless of whether or not they were treated or what kind of treatment they received?

Among the natural history studies listed in Table 5.1, several have characterized survival among selected patients similar to those included in our hepatic resection series. These include the 1970 and 1983 reports by Cady *et al.*, the Goslin *et al.* study published in 1982, and the Finlay and McArdle study of occult hepatic metastases published in 1986. Patients with limited liver involvement described in these natural history series are more analogous to those on whom we operate. The benefits of our surgical therapy should be evaluated by a comparison with these historical non-treated controls if prospective non-treatment controls

Table 5.1 Liver metastases from colorectal cancer: natural history series

Authors	Journal
Pestana C, Reitemeier RJ, Moertel CG *et al.*	*Am J Surg* 1964; 108: 826–829
Jaffe BM, Donegan WL, Watson F *et al.*	*Surg Gynecol Obstet* 1968; 127: 1–11
Bengmark S & Hafstrom L	*Cancer* 1969; 23: 198–202
Oxley FM & Ellis H	*Br J Surg* 1969; 56: 149–152
Cady B, Monson DO & Swinton NW	*Surg Gynecol Obstet* 1970; 131: 697–700
Abrams MS & Lerner HJ	*Dis Colon Rectum* 1971; 14: 431–434
Neilson J, Balslev & Jensen H-E	*Acta Chir Scand* 1971; 137: 463–465
Baden H & Anderson B	*Scand J Gastroenterol* 1975; 10: 221–223
Wood CB, Gillis CR & Blumgart LH	*Clin Oncol* 1976; 2: 285–289
Welch JP & Donaldson GA	*Am J Surg* 1978; 135: 505–511
Bengsson G, Carlsson G, Hafstrom L *et al.*	*Am J Surg* 1981; 141: 586–589
Goslin R, Steele G Jr, Zamcheck N *et al.*	*Dis Colon Rectum* 1982; 25: 749–754
Levine AN, Donegan WL & Irwin M	*JAMA* 1982; 247: 2809–2810
Cady B	*Semin Oncol* 1983; 10: 127–133
Lahr CJ, Scong S-J, Cloud G *et al.*	*J Clin Oncol* 1983; 1: 720–726
Wagner JS, Adson MA, Van Heerden JA *et al.*	*Ann Surg* 1984; 199: 502–507
Wood CB. In: Van de Velde CJH & Sugarbaker P (eds)	*Natural History of Liver Metastases*, Dordrecht: Martinus Nijhoff 1984; 47–54
Finan PJ, Marshall RJ, Cooper EH *et al.*	*Br J Surg* 1985; 72: 373–377
Fujimoto S, Miyazaki M, Kitsukawa Y *et al.*	*Dis Colon Rectum* 1985; 28: 588–591
Finlay IG & McArdle CS	*Br J Surg* 1986; 73: 732–735

From Steele and Ravikumar (1989), with permission.

cannot be a part of any prospective study of liver metastasis resection.

In 1982, we analysed a series of 125 liver metastasis patients who had at least 5 years of known outcome. This was a consecutive group of patients seen with liver-only colorectal carcinoma metastases in whom treatment was either obviously ineffectual or was chosen not to be initiated until symptoms occurred, usually well after presentation. Median survival overall was 12.5 months. The majority of patients who had moderately to well-differentiated tumour morphology had a median survival of between 17 and 30 months. Those few patients ($n = 18$) who had predominantly poorly differentiated morphology not only died quickly (median survival 6 months after diagnosis of their metachronous hepatic metastases) but had a pattern of death which was quite different from the others – they had profuse extrahepatic disease spread usually only several months after their initial presentation with liver-only disease (Goslin *et al.*, 1982). Most of the patients who presented to us were without any functional debility whatsoever. They had no symptoms, so that any treatment goal here would be focused on increased survival, not palliation. And, when the patients finally did die, most died from one or another consequence of inexorable tumour growth in the liver. Thus, even though we felt that the use of historical controls could lead to the artificial overly optimistic survival outcomes that others had reported in the earlier single-institution hepatic artery infusion studies (Steele, 1987), there was no question that if growth of the tumour in the liver, at least for the moderate to well-differentiated morphology patients, could be slowed or, in fact, reversed, death might be postponed.

The results of our natural history series are shown in Figures 5.1–5.5 and form the basis for all of our subsequent regional therapy outcome analyses.

Our first group of liver metastasis resection patients (Steele *et al.*, 1984) was a highly select group of patients who presented with no symptoms and with fewer than four liver metastases. Each of the patients was thought to have resectable liver metastases (prior to surgery) and the expected survival in this group of patients could be calculated as at least equal to the expected survival in the group of patients defined in the Goslin *et al.* (1982) natural history study. In fact, the 50% expectation for 5 year survival that we published (Fig. 5.6) was similar to that which we found in patients who had resectable hepatocellular carcinoma primaries in non-cirrhotic livers. This 50% expec-

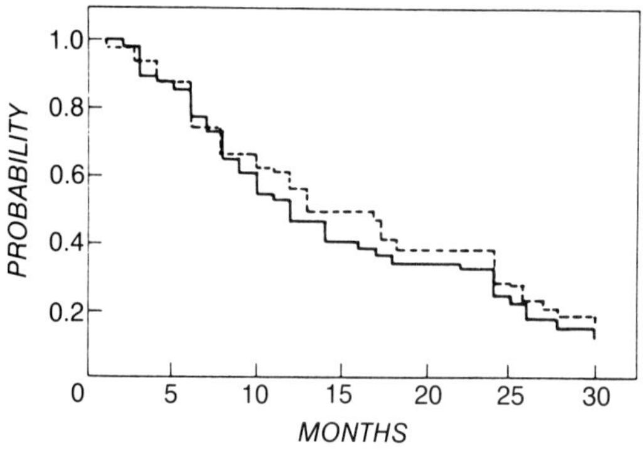

Sex		Alive	Dead	Total	Median
M	——	6	43	49	12
F	----	12	64	76	13

Figure 5.1 Overall survival for men and women. From Goslin *et al.* (1982), with permission.

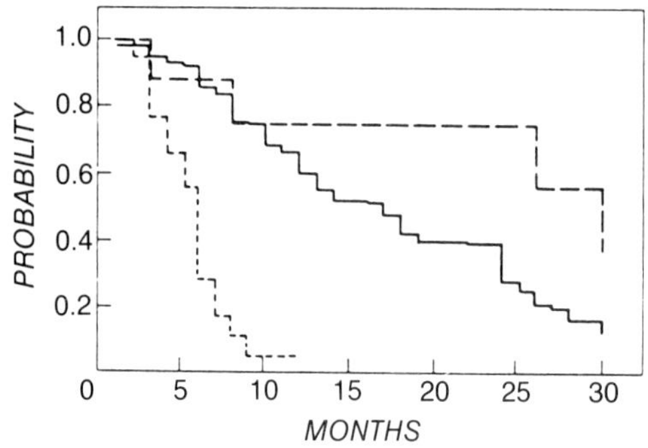

Degree of Differentiation		Alive	Dead	Total	Median
Moderate	——	14	85	99	17
Poor	----	0	18	18	6
Well	— —	4	4	8	30

Figure 5.2 Survival and histology of primary tumour. From Goslin *et al.* (1982), with permission.

tation for 5-year survival was not dissimilar to other single institution experiences, and the mortality and morbidity from the acute surgical procedure were also quite similar to other tertiary care environments (i.e. significantly less than 5% postoperative death rate). Several basic questions, however, remain unanswered. First, was the outcome purely a matter of our selecting 'good biology' patients, or was the surgery actually curing some? And second, were the low morbidity and mortality that were

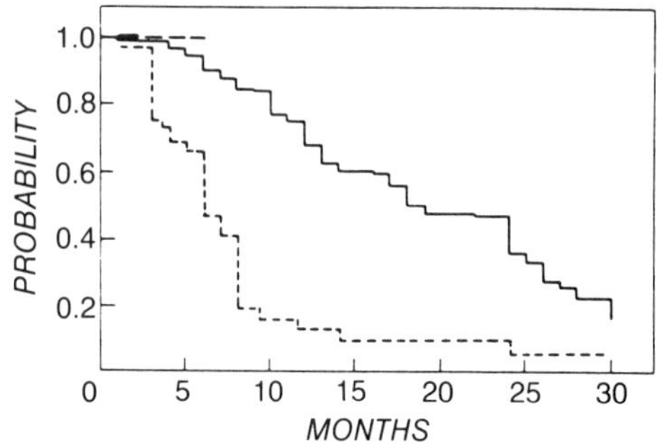

Performance Status		Alive	Dead	Total	Median
0	——	17	74	91	18
1	----	1	31	32	6
2	——	0	1	1	Undef
3	— —	0	1	1	Undef

Figure 5.3 Survival and performance status at presentation. From Goslin *et al.* (1982), with permission.

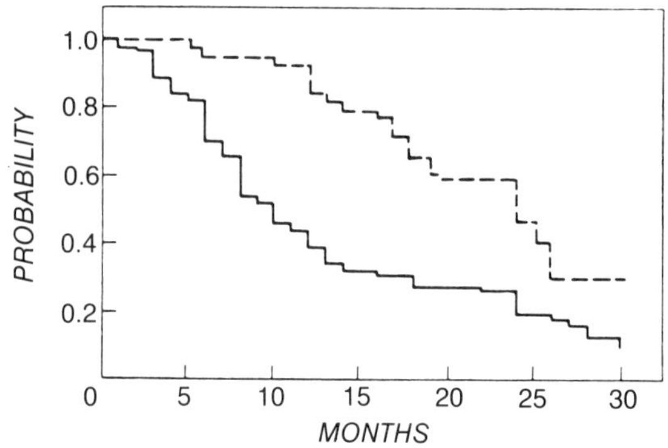

# of Liver Nodules		Alive	Dead	Total	Median
≥ 4	——	8	79	87	10
≤ 3	— — —	10	28	38	24

Figure 5.4 Survival and number of liver nodules. From Goslin *et al.* (1982), with permission.

being reported exportable to other primary or secondary care environments?

As our own experience extended, and as our indications for operation widened, both the overall as well as the disease-free survival diminished, and the intellectual exercise of retrospectively defining good-risk and bad-risk groups to predict subsets of good outcome (Fig. 5.7) could be clinically justified only if such predictors were applicable prospectively. Unfortunately, most could not be applied pro-

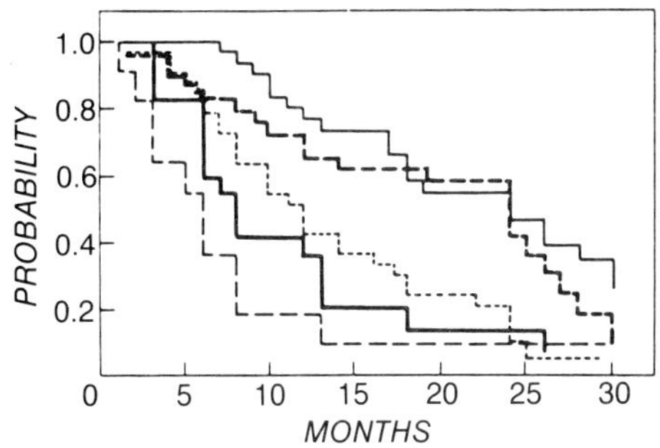

# of Elevated LFTs		Alive	Dead	Total	Median
0	——	6	24	30	24
1	– – –	7	22	29	24
2	-----	2	31	33	12
3	——	3	19	22	8
4	– –	0	11	11	6

Figure 5.5 Survival and abnormal liver function tests (LFTs). From Goslin *et al.* (1982), with permission.

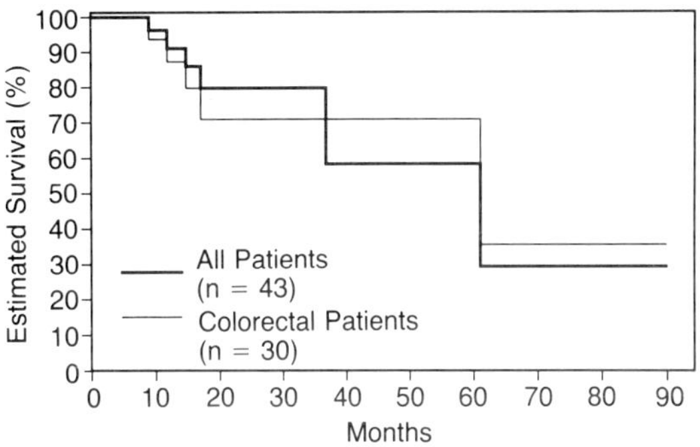

Figure 5.6 Major liver resections: cumulative survival (Kaplan-Meier). From Adson *et al.* (1984), with permission.

spectively in order to choose which patients should undergo resection and which should not.

Until the recent Gastrointestinal Tumor Study Group (GITSG) multi-institutional prospective treatment plan, the best look at *real* survival after hepatic metastasis resection came from the three papers presented by Hughes and Sugarbaker (Hughes *et al.* 1986, 1988a, 1988b) on their analysis of a North American registry of hepatic metastases. These investigators and numerous coworkers collected over 800 patients who had undergone hepatic metastasis resection for colon and rectum adenocarcinoma. The surgical procedures were done over approximately a 10-year period with at least 5 years of follow-up. One must remember that

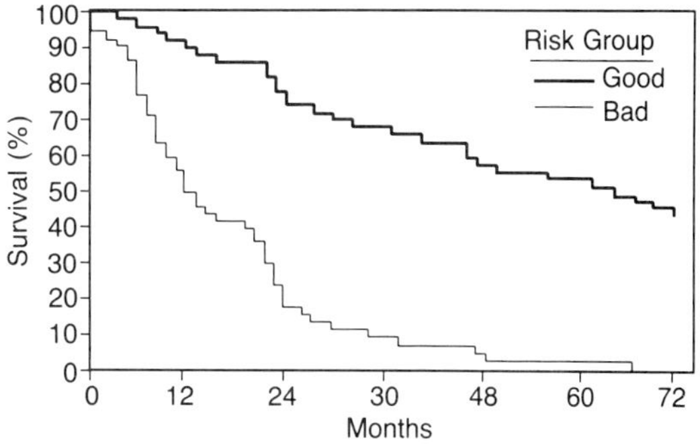

Figure 5.7 Projected disease-free survival for good- and bad-risk groups. The risk group is based on margin, disease-free interval and number of nodules good (all favourable) versus bad (all unfavourable).

the registry represents nothing more than an accumulation of retrospective single-institution series, most of which had already been published. Nevertheless, as shown in Figure 5.8, two important points are evident. First, the overall, as well as disease-free, survival was generally lower than in most of the single-institution series. This undoubtedly is a function of greater numbers of patients being looked at – less selection. And second, there is at least an implication of a survival plateau; in other words, surgery might actually be curing some of these patients. It should be stressed that if surgery cures some of these patients, this is the only evidence of any curative therapeutic approach for any patients with recurrent or disseminated colon and rectum carcinoma.

The main problem with the retrospective analysis of Hughes and Sugarbaker was, of course, that there was and still is no real way of defining the contribution of the selection process in determining outcome versus the actual

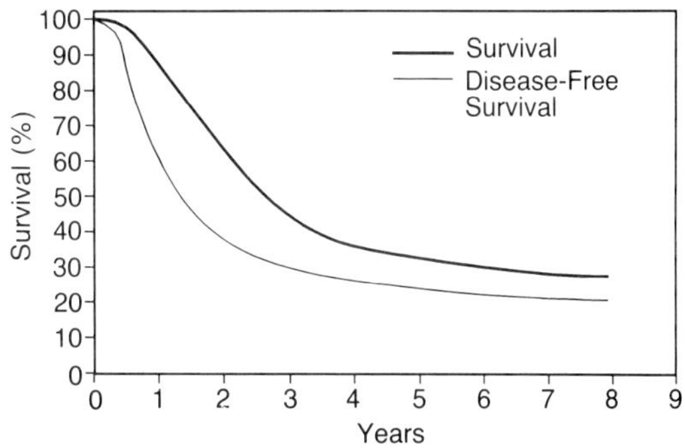

Figure 5.8 Registry of hepatic metastases. From Hughes *et al.* (1986), with permission.

benefit of the surgery itself. Furthermore, the validity of the survival plateau in the Hughes and Sugarbaker analysis is compromised by the fact that if patients are lost to follow-up, the end of the survival curve (particularly at the point of implied plateau) may be artificially optimistic.

For all of the above reasons, an attempt was made at the end of the GITSG's funding cycle to define prospectively the outcome (both acute and chronic morbidity) in a multi-institutional setting for patients who were felt preoperatively to have resectable adenocarcinoma metastases isolated to the liver from colon or rectum adenocarcinoma primaries. Although the pristine academic approach would have been to stage patients preoperatively, operate on the patients and restage them operatively, and then randomize between resection and simply follow-up, this approach was neither practical nor ethical. Thus, the treatment plan derived in this 15-institution, 150-patient series was one-armed and had the following objectives:

1. To determine the proportion of explored patients actually found to have resectable lesions, compared to the preoperative staging.
2. To identify important prognostic variables.
3. To evaluate the surgical morbidity and mortality in a multi-institutional setting.
4. To estimate survival among the curatively resected patients, the patients who were thought to be curatively resected by the surgeons but found by the pathologists to have tumour at the margins of resection, and the patients who were found at surgery not to have resectable disease, either because of unsuspected profuse disease in the liver or unsuspected extrahepatic disease.

As was the case in most of the single-institution studies defined in Table 5.2, almost 90% of the patients in this prospective trial had no debility whatsoever when they presented with either metachronous or synchronous liver metastases. Thus, the goal here, as was the case in the institutional series, was cure, not palliation, since there were no symptoms to palliate.

Of the 150 patients who presented from the 15 institutions, there was the usual demography of metastasis presentation with the disease in the right lobe being much more prevalent, probably on the basis of tissue-at-risk (Steele *et al.*, 1991). Over 80% of the patients presented with metachronous as opposed to synchronous metastases. There were no preoperative laboratory indicators as to how the patients were going to do postoperatively, including carcinoembryonic antigen, alkaline phosphatase, serum glutamic or bilirubin levels.

There was a good variety of major as well as relatively limited resections, so that no bias existed in analysing outcome simply because patients were having predominantly minor hepatic surgery. Even at the relatively early time of this study (1984–1986), there was remarkably little morbidity as defined by several important assessments of outcome. First, the median number of units of blood used for those who underwent resection had dropped to between three and four. Median hospital length of stay was only between 2 and 2.5 weeks, which was, in fact, exactly the same length of stay as for patients who underwent exploration but had no liver resection. This represents a dramatic decrease in morbidity from what our experience had been only 10 years before.

The data on preoperative staging were surprising. Despite predictions of resectability, half of the 150 patients were found not to have resectable disease at surgical exploration and, as shown in Table 5.3, the computed tomographic (CT) scan was inadequate for a variety of reasons. Of those not resected, two-thirds could not be resected because of disease that was either too profuse in the liver or was located in an anatomical position within the liver that the surgeon at the time of operation felt would not allow for an adequate margin. The other third of the patients not resected were found to have previously unsuspected disease outside the liver, usually in a periportal node or periaortic or mesenteric nodes below the resolution capacity of the CT scan or ultrasound. There is no question that even at present the resolution capacity for all but CT portography is inadequate, with approximately 1 cm diameter tumour threshold for disease in the right lobe and perhaps an even greater size as the resolution capacity is limited for lesions in the left lobe of the liver (Clarke *et al.*, 1989).

Since this is the only multi-institutional series looking at liver resection, the morbidity–mortality figures are as meaningful as one can get in defining whether institutional 'advertisements' of low morbidity and mortality are really applicable to non-specialized institutions. In fact, the morbidity was quite low, with only 13% of

Table 5.2 Single-institution series of colorectal cancer liver metastasis resection

Authors	Journal
Memorial	
Pack GT & Brasfield RD	*Am J Surg* 1955; 90: 704–716
Attiyeh F, Wanebo HJ & Sterns MW	*Dis Colon Rectum* 1978; 21: 160–162
Wanebo JH, Semoglov C, Attiyeh F *et al.*	*Am J Surg* 1978; 135: 81–85
Fortner JG, Silva JS, Golbey RB *et al.*	*Ann Surg* 1984; 198: 306–316
Butler J, Attiyeh F & Daly JM	*Surg Gynecol Obstet* 1986; 162: 109–113
Fortner JG	*Am J Surg* 1988; 155: 378–382
Hartford	
Flanagan L & Foster JH	*Am J Surg* 1967; 113: 551–557
Foster JH	*Cancer* 1970; 26: 493–502
Foster JH	*Am J Surg* 1978; 135: 389–394
Foster JH & Lundy J	*Curr Probl Surg* 1981; 18: 161–202
Mayo	
Wilson SM & Adson MA	*Arch Surg* 1976; 111: 330–334
Adson MA & Van Heerden JA	*Ann Surg* 1980; 191: 576–583
Adson MA, Van Heerden JA, Adson MA *et al.*	*Arch Surg* 1984; 119: 647–651
Adson MA	*World J Surg* 1987; 11: 511–520
University of California at Los Angeles	
Logan SE, Meier SJ, Ramming KP *et al.*	*Arch Surg* 1982; 117: 25–28
Thompson HH, Tompkins RK & Longmire WP	*Ann Surg* 1983; 197: 375–388
Toronto	
Taylor B, Langer B, Falk RE *et al.*	*Can J Surg* 1983; 26: 215–217
Coburn CS, Makowka L, Langer B *et al.*	*Surg Gynecol Obstet* 1987; 165: 239–246
Boston	
Steele G Jr, Osteen RT, Wilson R *et al.*	*Am J Surg* 1984; 147: 554–559
Cady B & McDermott WV	*Ann Surg* 1985; 201: 204–209
Cady B, Saenz N, Steele G Jr *et al.*	*Surg Clin North Am* 1989; 69: 361–370
Lund	
Ekberg H, Tranberg K-G, Andersson R *et al.*	*Br J Surg* 1986; 73: 727–731
Ekberg H, Tranberg K-G, Andersson R *et al.*	*World J Surg* 1987; 11: 541–547
Quattlebaum JK	*Surg Clin North Am* 1962; 42: 507–518
Woodington GF & Waugh JM	*Am J Surg* 1963; 105: 24–29
Boey J, Choi TK, Wong T *et al.*	*Surg Gynecol Obstet* 1981; 153: 844–848
Blumgart LH & Allison DJ	*World J Surg* 1987; 6: 320–345
Morrow CE, Grage TB, Sutherland DER *et al.*	*Surgery* 1982; 92: 610–614
Rajpal S, Dasmahapatra KS, Ledesma EJ *et al.*	*Surg Gynecol Obstet* 1982; 155: 813–816
Iwatsuki S, Byers WS Jr & Starzl TE	*Ann Surg* 1983; 197: 247–253
Kortz WJ, Meyers WC, Hanks JB *et al.*	*Ann Surg* 1984; 199: 182–186
Nims TA	*Surg Gynecol Obstet* 1984; 158: 46–48
Tomas de la Vega JE, Donahue JS, Doolas A *et al.*	*Surg Gynecol Obstet* 1984; 159: 223–228
August DA, Sugarbaker PH, Ottow RT *et al.*	*Ann Surg* 1985; 201: 210–218
Coppa GF, Eng K, Ranson JHC *et al.*	*Ann Surg* 1985; 202: 203–208
Fegiz G, Bezzi M, DeAngelis R *et al.*	*Ital J Surg Sci* 1985; 15: 259–265
Petrelli NJ, Nambisan RN & Herrera L	*Am J Surg* 1985; 149: 205–209
Gennari L, Doci R, Bozzetti F *et al.*	*Ann Surg* 1986; 203: 49–54
Bozzetti F, Bignami P, Morabito A *et al.*	*Ann Surg* 1987; 205: 264–270
Nordlinger B, Quilichini MA, Parc R *et al.*	*Ann Surg* 1987; 205: 256–263
Sesto ME, Vogt DP & Hermann RE	*Surgery* 1987; 102: 846–851
Brown DA, Pommier RF, Woltering EA *et al.*	*Arch Surg* 1988; 123: 1063–1066
Stephenson ICR, Steinberg SM, Hughes KS *et al.*	*Ann Surg* 1988; 203: 679–687

From Steele and Ravikumar (1989), with permission.

the patients having major complications postoperatively. The most prevalent complication was biloma, and most of the patients who experienced this had drainage via a percutaneously guided pigtail catheter placement, obviating the need for reoperation. Often this

Table 5.3 Preoperative versus surgical staging (supplemental data on 139–144 patients)

Computed tomography	
Missed hepatic disease completely	10/139
Missed extrahepatic disease	17/144
Underestimated liver involvement	46/139
Overestimated liver involvement	5/139

Modified from Steele *et al.* (1991).

was done with a 1-day hospital stay or as an outpatient procedure. Thirty-day mortality was under 5% – again a surprisingly good figure given that this was the first multi-institutional experience reported for major liver resection.

The initial analysis of chronic outcome occurred at a median follow-up of slightly less than 2 years and was published in the *Journal of Clinical Oncology* in 1991 (Steele *et al.*, 1991). Overall survival and disease-free survival of the entire group are shown in Figure 5.9; survival for the subgroups is shown in Figure 5.10. At the time of initial publication, we showed that curative resection patients had a median of 36 months of survival, which was significantly different from the other two groups – the non-curative resection patients had a median of 21.3 months and the unresectable group (those who were simply followed after exploration) 19.5 months. Non-curative resection in this series was defined as the surgeon thinking that he had removed all of the tumour, but the pathologist showing that there was microscopic evidence of disease at the surgical margin. Curative resection was defined as both the surgeon and the pathologist having agreed that all tumour was removed.

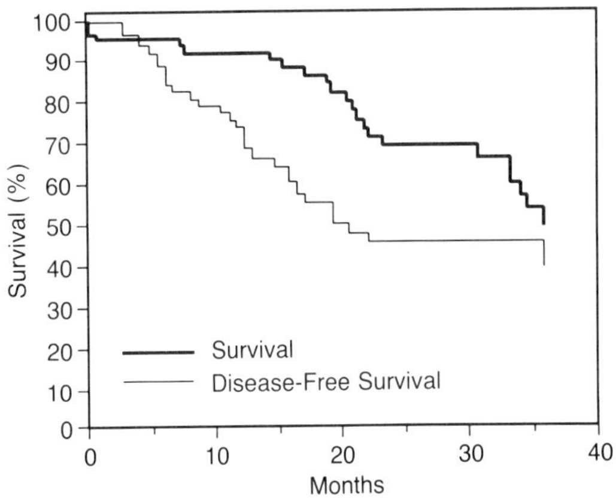

Figure 5.9 Probability of survival and disease-free survival of curatively resected patients. From Steele *et al.* (1994a), with permission.

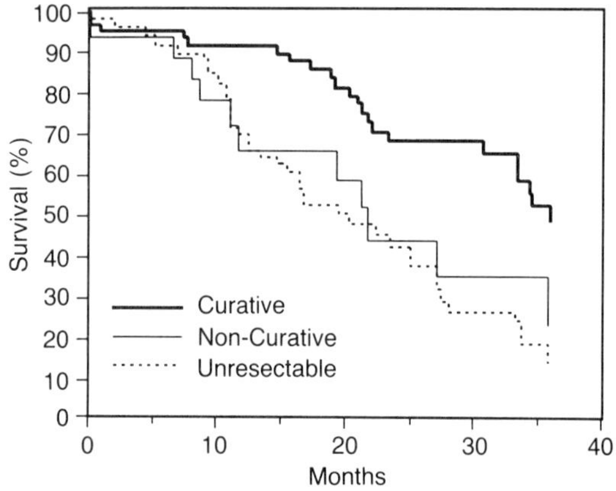

Figure 5.10 Probability of survival by resection type. From Steele *et al.* (1994a), with permission.

The take-home message at the time of this initial analysis was straightforward. None of the groups had yet shown even the implication of a survival plateau. And, patients who did not end up with tumour-free margins (defined by both surgeon and pathologist) should not be operated on and certainly should not be resected after exploration since there was no difference in survival between the non-curative resection group and the unresectable patients. Finally, the entire group did remarkably well (as predicted from our original natural history series), again showing that this experience focuses on a relatively small and biologically select group of patients who will have a long and asymptomatic expected survival regardless of the therapy that is offered and perhaps regardless of whether or not therapy is offered.

More recent follow-up of GITSG 6584 was presented at the 1993 New England Surgical Society and shows the three groups continuing to degenerate (Fig. 5.11; Steele *et al.*, 1994). In fact, the patients who were unresected are all dead. The patients who were non-curatively resected have few survivors. Even the patients in the curatively resected group continued to recur and will probably show a survival plateau of less than 20%.

The fact is that, in this single prospective look, although the acute morbidity and mortality of liver resection are quite low and undoubtedly is lower now than it was even at the

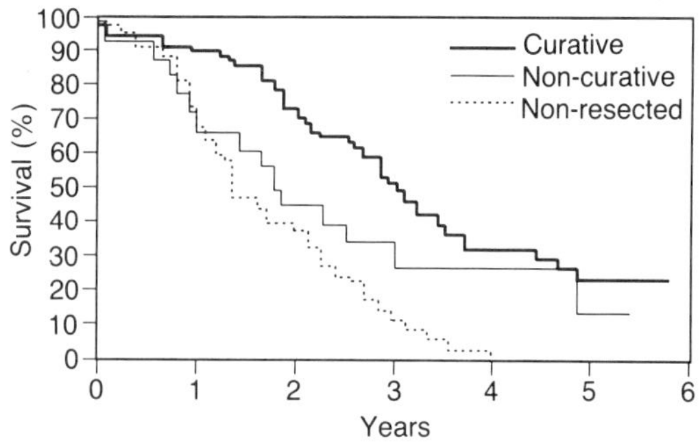

Figure 5.11 Probability of survival by resection type. From Steele *et al.* (1994a), with permission.

conclusion of this GITSG trial, the number of patients who are cured is small.

At present, a total of 115 deaths have been reported, including 44 of 69 on the curative resection arm (64%), 14 of 18 on the non-curative resection arm (78%) and 57 of 63 on the non-resected arm (90%). Median survival times for patients receiving curative and non-curative resections and those receiving no resection are estimated to be 35.7, 21.2 and 16.5 months, respectively. No statistically significant difference in the survival distribution of the latter two groups is observed. The survival distribution of curatively resected patients remains statistically superior to the distribution of non-curatively resected patients and those receiving no resection (P=0.01). Sixteen of the 25 surviving patients who underwent curative resection remain free of disease. Minimum follow-up on all surviving patients on this arm is 2.2 years and median follow-up is 3.2 years. Six patients are alive on this arm more than 5 years postsurgery; 2 of these patients remain disease-free. The longest survivor reported to date is 5.7 years, and the last death reported was at 4.8 years. An estimate of 5-year survival probability for patients who underwent curative resection is 23% (95% confidence interval (10%, 36%)).

These data are, perhaps, the most rational justification for several of the more recent improvements in diagnostic and therapeutic techniques that form the basis of this book. First, the application of the intraoperative ultrasound at the time of exploration and prior to hepatic resection for presumed isolated liver metastases has opened up a vast new area of staging and has allowed us to define lesions that are only 3–4 mm in diameter, at least three times better in resolution threshold capacity compared to any of our other preoperative or intraoperative staging techniques (Clarke *et al.*, 1989). This allows greater exclusion of patients who might have insidious disease in their residual unresected liver and would very shortly after resection be shown to have recurrence (or, more accurately, residual tumour growth). The application of such intraoperative ultrasound staging is presently being transformed in order to allow laparoscopic exploration to rule out extrahepatic disease and at the same time placement of a translaparoscopic transducer to allow examination of the liver (Kane *et al.*, 1994). At present, we are accumulating a prospective series in such patients, hopefully obviating full laparotomy in the 50% of patients who will be found not to benefit from liver resection.

And finally, the continuing maturation of our own and several other major studies using cryosurgical ablation has shown no difference in efficacy (for properly selected patients) when successful surgical cryoablations are compared to surgical resection (Fig. 5.12), but a definite decrease in morbidity and mortality is apparent. There has been no mortality in our series and, with well over 200 patients in the Morris and Ravikumar series (personal communication), morbidity is also considerably lower, with median lengths of stay in hospital of only 5–7 days. Thus, with the decreased risk of this newer technique, the fact that few, if any, of these patients are cured should, at the very least, be less guilt-producing for those of us who are committed to continue to try and take advantage of the good biology in an asympto-

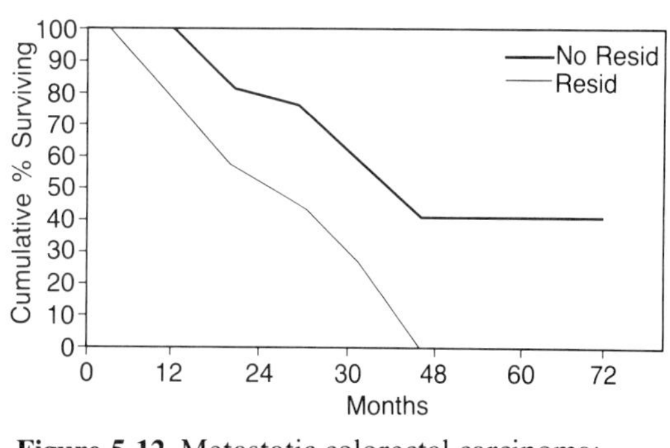

Figure 5.12 Metastatic colorectal carcinoma: cryosurgical treatment: impact of residual (Resid) disease. From Steele (1994a), with permission.

matic group of patients with isolated-target single-organ metastases, at least until some type of effective systemic therapy is at hand for the 75–80% of patients with insidious systemic disease present at the completion of successful liver resection or cryoablation.

References

Adson MA (1983) Cannon Lecture: hepatic metastases in perspective. *AJR* **140**, 695–700.

Adson MA (1987) Resection of liver metastases – when is it worthwhile? *World J. Surg.* **11**, 511–520.

Adson MA, Van Heerden JA, and Adson MH (1984) Resection of hepatic metastases from colo-rectal cancer. *Arch. Surg.* **119**, 647–651.

Boring CC, Squires TS & Tong T (1993) Cancer statistics, 1993. *CA-A Cancer J. Clinicians* **43**, 7–26.

Cady B, Monson DO & Swinton NW (1970) Survival of patients after colonic resection for carcinoma with simultaneous liver metastases. *Surg. Gynecol. Obstet.* **131**, 697–700.

Clarke MP, Kane RA, Steele G Jr, *et al.* (1989) Prospective comparison of preoperative imaging and intraoperative ultrasound in the detection of liver tumors. *Surgery* **106**, 849–855.

Forse RA, Babineau T, Bleday R, *et al.* (1993) Laparoscopy/thoracoscopy for staging: I. staging endoscopy in surgical oncology. *Semin. Surg. Oncol.* **9**, 51–55.

Foster JH & Berman MM (1977) Solid liver tumors. In: Ebert PA (ed) *Major Problems in Clinical Surgery*, pp. 1–342, Philadelphia, PA: WB Saunders.

Gastrointestinal Tumor Study Group (1984) Adjuvant therapy of colon cancer – results of a prospectively randomized trial. *N. Engl. J. Med.* **310**, 737–743.

Gastrointestinal Tumor Study Group (1985) A controlled trial of adjuvant chemotherapy, radiation therapy or combined chemo-radiation therapy following curative resection for rectal carcinoma. *N. Engl. J. Med.* **312**, 1465–1472.

Goslin R, Steele G Jr, Zamcheck N *et al.* (1982) Factors influencing survival in patients with hepatic metastases from adenocarcinoma of the colon and rectum. *Dis. Colon Rectum* **25**, 749–754.

Hughes KS, Simon R, Songhorabodi S *et al.* (1986) Resection of the liver for colorectal carcinoma metastases: a multi-institutional study of patterns of recurrence. *Surgery* **100**, 278–284.

Hughes KS, Simon R, Songhorabodi S *et al.* (1988a) Resection of the liver for colorectal carcinoma metastases: a multi-institutional study of long term survivors. *Surgery* **100**, 278–288.

Hughes KS, Simon R, Songhorabodi S *et al.* (1988b) Resection of the liver for colorectal carcinoma metastases: a multi-institutional study of indications for resection. *Dis. Colon Rectum* **31**, 1–4.

Kane RA, Roizental M, Jenkins R *et al.* (1994) Preliminary investigation of liver and biliary imaging with a dedicated laparoscopic ultrasound system. *Int. Hepato-Biliary Assoc.* (in press).

Pestana C, Reitemeier RJ, Moertel CG *et al.* (1964) The natural history of carcinoma of the colon and rectum. *Am. J. Surg.* **108**, 826–829.

Steele G Jr (1987) Pattern of recurrence in liver resection for colorectal secondaries. Invited commentary. *World J. Surg.* **11**, 546–547.

Steele G Jr (1994a) Advances in the treatment of early to late stage colorectal cancer: 20 years of progress. *Ann. Surg. Oncol.* **2**(11), 17–88.

Steele G Jr (1994b) Colorectal cancer. In: McKenna RJ & Murphy GL (eds) *Cancer Surgery*, pp. 128–184. Philadelphia, PA: JB Lippincott.

Steele G Jr & Ravikumar TS (1989) Resection of hepatic metastases from colorectal cancer: biologic perspectives. *Ann. Surg.* **210**, 127–137.

Steele G Jr, Osteen RT, Wilson RE *et al.* (1984) Patterns of failure after surgical cure of large liver tumors. *Am. J. Surg.* **147**, 554–559.

Steele G Jr, Bleday R, Mayer RJ *et al.* (1991) A prospective evaluation of hepatic resection for colorectal carcinoma metastases to the liver: Gastrointestinal Tumor Study Group protocol 6584. *J. Clin. Oncol.* **9**, 1105–1112.

Steele G Jr, Mayer R, Lindblad A (1994) A prospective evaluation of hepatic resection for colorectal carcinoma metastases to the liver: follow-up report. *Journal of Hepato-Biliary-Pancreatic Surgery* (in press).

Weiss GR, Garnick MB, Osteen RT *et al.* (1983) Long-term hepatic arterial infusion of 5-fluorodeoxyuridine for liver metastases using an implantable pump. *J. Clin. Oncol.* **1**, 337.

6

Intra-arterial chemotherapy: surgical approach

Colin S. McArdle

Regional chemotherapy for patients with colorectal liver metastases is based on the premiss that cytotoxic drugs delivered via the hepatic artery will produce a greater tumour response than the same agents administered systemically.

Since the observation by Bierman and his colleagues in 1951 that tumour blood vessels could be demonstrated by arteriography in patients with metastatic liver disease, evidence has continued to emerge, confirming that established hepatic metastases derive their blood supply predominantly from the hepatic artery (Ridge *et al.*, 1987). However, early experience with hepatic arterial catheters, inserted surgically and then exteriorized, proved disappointing. Although higher response rates and reduced systemic toxicity were reported, these potential benefits were negated by the high incidence of catheter-related complications, including catheter blockage, leakage or displacement, hepatic arterial thrombosis, sepsis, peptic ulceration and gastrointestinal haemorrhage.

More recently, technological developments and the continuing failure of systemic chemotherapy have contributed to a resurgence of interest in hepatic arterial perfusion therapy. The introduction of inert silicon catheters and subcutaneous injection ports and improved surgical techniques have reduced the high mortality and morbidity previously associated with hepatic arterial access.

Surgical procedure

Prior to surgery, chest X-ray and computed tomographic (CT) scan of chest and abdomen should be performed to exclude extrahepatic disease and measure the extent of hepatic replacement. The presence of locoregional recurrence should be excluded by barium enema, colonoscopy or CT scan of pelvis, as appropriate. Histological confirmation of liver metastases should be obtained by ultrasound or CT-guided fine-needle aspiration or Tru-cut biopsy. Approximately one-third of patients have abnormal vascular anatomy (Table 6.1); selective coeliac axis and superior mesenteric angiography is therefore advisable (Anderson *et al.*, 1992).

In patients with classical anatomy, the

Table 6.1 Anatomy in first 100 patients treated

Normal	65
Abnormal	35
Trifurcation	9
Gastroduodenal arises from right hepatic artery	3
Common coeliac axis/superior mesenteric artery	3
Common hepatic artery arises from superior mesenteric artery	2
Right hepatic artery arises from superior mesenteric artery	14
Left hepatic artery arises from left gastric	4

common hepatic artery arises from the coeliac axis and gives off the gastroduodenal branch before dividing into right and left hepatic arteries. At laparotomy, the common hepatic artery can be located by dividing the gastrohepatic ligament and mobilizing the pylorus and the first part of the duodenum. In most patients, the hepatic artery and its gastroduodenal branch are easily palpated. The vascular anatomy of the region is displayed by dissecting the common hepatic, right and left hepatic and gastroduodenal arteries completely. Any other branches, in particular the right gastric artery, should be ligated to avoid unwanted perfusion of the lesser curve of stomach and adjacent organs. To avoid the possibility of chemical cholecystitis, cholecystectomy is performed.

A subcutaneous pocket over the lower ribs is then prepared, the port is sutured in position and the catheter passed through the anterior abdominal wall.

The gastroduodenal artery should be ligated 2–3 cm from its origin and the tip of the beaded catheter inserted retrogradely into the vessel so that the tip of the catheter lies at its origin from the hepatic artery, thereby gaining access to the hepatic artery without compromising hepatic arterial flow (Fig. 6.1). The beaded tip of the catheter is held in position by non-absorbable silk or linen ties. The adequacy of liver perfusion can then be checked by injecting patent bleu through the port. Postoperatively the patency of the catheters is maintained by flushing weekly with heparinized saline.

In patients with a trifurcation, where the gastroduodenal branch originates less than 2 cm from the bifurcation of the common hepatic artery, cannulation of the gastroduodenal artery often leads to poor mixing of injec-

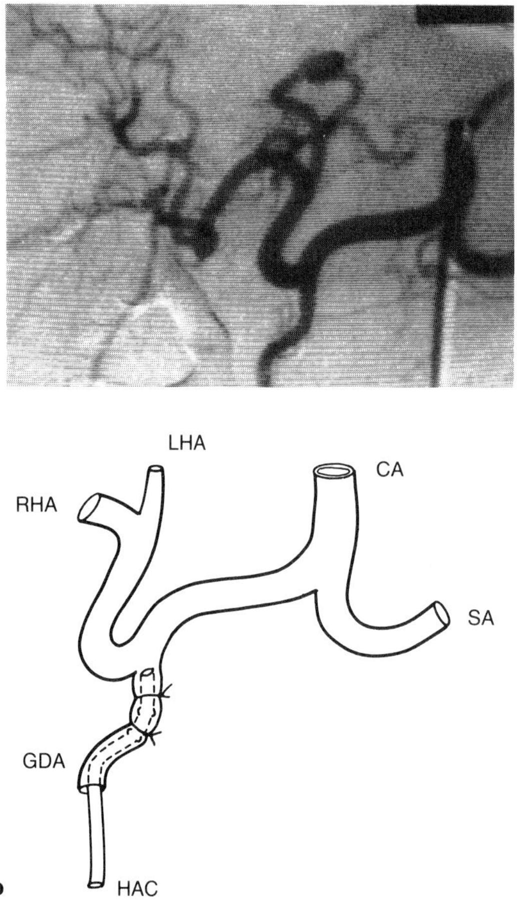

Figure 6.1 Normal anatomy.(a) Digital subtraction selective hepatic angiogram demonstrating normal arterial anatomy. (b) Hepatic artery catheter (HAC) inserted into the gastroduodenal artery (GDA). LHA and RHA = left and right hepatic artery; CA = coeliac axis; SA = splenic artery.

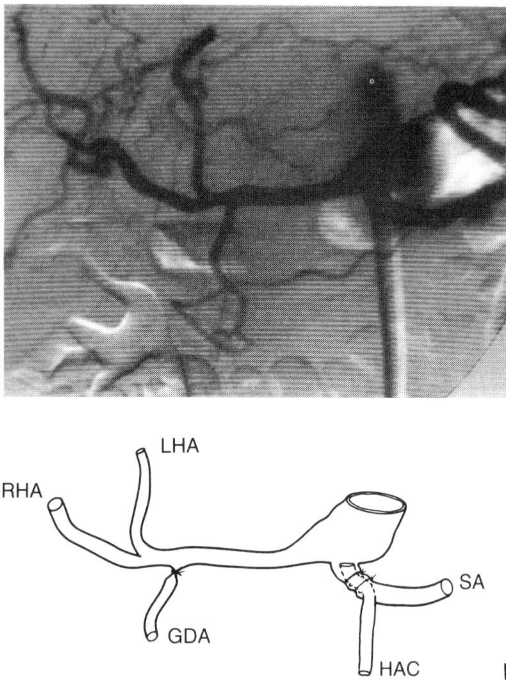

Figure 6.2 Trifurcation. (a) Digital subtraction selective hepatic angiogram. (b) Hepatic artery catheter (HAC) inserted retrogradely into the splenic artery (SA); the gastroduodenal artery (GDA) is ligated. LHA and RHA = left and right hepatic artery.

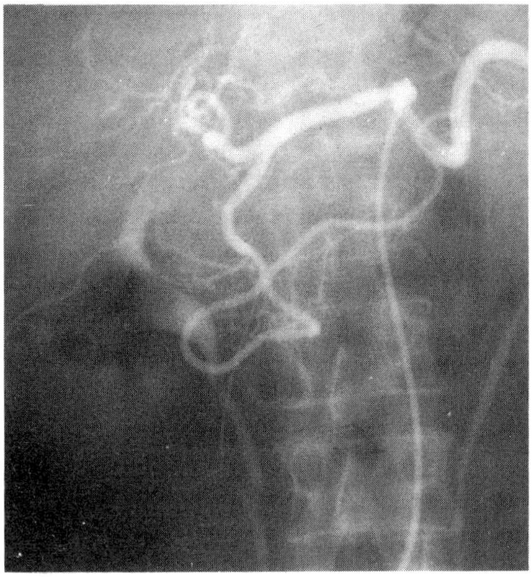
a

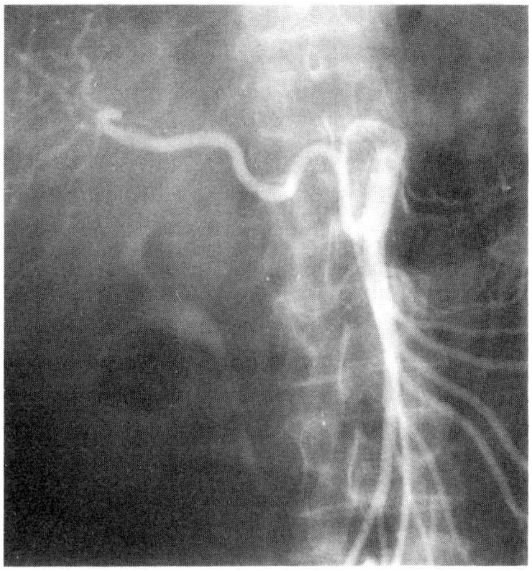
b

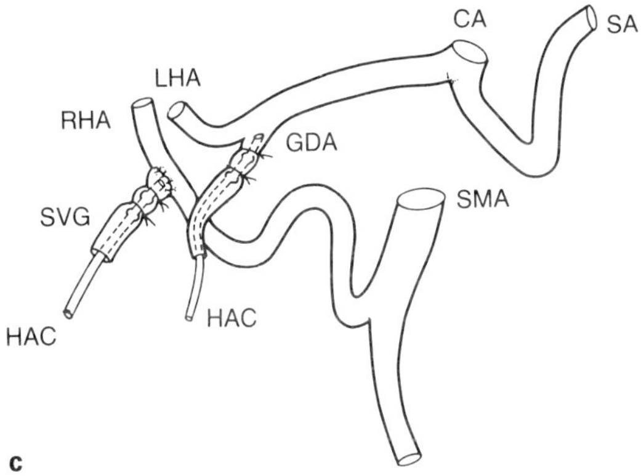

c

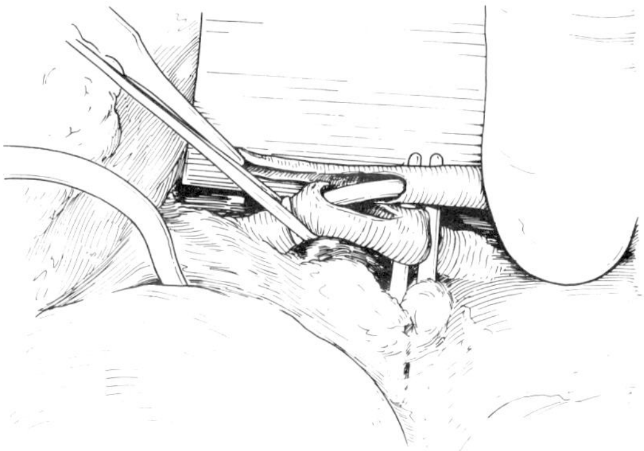
d

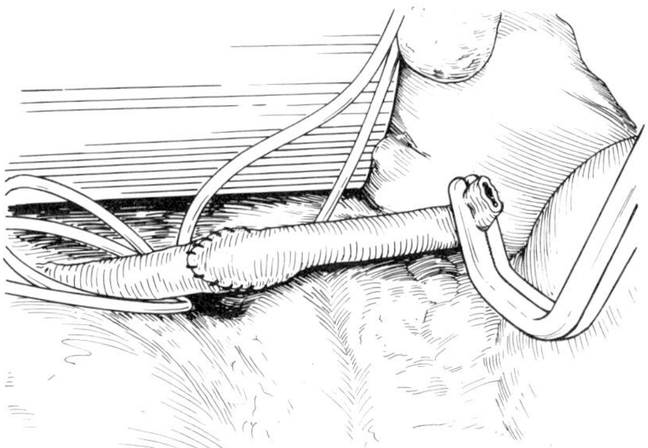
e

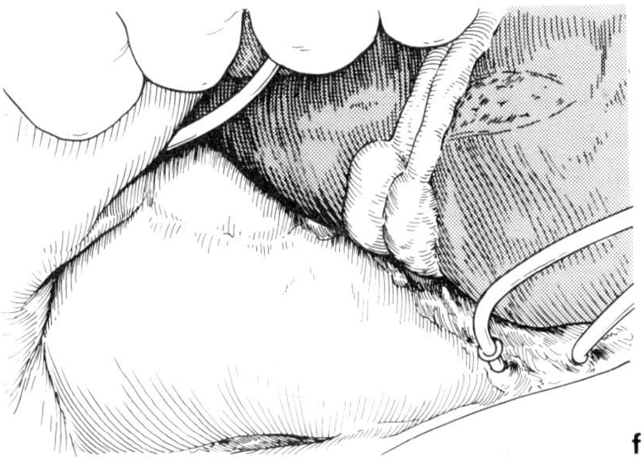
f

Figure 6.3a, b, c, d, e, f (*continued overleaf*)

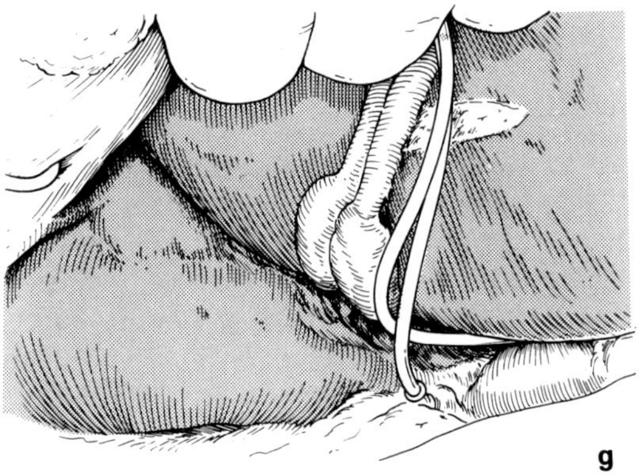

Figure 6.3 Injection of methyl blue to confirm distribution of flow in patient with dual blood supply; (a) The left hepatic artery with a gastroduodenal branch arising from the coeliac axis; (b) the right hepatic artery arising from the superior mesenteric artery; (c) the hepatic artery catheters (HAC) inserted into the gastroduodenal branch of the left hepatic artery and into the saphenous vein graft (SVG) anastomosed to the unbranching right hepatic artery (RHA and LHA = right and left hepatic arteries; CA = coeliac axis; SA = splenic artery; GDA = gastroduodenal artery; SMA = superior mesenteric axis); (d) the saphenous vein graft; formation of anastomosis; and (e) the saphenous vein graft completed anastomosis. The hepatic artery catheter would be inserted into the saphenous vein graft so that the tip of the catheter would lie at the level of the anastomosis, thereby gaining access to right hepatic arterial flow; (f) injection via LHA to perfuse left lobe; (g) subsequent injection via RHA to perfuse both lobes.

tate in the hepatic arterial flow and uneven distribution within the liver due to streaming. In these patients it is possible to cannulate the splenic artery retrogradely to gain access to the common hepatic artery; at the same time the gastroduodenal artery should be ligated (Fig. 6.2). A similar approach can be used on patients where the left gastric artery arises proximal to the gastroduodenal artery or where the gastroduodenal artery arises from or other hepatic branch. Alternatively a saphenous vein graft can be applied proximal to the trifurcation of the common hepatic artery to act as a conduit for the catheter.

Approximately 20% of patients will have a dual blood supply. Most commonly, the right hepatic artery arises from the superior mesenteric artery whilst the left hepatic artery (with its gastroduodenal branch) originates from the coeliac axis. In patients with a non-dominant right hepatic artery, adequate perfusion can usually be obtained by ligating the right hepatic artery and inserting a catheter into the gastroduodenal branch of the left hepatic artery and allowing cross-perfusion.

In patients with a dominant right hepatic artery, adequate perfusion can be achieved by inserting two catheters, one into the gastroduodenal artery to perfuse the left lobe and a second into the right hepatic artery using a saphenous vein graft (Fig. 6.3). The right hepatic artery should be identified as it lies behind the common bile duct and portal vein in the foramen of Winslow. A segment of long saphenous vein is prepared and anastomosed end-to-side to the right hepatic artery (Goldberg *et al.*, 1989). The catheter is then introduced into the vein graft so that the tip lies at the anastomosis. In this way, the saphenous vein graft acts as a conduit for the catheter.

Less frequently, the left hepatic artery will arise from the left gastric artery whilst the right hepatic artery, with its gastroduodenal branch, arises from the coeliac axis. In these patients it is usually possible to achieve adequate liver perfusion by ligating the non-dominant left hepatic artery (or the left gastric) and inserting a catheter into the gastroduodenal branch of the dominant right hepatic artery. Rarely, it may be necessary to insert a catheter into the left gastric artery.

Postoperatively all patients receive prophylactic H_2 antagonists to reduce the potential for gastroduodenal ulceration.

Postoperative complications

Subsequent problems are uncommon. Inevitably, with time, spontaneous thrombosis of the catheter may occur. If suspected, it can be confirmed radiographically by injecting contrast medium via the port. Angiography should be performed to demonstrate the site of occlusion and confirm that the hepatic artery remains patent (Fig. 6.4). If it is deemed appropriate, a replacement catheter can be inserted proximal to the blocked catheter using a saphenous vein graft (Goldberg *et al.*, 1988). At laparotomy the common hepatic artery is mobilized proximal to the insertion of the blocked catheter and a segment of vein anastomosed end-to-side to the hepatic artery. The replace-

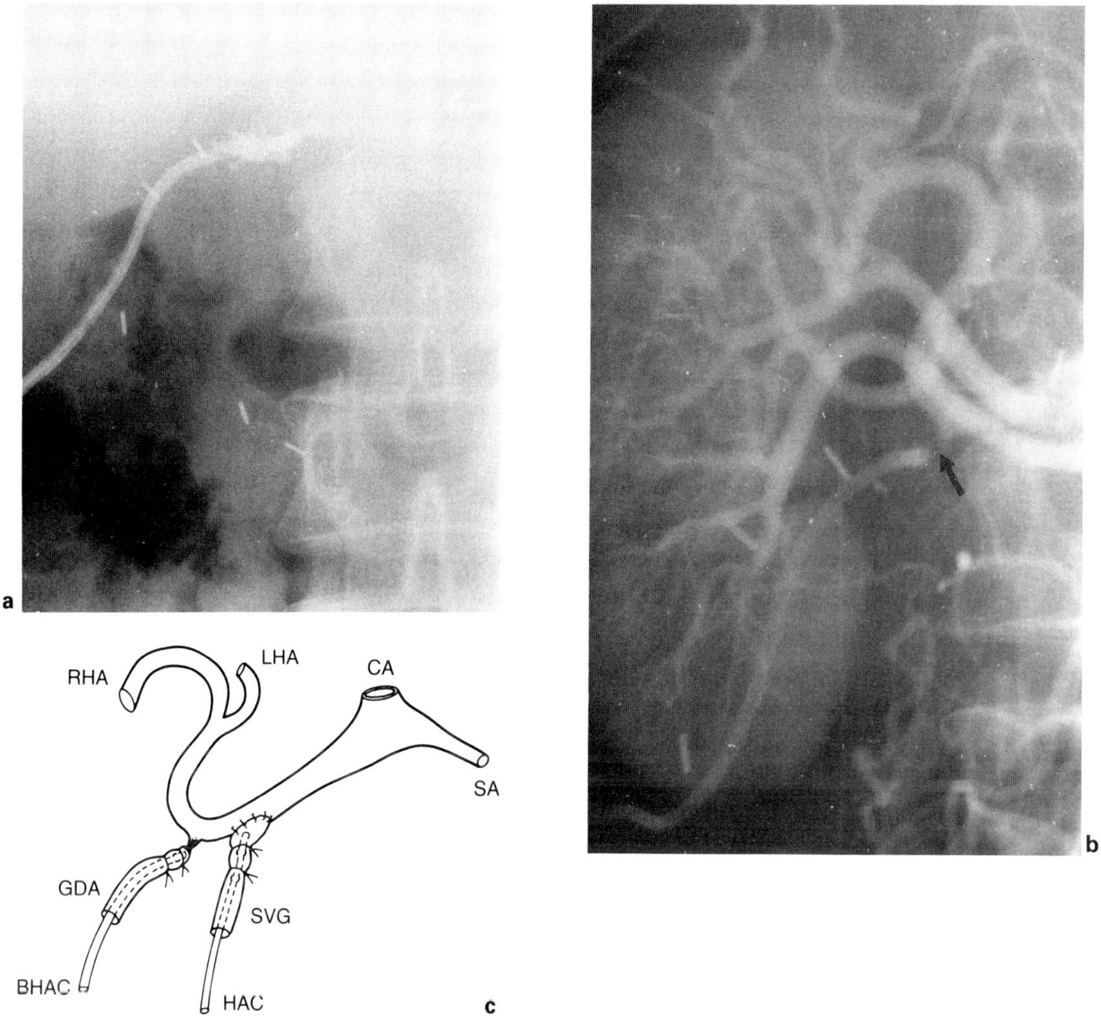

Figure 6.4 Blocked catheter. (a) Catheter blockage, demonstrated by injection of contrast into port. (b) Angiography performed to exclude hepatic artery thrombosis prior to catheter replacement. The site of blockage is indicated by the arrow. (c) Hepatic artery catheter (HAC) inserted proximal to the blocked catheter, using saphenous vein graft (SVG). RHA and LHA = right and left hepatic artery; CA = coeliac axis; SA = splenic artery; GDA = gastroduodenal artery; BHAC = blocked hepatic artery catheter (reproduced with permission from the *British Journal of Surgery*).

ment catheter is then inserted into the vein graft so that the tip lies flush with the hepatic artery. Alternatively a replacement catheter can be inserted retrogradely into the splenic artery.

Minor upper gastrointestinal bleeds may occur. Endoscopy usually confirms the presence of duodenitis or an area of gastritis on the lesser curve aspect of the antrum. Frank ulceration is seldom present. Further intervention is seldom required and the bleeding usually settles spontaneously. Further bleeding can be prevented by the addition of omeprazole to the H_2 antagonist therapy.

If the subcutaneous port becomes infected during the immediate postoperative period, the collection should be drained and packed. Eventually the port will be extruded from the granulating subcutaneous 'pocket'. With care the catheter can still be used for treatment by soaking the extruded port in antiseptic for 20 min prior to injection of chemotherapy, and simply wrapping it in a dry dressing when not in use. Three months later, the extruded port and exposed segment of the catheter can be excised, leaving the distal end *in situ*. A new port and catheter can be positioned at a fresh site and a double-ended male metal connection piece (male double-ended catheter connector) used to join the two free ends of catheter. In these patients, successful repositioning of the injection port can usually be achieved.

References

Anderson JH, Goldberg JA, Leiberman DP, Stewart I, Cooke TG & McArdle CS (1992) Saphenous vein grafts for anatomical variations encountered at surgical insertion of a hepatic artery catheter. *Eur. J. Surg. Oncol.* **18**, 484–486.

Bierman HR, Miller ER, Byron RL *et al.* (1951) Intra-arterial catheterisation of viscera in man. *AJR* **66**, 555–568.

Goldberg JA, Leiberman DP & McArdle CS (1988) Salvage of blocked hepatic artery infusion catheter for regional therapy of metastatic liver disease. *Br. J. Surg.* **75**, 466.

Goldberg JA, Leiberman DP & McArdle CS (1989) A useful maneuver for hepatic arterial catheterization in patients with metastatic hepatic disease and abnormal vascular anatomy. *Surg. Gynecol. Obstet.* **169**, 71–72.

Ridge JA, Bading JR, Gelbard AS *et al.* (1987) Perfusion of colorectal hepatic metastases. Relative distribution of flow from the hepatic artery and portal vein. *Cancer* **59**, 1547–1553.

7

Results of systemic chemotherapy for the treatment of hepatic metastases from colorectal cancer

Philip R. Clingan

Colon cancer is the commonest cause of cancer death in non-smokers in the USA, UK and Australia. Two-thirds of all patients with colorectal cancer will die of their cancer. Metastases to the liver are one of the commonest means of spread and almost all patients with liver metastases will die of their disease (Van de Velde & De Brauw, 1989). Several factors influence the patient's survival once they have developed metastases. These include the percentage of liver involvement, performance status, serum albumin and lactate dehydrogenase (Kemeny *et al.*, 1989). Diploid tumours have been shown to have a longer survival than aneuploid tumours (Scott & Beart, 1988). The percentage of liver involvement is a major determinant of survival. The median survival of patients with less than 25% liver involvement is 6.2 months; 27–75% involvement is 5.5 months and with greater than 75% is reduced to 3.4 months (Stehlin *et al.*, 1988; Hughes *et al.*, 1989). The majority of patients with liver metastases are unsuitable for surgery, with only 20% of patients with liver metastases suitable for resective surgery (Saenz *et al.*, 1989). In the remaining group of patients the only alternative for treatment is chemotherapy given either systemically or intra-arterially.

Chemotherapy has been used as a palliative treatment for liver metastases over the last 30 years. There is still a large controversy as to the optimum scheduling of treatment, the combination of drugs and the influence of treatment on patient survival and quality of life (Kemeny and Seiter, 1991; Wirth *et al.*, 1992).

Cancer of the colon responds rather poorly to systemic chemotherapy and the tumour remains highly resistant. The reasons for resistance of large bowel cancer to chemotherapy are multifactorial (Carter, 1976; Allen-Mersh, 1989; Grem, 1991). The kinetics of the growth of colorectal cancer make it relatively unsuitable for treatment with chemotherapy. Table 7.1 summarizes the kinetics of colorectal cancer. Colorectal cancer has a low labelling index with a long cell cycle time of 3 days and a tumour-doubling time averaging 83 days. The average cell turnover is approximately 2% in any one day, with a low growth fraction of 6%. Chemotherapy is effective against growing cells and, as colorectal cancer has a slow growth fraction, most cells will not be exposed to the

Table 7.1 Kinetics of colorectal cancer

Labelling index	3%
Cell cycle time	3.0 days
Duration of DNA synthesis	17 h
Doubling time	83 days
Daily tumour cell turnover	2%
Cell loss	71%
Growth fraction	6%

Adapted from Tannock (1987).

drugs used and will be unaffected by the treatment (Tannock, 1987).

There are a number of important factors in deciding whether to treat a patient with metastatic liver cancer. Although systemic cytoreductive treatment has been widely used for palliation, the true benefit of chemotherapy is often disputed. Quality of life of all cancer patients is of prime importance. The goal of chemotherapy can include improvement in quality of life as well as quantity of life.

A recent review in the *Journal of Clinical Oncology* (June 1992) suggested, in a trial performed by the Nordic Gastrointestinal Tumour Adjuvant Therapy Group, that patients who were randomized to expectant treatment, compared to those who were treated with chemotherapy from the time of diagnosis, had an improved survival over patients who waited to develop symptoms before chemotherapy was started. In this study, there was a modest improvement in survival. The median survival in this group of patients was 8 months longer than the patients who did not receive treatment from the initial diagnosis. It was also interesting to note that the symptom-free period in the expectancy group was rather short, usually being less than 6 months. This study has added weight to the use of palliative chemotherapy in asymptomatic patients.

The traditional treatment of colorectal cancer has usually relied on combinations including 5-fluorouacil (5-FU). There is continuing research into the optimum combination of chemotherapy for colorectal cancer (Bleiberg, 1989). This chapter will attempt to define some of the new advances in the treatment of colorectal cancer.

Chemotherapy with 5-fluorouracil as a single agent

5-FU was manufactured by Heidelberger *et al.* in 1957. It was specifically designed as an antitumour agent. The comments at its introduction in 1957 were that this compound exhibited a higher order of tumour-inhibitory activity which warrants further exploration.

Over the next 30 years, scientists have continued to explore the use of this compound and have found it to be highly active in treating colorectal cancer, breast cancer and ovarian cancer. Surprisingly, despite 30 years of usage, there is still controversy as to the optimal scheduling and dosage of this drug. Currently, several routes of administration are used; including oral, intravenous bolus, continuous infusion over several days and protracted infusion via an ambulatory pump for 1 or 2 weeks or longer.

Pharmacology

The pharmacology of 5-FU has been widely studied. The drug is inactive until metabolized. It enters the cell by a carrier-mediated transport mechanism, which may have a saturation capacity. It is then metabolized to a number of nucleotides. Figure 7.1 shows the pathways involved in 5-FU metabolism. Several enzymes are involved in its activation; these enzymes are part of the pyrimidine pathway.

5-FU has a rapid volume of distribution and elimination. The half-life of a single bolus injection varies between 10 and 20 min, with the average clearance rate being 11 min. Catabolism eliminates more than 80% of the administered drug, with the remaining drug being eliminated by the kidneys. The enzyme responsible is dihydrofluorouracil dehydrogenase and has its highest concentration in the liver; some elimination occurs from the lungs.

5-FU is an antimetabolite. Its major cytotoxicity occurs during the S phase of the cell cycle.

5-FU has four main actions on the cell:

1. Inhibition of thymidylate synthetase.
2. Incorporation into RNA.
3. Incorporation into DNA.
4. Interaction with cellular membrane.

Resistance to 5-FU can develop from any of the various steps, from entry into cell to interac-

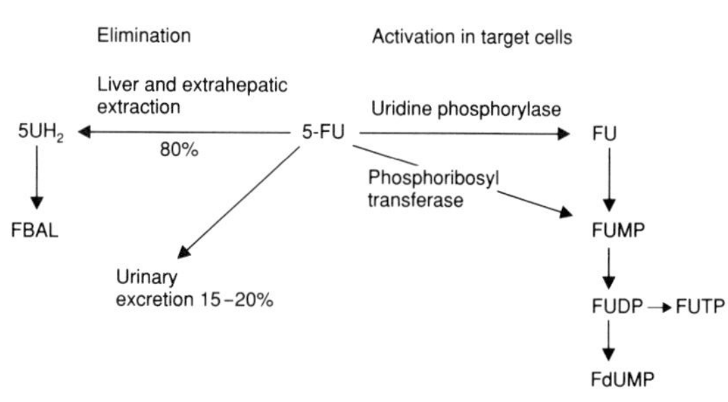

Figure 7.1 Metabolic fate of 5-fluorouracil (5-FU) in humans. Adapted from Diasio and Harris (1989).

Table 7.2 Determinants of response to 5-FU and FUDR

The intracellular concentrations of FdUMP and its normal counterpart dUMP
Extent and duration of inhibition of thymidilate synthatase
Level of thymidylate synthetase
Amount of drug incorporated into cellular RNA and DNA
Levels of activating enzymes (TK, ribonucleotide reductase, phosphoribosyl transferase) and cofactors (ribose-1-phosphate, deoxyribose-1-phosphate and 5-phosphoribosyl-1-pyrophosphate)
Pre-existing intracellular total CH_2 H_4 $PteGlu_n$ (leucovorin) concentration and polyglutamate chain length distribution

5dUrd = 5-fluoro-2′deoxyuride; FdUMP = 5-fluoro-2′-deoxyuridine-5′-monophosphate; dUMP = deoxyuridine monophosphate; TK = thymidine kinase.
Adapted from Zhang *et al.* (1992).

tion with the intracellular target responsible for toxicity to a particular cell.

Table 7.2 summarizes cellular factors affecting the response to 5-FU. Table 7.3 summarizes the mechanisms of resistance to 5-FU (Pinedo & Peters, 1988; Diasio & Harris, 1989; Didolkar *et al.*, 1989; Greenhalgh & Parish, 1989).

Table 7.3 Factors affecting resistance to 5-fluorouracil (5-FU)

Deficiency of 5-FU anabolism
Deficiency of 5-FU transport
Depletion of essential cosubstrates
Enhanced catabolism of 5-FU, FUMP or FdUMP
Enhanced intracellular uridine concentrations
Altered dTTP levels
Alterations in thymidylate synthase
Altered enzyme kinetics
Enhanced dUMP accumulation
Decreased FdUMP retention
Rapid recovery of new enzyme synthesis
Gene amplification
Decreased stability of ternary complex
Depletion of folates
Decreased polyglutamylation of folates

dTTP = Deoxythymidine triphosphate; FUMP = 5-fluorouridine-5′-monophosphate; FdUMP = 5-fluoro-2′-deoxyuridine-5′-monophosphate.
Adapted from Pinedo and Peters (1988)

Single agent – 5-fluorouracil

5-FU demonstrates a narrow toxic margin. The bioavailability of oral 5-FU is variable, with a range from 28 to 100%, due to initial first-pass metabolism in the liver and because of this factor, is not commonly given orally. With single IV bolus 5-FU the reported response rate is approximately 15%. On this scheduling, there is no effect on the patient's overall survival. The initial dosage recommended when 5-FU was first introduced was a loading dose schedule of 15 mg/kg over five days, then reducing to 7.5 mg/kg for eleven doses. Using this particular regimen of 5-FU, the average response varied from 15 to 25%, with an average duration of response from seven to eight months. This proved to be an extremely toxic regime, with a 3% death rate. It was subsequently modified to 12 mg/kg loading dose and 6 mg/kg on alternate days for five to eleven doses (Ansfield *et al.*, 1977; Baker *et al.*, 1976). Table 7.4 shows the toxicity and response rates to 5-FU used as a single agent in different scheduling.

The dose intensity of 5-FU is an important variable in predicting response rate and toxicity. There is a steep dose response curve from 500 mg/m^2 to 600 mg/m^2 per week, with a change in response rate from 20% to 29% when the dosage of 5-FU is increased from 500 mg/m^2 to 600 mg/m^2 per week. In the study by Hyriniuk, looking at dose intensity, seventeen cases at a dose intensity of 800 mg/m^2 per week yielded the highest response rate of 29%. The lowest response rate was recorded at a dose intensity of 300 mg/m^2 per week, with only 4% of patients responding to treatment (Hryniuk and Pater 1987; Hryniuk *et al.* 1987).

Infusion of 5-fluorouracil

In an attempt to improve therapeutic advantages of 5-FU, several infusional regimes have been studied. The maximum safe infusional level of 5-FU over twenty-four hours has been

Table 7.4 Comparison of response rate and toxicity of 5-fluorouracil (5-FU) in different schedules

Scheduling	Bolus	Short infusion (1–5 days)	Protracted infusion
Dosage Maximum tolerated Response rate	12 mg/kg × 5 days then 6 mg/kg 15%	1000 mg/m² Repeat 3-weekly 44%	300 mg/m² Continuous 38%
Survival advantage over 5-FU bolus	NS	NS	NS
Steady-state plasma level of 5-FU	1 μmol/l	0.5 μmol/l	0.13–1.16 μmol/l
Toxicity			
Leukopenia	20%	4%	1%
Mucositis	30%	22%	23%
Diarrhoea	15%	8%	17%
Hand–foot syndrome	0	0	23%

NS = Not significant.

shown to be 2.6 g/m^2 per day given weekly (Ardalan *et al.*, 1988), the dose-limiting toxicity being mucositis and haematological toxicity. The maximum 5-day infusional dose of 5-FU is 1000 mg/m^2 per day once every 3 weeks, with mucositis being the dose-limiting toxicity (Lokich, 1985). If prolonged infusion is used, 300 mg/m^2 per day continuously is the maximum tolerated dose (Lokich *et al.*, 1989). At a dose rate of 300 mg/m^2 per day, there has been a recorded response rate as high as 38%. Lokich *et al.* compared a dose of 300 mg/day IV infusion to IVI 500 mg bolus over 5 consecutive days and found that there was a higher response rate in the infusional group compared to the bolus group, with a total response rate of 30% in the infusional versus 7% in the bolus group.

The toxicities between the different methods of administration were quite different. The patients who received bolus therapy had mainly bone marrow suppression, particularly leukopenia, as well as severe stomatitis. The hand–foot syndrome was only observed in the infusion group, where it occurred in approximately 24% of patients. This syndrome is peculiarly associated with protracted infusions of 5-FU and consists of palmar-plantar erythrodysaesthesia, which is a rash and change in sensation and feeling of the palms and soles of the feet. Rapid recognition and dose adjustment result in prompt resolution of the syndrome (Lokich *et al.*, 1989).

Although there is a higher response rate with infusional 5-FU, the impact on survival has only been modest at best, with one study showing an improvement in survival from 2 to 8 months (Seifert *et al.*, 1975; Barbounis *et al.*, 1989; Hansen *et al.*, 1989a, 1989b).

The advantage of infusional therapy may lie in the different spectrum of toxicity from bolus treatment. There are other unusual complications which can occur from 5-FU infusion. 5-FU infusion can cause some cardiac toxicity. In a study of patients during infusion of 5-FU, 25% of patients were found to have abnormal electrocardiograms prior to infusion. A further 53% developed ST-T wave changes during the infusion. There have also been reports of sudden death and arrhythmias in patients who receive infusional 5-FU. This has been more common in patients with pre-existing coronary artery disease (Rezkalla *et al.*, 1989). Overall, there has been little impact on patient survival in colorectal cancer patients using 5-FU as a single agent.

Although there is controversy as to the ultimate scheduling of both intravenous and bolus treatment, it is generally agreed that 5-FU, if used alone, should be given until moderate toxicity reactions occur. Severe toxicity should be avoided and dosage modified according to the patient's reactions.

Table 7.5 shows the maximum tolerated dosage of 5-FU and their toxicities.

Table 7.5 Maximum tolerated dosage of 5-fluorouracil

Schedule	Dosage	Response rate	Toxicity
24 h (Adralan *et al.*, 1988)	2.6 g/m^2 per day every 7 days	15–20%	Neurological Mucositis Haematological
Infusion 5 days (Seifert *et al.*, 1975)	1000 mg/m^2 per day or 30 mg/kg per day	20–40%	Mucositis
Continuous (Lokich *et al.*, 1981)	300 mg/m^2 per day		Mucositis

Biomodulation

Folinic acid is an agent that is known to affect the drug 5-FU. The activation of the drug 5-FU is dependent on the concentration of reduced folate in the cell. This affects thymidylate synthetase, a key enzyme in DNA synthesis. The combination of 5-FU and folinic acid has held a greater hope for improvement of survival in patients with metastatic colorectal cancer (Einhorn, 1989). 5-FU and folinic acid are known to react with each other on a cellular basis, resulting in increased binding of the enzyme thymidylate synthetase and formation of a tertiary complex with 5-FU and folinic acid, which increases the cytotoxicity of 5-FU. This effect is due to the formation of a ternary complex involving thymidylate synthetase (DTMP synthetase), the coenzyme 5,10-methylenetetrahydrafolate and a metabolite of 5-FU, fluoroxydioxyuridine-5-fluoro-2′deoxyuridine-5′-monophosphate. This covalently bound complex dissociates in the presence of low concentrations of 5,10-methylhydrofolate (or 5-methyltetrahydrofolate metabolate of folinic acid) and its synergistic activity is enhanced by increasing concentration of the coenzyme. There have been various different schedules of 5-FU and folinic acid used together, demonstrating a quite dramatic difference in response rates (Van der Wilt *et al.*, 1992; Zhang *et al.*, 1992). There have been a number of encouraging clinical studies (Ardalan *et al.*, 1991).

Folinic acid has been shown to be effective in both high-dose and low-dose intravenous schedules. A number of different studies have been undertaken to try and determine the optimum schedule and dosing of 5-FU and folinic acid. The scheduling of 5-FU and folinic acid has varied with basically two main scheduling regimes being used – one, a weekly regime using 5-FU/folinic acid and the other, using a 5-day schedule of 5-FU together with folinic acid. The combination of 5-FU and folinic acid results in increased toxicity with the dose-limiting toxicities being mucositis and diarrhoea. Continuous infusions and bolus infusions of 5-FU and folinic acid have shown similar response rates. Both high- and low-dose folinic acid have been shown to be additive to the response rate of 5-FU alone, with the high-dose regime using 500 mg/m^2 and low doses using 25 mg/m^2. Most published studies have claimed a tripling of the response rate for patients who are given a combination (Kohne-Wompner *et al.*, 1992). Two studies have demonstrated an improved survival. Firstly the Princess Margaret study showed a significant survival advantage with a median survival of 9.6 months with 5-FU alone, compared with 12.6 months with combined 5-FU/folinic acid (Erlichman *et al.*, 1988). Secondly the North Central Oncology Group showed a median survival of 7.5 months with 5-FU alone compared to 12.3 months with the high dose and a 13.8-month survival with low-dose folinic acid (Poon *et al.*, 1989). It is obvious that both high-dose and low-dose folinic acid improve the response rate of 5-FU and both high- and low-dose regimes have been shown to improve the survival of patients. The prolongation of survival has been questioned by some groups and, recently, meta-analysis was performed by the Advanced Colorectal Cancer Meta-Analysis Project and published in the *Journal of Clinical Oncology* in June 1992. This study analysed 10 published studies where randomized intravenous 5-FU was given compared to intravenous 5-FU/folinic acid. It included 1500 patients, with six out of 10 trials reporting a higher

Table 7.6 Response rate of 5-fluorouracil (5-FU) and folinic acid for weekly and daily schedule in untreated patients.

	Dose (mg/m^2)				Toxicity		
Reference	5-FU	Folinic acid	Response (PR + CR)	Median survival (weeks)	>Grade II leukopenia	>Grade I mucositis stomatitis	>Grade I diarrhoea
Daily							
Poon *et al.* (1989)	370, days 1–5, i.v. push q, 5 weeks	200, days 1–5 i.v. push q, 5 weeks	26%	53	19%	30%	9%
Poon *et al.* (1989)	425, days 1–5, i.v. push q, 5 weeks	20, days 1–5 i.v. push q, 5 weeks	43%	52	21%	26%	14%
Erlichman *et al.* (1988)	370, days 1–5, i.v. push q, 5 weeks	200, days 1–5 i.v. push q, 5 weeks	33%	54	22%	17%	19%
Valone *et al.* (1989)	400, days 1–5 15-min infusion q, 4–5 weeks	200, days 1–5 i.v. push q, 5 weeks	19%	46	12%	46%	32%
Doroshow *et al.* (1990)	370, days 1–5 push q, 4–5 weeks	500 continuous infusion for 5.5 days	44%	62	9%	47%	31%
Weekly							
Petrelli *et al.* (1989)	600 i.v. weekly × 6 q, 8 weeks	500, 2-h infusion, start 1 h prior to 5-FU	30%	55	8%	4%	25%
Petrelli *et al.* (1989)	600 i.v. weekly × 6 q, 8 weeks	25, 10-min infusion	19%	45	4%	0%	13%
Sobrero *et al.* (1989)	600 i.v. weekly × 6 q, 8 h	500, 2-h infusion, start 1 h prior to 5-FU	28%	50	0%	9%	20%

PR = Partial response; CR = complete response
From Zhang *et al.* (1992), with permission.

tumour response rate. These results confirmed the advantage of higher response rate with 5-FU plus folinic acid. Patients who received folinic acid either as a weekly or monthly regime showed a significantly higher response rate of 23% versus 11% compared to 5-FU alone. However, the overall survival from all studies was not significantly improved. Some of the patients who failed were crossed over to 5-FU and folinic acid, which may have influenced the survival analysis of patients in this study. There is no doubt that there is a higher response rate using this regime, with survival being improved in some studies (Valone *et al.*, 1989). Table 7.6 summarizes some of the studies of the combination of 5-FU and folinic acid (Arbuck, 1989; Petrelli *et al.*, 1989; Sobrero *et al.*, 1989; Valone *et al.*, 1989; Doroshow *et al.*, 1990).

Other biochemical modulations of 5-fluorouracil

Methotrexate/5-fluorouracil

Methotrexate pretreatment inhibits the *de novo* purine synthesis causing expansion of phosphoribosylpyrophosphate (PRPP) pools and increases the incorporation of 5-FU into RNA. The combination has an improved response rate compared to 5-FU alone. Methotrexate must be given at least 24 h before 5-FU for maximum enhancement to be seen.

Methotrexate pretreatment causes expansion of PRPP pools, which reach a maximum at 24 h, resulting in maximum modulation of biochemical interference with RNA and DNA synthesis.

A trial performed by the Piedmont Oncology Association showed a significantly higher response rate of 29% versus 14% in the pretreated patients who received methotrexate. This was associated with an improvement in survival from 5.9 to 9.9 months. They compared a 1-h interval with a 24-h interval in the sequential application of methotrexate and 5-FU. In this study, a sufficient number of patients were treated in both arms and a significantly improved response rate was seen with the 24 h interval. They also demonstrated a significant prolongation of survival from 11.4 to 15.3 months (Nordic Gastrointestinal Tumor Adjuvant Therapy Group; Marsh *et al.*, 1991). It would appear from the studies which have been performed so far, that 5-FU and methotrexate may produce similar response rates to 5-FU and folinic acid.

Other biochemical modulations have been attempted using different substances.

PALA

Enhancement of 5-FU can be achieved by biochemical modulation to produce the selective enhancement of 5-FU's antitumour effect. *N*-phospho-acetyl-L-aspartate aspartic acid (PALA) is a biochemical modulating agent for 5-FU. PALA is an inhibitor of the *de novo* pyrimedine biosynthesis. 5-FU competition with urocil nucleotides provided opportunity for the administration of PALA prior to 5-FU to enhance 5-FU anticancer activity by lowering the intracellular uridine pools.

However, in clinical studies, there have been conflicting results. High-dose PALA, 1–2 g/m^2, was not tolerated; 84% of patients needed a reduction in their dosage to half the calculated dose of 5-FU to enable them to tolerate the combination. With this combination of high-dose PALA and 5-FU, the results were suboptimal (Martin & Kemeny, 1992).

Low-dose PALA and 5-FU may be beneficial and as yet further studies are needed to see whether low-dose PALA and standard-dose 5-FU may be more acceptable. A phase II study published in the *Journal of Clinical Oncology* in September 1990 of PALA given at a dose of 25 mg/m^2 given on day 1, followed by a 24-h infusion of 5-FU at 2600 mg/m^2. Repeated weekly, given to 37 patients achieved a partial response of 43% with a median duration of response of 5 months (O'Dwyer *et al.*, 1990).

Using maximum tolerated doses of 5-FU, folinic acid and PALA 250 mg/m^2, Ardalan *et al.* (1992) reported a response rate of 86% in previously untreated patients. The major toxicities were diarrhoea and stomatitis.

Kemeney *et al* (1992) used oral uridine in combination with 5-FU and PALA in an attempt to reduce toxicity but could only achieve a low response rate, and theorized that the tumour cells may also have been rescued by the uridine. The use of PALA and 5-FU is an area where there will be continued advancements. Further studies are awaited.

Table 7.7 lists the potential interactions with 5-FU and other biomodulators.

Dipyridamole alters 5-FU metabolism, producing a selective increase in fluorodeoxyuridine monophosphate levels by blocking the efflux of fluorodeoxyuridine. This interaction may increase the intracellular effect of 5-FU. However, the optimum scheduling and dosing of these two compounds are still under investigation (Trump *et al.*, 1991).

Other chemotherapeutic drugs used in colorectal cancer

There have been a number of other drugs tried in colorectal cancer. All have a relatively low response rate, in the vicinity of 15–20%. Some have been used in combination with 5-FU. Table 7.8 summarizes the single-agent response rates to a number of drugs tried in colorectal cancer (Davis, 1982).

Mitomycin C

The response rate to Mitomycin C has varied from 11% to 33%, with the highest response rate recorded with intermittent high-dose treatment of 20 mg/m^2 every 8 weeks. Results suggest that, at best, there is a moderate response. Complete responses are rarely obtained and no prolongation of survival has been demonstrated

Table 7.7 Biochemical modulation of 5-fluorouracil (5-FU)

Modulating agent	Postulated mechanism
Purine inosine	Increased rib-I-P might lead to increased anabolism
Guanosine	Similar to inosine
GMP	Similar to guanosine after conversion of GMP to guanosine
Deoxyinosine	Increased dRib-I-P leads to enhanced FdUMP
Pyrimidines – thymidine	Inhibition of 5-FU breakdown
Uridine	Rescue of normal tissue by competition of UTP with FUTP
Cytidine	Similar to uridine
Antimetabolites – methotrexate	Increased 5-FU anabolism due to enhanced PRPP
PALA	Decrease of uracil nucleotides leads to enhanced anabolism
Allopurinol	Postulated differential metabolism of 5-FU in tumours and normal tissues is used; decreased toxicity
Hydroxyurea	Inhibition of ribonucleotide reduction prevents rescue by normal nucleotides
Dipyridamol	Prevention of efflux of FUR and FUdR
Leucovorin	Enhanced retention of FdUMP binding to thymidylate synthetase in tumours

Rib-I-P = Ribose-I-P; dRib-I-P = deoxyribose-I-P; GMP = guanosine-5′-phosphate; PRPP = phosphoribosylpyrophosphate; PALA = *N*-phospho-acetyl-L-aspartate aspartic; FdUMP = 5-fluoro-2′deoxyuridine-5′-monophosphate; UTP = uridine triphosphate; FUTP = fluorouridine 5′-triphosphate; FUR = 5-fluorouridine; FUdR = 5-fluoro-2′ deoxyuridine. Adapted from Pinedo and Peters (1988).

Table 7.8 Response rate of colorectal cancer to single-agent chemotherapy

Drug	Response rate
5-Fluorouracil	15–25%
5-FUdR	21–22%
Methotrexate	17%
Mitomycin C	12–16%
Methyl-CCNU	18%
Doxorubicin	7%

5-FUdR = 5-fluoro-2′ deoxyuridine

either alone or in combination with other drugs (Ogawa *et al.*, 1981).

Combination chemotherapy for colorectal cancer

Mortel *et al.* (1975) compared MOF (methyl-nitrosourea, vincristine and 5-FU) with 5-FU alone and showed a higher response rate of 43% compared to 19%. Although the patients had a higher response rate to this regime, this was a preliminary observation and no survival advantage was demonstrated. Subsequent problems with leukaemia from CCNU have been of concern. Carmustine (BCNU) has also been used in a similar combination, with no significant improvement in survival (Moertel *et al.*, 1975).

Einhorn and colleagues (1975) have also used a combination of methyl-CCNU and 5-FU infusions and likewise showed a partial response rate of 29%, with a median duration of response of 6 months with minimal toxicity.

Baker *et al.* (1975) reported a study of 5-FU versus 5-FU plus methyl-CCNU, showing a response rate of 31% in 294 patients. Similarly, Lokich *et al.* (1977) compared 52 patients with 5-FU versus 5-FU, methyl-CCNU and vincristine and showed that 84% of patients receiving the combination had progression of their symptoms by 4 months after one and a half cycles of therapy.

In all of these studies, the combination of 5-FU with these drugs did not produce any superior survival rate compared to 5-FU alone.

Cis-platinum and 5-fluorouracil

After initial early enthusiasm for the combination of 5-FU and cis-platinum, subsequent studies have revealed that the initial findings were unable to be repeated.

The original study was published in June in *Cancer Treatment Reports* (Cantrell *et al.*, 1987). This study compared the combination of continuous infusion of 5-FU and weekly cis-platinum in advanced colorectal patients. Thirty-five patients were included in the study and the response rate was reported to be 63% with mild toxicity.

Kemeney *et al.* (1990a) compared a dose of 5-FU of 1 g/m^2 per day for 5 consecutive days every 4 weeks, with the same dose of 5-FU plus cis-platinum 20 mg/m^2 intravenously on days 1–5 of each cycle. The response rate was 25% for the combination versus 3% for the single agent. However, the duration of response was only 6 months for the combination and 4.7 months for the 5-FU alone, with the median survival being 10 and 12 months respectively.

A similar study was conducted by Loehrer *et al.* (1988), using a dose of 15 mg/kg per week of 5-FU alone versus the same dose of 5-FU plus cis-platinum, 60 mg/m^2 every 3 weeks. In 132 evaluated patients there was a 19% response rate for the 5-FU-alone arm and a 22% response rate for the 5-FU plus cis-platinum group. There was no difference in the median survival times of 40 and 39 weeks respectively.

The combinations of cis-platinum and 5-FU have not produced any significant survival advantage over 5-FU alone. These combinations have increased toxicity, particularly haematological toxicity, which is much more severe than 5-FU alone.

In summary, it seems that all the combinations of 5-FU and other cytotoxic agents have proved to be more toxic but not more beneficial than 5-FU alone.

Combination of 5-fluorouracil with biomodulators

5-fluorouracil and biological response modifiers

Preclinical data suggested that interferon and 5-FU have a synergistic cytostatic effect upon cultured colorectal cells. The uptake of 5-FU is increased, resulting in increased concentration of an active 5-FU metabolite at its intracellular target. α-Interferon may also enhance the inhibition of thymidylate synthetase (Wadler *et al.*, 1989).

Because of this synergism, it was felt that the combination of interferon and 5-FU may result in improved results in colorectal cancer. The initial treatment consisted of 5-FU as a continuous infusion, 750 mg/m^2 per day for 5 days, followed by weekly intravenous bolus doses of 750 mg/m^2 of 5-FU commencing on day 15. Interferon was commenced on day 1 of the treatment regime and given at a dose of 9 million units for each day. The reported response rate in this regime was 76%. There was quite marked toxicity, with virtually all patients complaining of fever and fatigue, which resolved on reduction of the dose of interferon. Three of 32 patients had grade III leukopenia and diarrhoea and 3 out of 32 had grade III mucusitis (Ernstoff *et al.*, 11989; Wadler *et al.*, 1989; Wadler & Wiernik, 1990).

A phase 2 study of 38 previously untreated metastic colorectal patients used the same regime as above with the same dose of inteferon. Only 26% achieved a partial response, lasting a median of 7.5 months; the median survival was 13 months. Toxicities were stomatitis in 52% of patients and diarrhoea in 43%. Neurotoxicity was seen in 34% of patients. A total of 84% required reduction in the interferon dosage by at least 50% and 63% required a reduction of 5-FU by at least 25%. The authors concluded that, although this regime had a higher response rate, the toxicity was substantial and the responses were not significantly superior to 5-FU alone (Kemeny *et al.*, 1990b).

A similar study undertaken by the M.D. Anderson Hospital and Pazdur *et al.* (1990) assessed 45 patients and demonstrated a response rate of 35%. A total of 25% developed toxicity and 82% had grade III toxicity or greater. The median survival of the group was 16 months (Pazdur *et al.*, 1990).

Table 7.9 summarizes some studies of 5-FU and interferon.

In conclusion, the role of systemic chemotherapy in treating advanced colorectal cancer is often debated. However, improvement in quality of life and survival may be obtained in some patient groups. The optimum scheduling and combination of drugs are still to be discovered, but there are encouraging results from

Table 7.9 5-Fluorouracil with interferon

	Einstein	M.D. Anderson	MSKCC
Evaluable patients	32	45	35
Responses	20	16	9
Response rate	63%	35%	26%
95% confidence interval	(46–79%)	(22–50%)	(11–41%)

From Kemeney and Younes (1992), with permission.

some of the trials with biomodulation of 5-FU, folinic acid and interferon. Future studies to find the optimum scheduling of PALA, dipyridamole and the new investigational studies of somatostatin and H_2 antagonists may lead to even better combinations, with the hope of continuing improvement in survival and quality of life of these patients.

References

Advanced Colorectal Cancer Meta-Analysis Project (1992) Modulation of fluorouracil by leucovorin in patients with advanced colorectal cancer: evidence in terms of response rate. *J. Clin. Oncol.* **10**;896–903.

Allen-Mersh TG (1989) Colorectal liver metastases: is 'no treatment' still best? *J. R. Soc. Med.* **82**, 2–3.

Ansfield F, Klotz J, Nealon T *et al.* (1977) A phase III study comparing the clinical utility of four regimens of 5-fluorouracil. *Cancer* **39**, 34–40.

Arbuck SG (1989) Overview of clinical trials using 5-fluorouracil and leucovorin for the treatment of colorectal cancer. *Cancer* **63**, 1036–1044.

Ardalan B, Singh G & Silverman H (1988) A randomized phase I and II study of short-term infusion of high-dose fluorouracil with or without *N*-(phosphonacetyl)-L-aspartic acid in patients with advanced pancreatic and colorectal cancers. *J. Clin. Oncol.* **6**, 1053–1058.

Ardalan B, Chua L, Tian E *et al.* (1991) A phase II study of weekly 24-hour infusion with high-dose fluorouracil with leucovorin in colorectal carcinoma. *J. Clin. Oncol.* **9**, 625–630.

Ardalan B, Donofrio K, Sridhar KS *et al.* (1992) Is there hope after 5-FU bolus? A phase II study of short term protracted infusion of high dose 5-fluorouracil (5-FU) with leucovorin (LV) and low dose phosphonacetyl-L-aspartic acid (PALA) in colorectal carcinoma. *Proc. ASCO* **11**, 186.

Baker LH, Mather R, Talley R *et al.* (1975) 5-FU versus 5-FU and MeCCNU in gastrointestinal cancers. A phase II study of the southwest oncology group. *Proc. Am. Assoc. Cancer Res.* **16**, 229.

Baker LH, Talley RW, Matter, R *et al.* (1976) Phase III comparison of the treatment of advanced gastrointestinal cancer with bolus weekly 5-FU vs methyl-CCNU plus bolus weekly 5-FU. A southwest oncology group study. *Cancer* **38**, 1–7.

Barbounis VP, Kalofonos HP, Munro AJ, McKenzie CG, Sackier JM & Epenetos AA (1989) Treatment of colorectal cancer and other malignancies with continuous infusion of 5-fluorouracil. *Anticancer Res.* **9**, 33–40.

Bleiberg H (1989) Treatment of advanced colorectal cancer. *Anticancer Res.* **9**, 1013–1016.

Cantrell JE, Hart RD, Taylor RF & Harvey JH (1987) Pilot trial of prolonged continuous-infusion 5-fluorouracil and weekly cisplatin in advanced colorectal cancer. *Cancer Treat. Rep.* **71**, 615–618.

Carter SK (1976) Large-bowel cancer – the current status of treatment. *J. Natl. Cancer Inst.* **56**, 3–10.

Davis HL (1982) Chemotherapy of large bowel cancer. *Cancer* **50**, 2638–2646.

Diasio RB & Harris BE (1989) Clinical pharmacology of 5-fluorouracil. Clinical pharmacokinetics, vol. 16, pp. 215–237. ADIS Press.

Didolkar MS, Jackson AJ, Covell DG, Walker AP & Eddington ND (1989) Influence of the routes of continuous intrahepatic infusion of 5-fluorouracil on its pharmacokinetics. *J. Surg. Oncol.* **41**, 187–193.

Doroshow JH, Multhauff P. Leong L *et al.* (1990) Prospective randomized comparison of fluorouracil versus fluorouracil and high-dose continuous infusion leucovorin calcium for the treatment of advanced measurable colorectal cancer in patients previously unexposed to chemotherapy. *J. Clin. Oncol.* **8**, 491–501.

Einhorn LH (1989) Improvements in fluorouracil chemotherapy. *J. Clin. Oncol.* **7**, 1377–1379.

Einhorn LH, Furnas BE, Bond WH *et al.* (1975) Combination chemotherapy with 5-day continuous infusion 5-FU and methyl CCNU in disseminated enteric adenocarcinoma. *Proc. Am. Assoc. Cancer Res.* **16**, 18.

Erlichman C, Fine S, Wong A *et al.* (1988) A randomised trial of fluorouracil and folinic acid in patients with metastatic colorectal carcinoma. *J. Clin. Oncol.* **3**, 469–475.

Ernstoff MS, Lembersky BC & Kirkwood JM (1989) Fluorouracil, interferon-alpha, and colon cancer: rational pursuit of synergism between antimetabolites and biologicals. *J. Clin. Oncol.* **7**, 1764–1765.

Greenhalgh DA & Parish JH (1989) Effects of 5-fluorouracil on cytotoxicity and RNA metabolism in human colonic carcinoma cells. *Cancer Chemother. Pharmacol.* **25**, 37–44.

Grem J, (1991) Current treatment approaches in colorectal cancer. *Semin. Oncol.* **18** (suppl 1), 17–26.

Hansen RM, Quebbeman E & Anderson T. (1989a) 5-Fluorouracil by protracted venous infusion. *Oncology* **46**, 245–250.

Hansen R, Quebbeman E. Ausman R *et al.* (1989b) Continuous systemic 5-fluorouracil infusion in advanced colorectal cancer: results in 91 patients. *J. Surg. Oncol.* **40**, 177–181.

Heidelberger C, Chaudhuri NK, Danneberg P *et al.* (1957) Fluorinated pyrimidines, a new class of tumour-inhibitory compounds. *Nature* **4561**, 663–666.

Hryniuk WM & Pater JL (1987) Implications of dose intensity for cancer chemotherapy. *Semin. Oncol.* **14** (suppl. 4), 43–44.

Hryniuk WM, Figueredo A & Goodyear M (1987) Applications of dose intensity to problems in chemotherapy of breast and colorectal cancer. *Semin. Oncol.* **14** (suppl. 4), 3–11.

Hughes K, Scheele J & Sugarbaker PH (1989) Surgery for colorectal cancer metastatic to the liver. Optimizing the results of treatment. *Surg. Clin. North Am.* **69**, 339–359.

Hunt TM & Taylor I (1989) The role of chemotherapy in the treatment and prophylaxis of colorectal liver metastases. *Cancer Surv.* **8**, 71–90.

Kemeney N & Seiter K (1991) Therapy for colorectal cancer. *Opinion Oncol.* **3**, 743–752.

Kemeny N & Younes A (1992) Alfa-2A interferon and 5-fluorouracil for advanced colorectal carcinoma. The Memorial Sloan-Kettering experience. *Semin. Oncol.* **19** (suppl. 3), 171–175.

Kemeny N, Niedzwiecki D, Shurgot B & Oderman P (1989) Prognostic variables in patients with hepatic metastases from colorectal cancer. Importance of medical assessment of liver involvement. *Cancer* **63**, 742–747.

Kemeney N, Israel K. Niedzwiecki D *et al.* (1990a) Randomized study of continuous infusion fluorouracil versus fluorouracil plus cisplatin in patients with metastatic colorectal cancer. *J. Clin. Oncol.* **8**, 313–318.

Kemeny N, Younes A, Seiter K *et al.* (1990b) Interferon alfa-2a and fluorouracil for advanced colorectal carcinoma: assessment of activity and toxicity. *Cancer* **66**, 2470–2475.

Kemeny N, Conti J, Martin D *et al.* (1992) Oral uridine (UR) protects from 5-fluorouracil (FU) toxicity in metastatic colorectal carcinoma: phase I/II trial of phosphonacetyl-L-aspartic acid (PALA) + FU with UR as a rescue agent. *Proc. ASCO* **11**, 171.

Kohne-Wompner CH, Schmoll HJ, Harstrick A & Rustum YM (1992) Chemotherapeutic strategies in metastatic colorectal cancer: an overview of current clinical trials. *Semin. Oncol.* **19** (suppl. 3), 105–125.

Loehrer P, Turner S, Kubilis P *et al.* (1988) A prospective randomized trial of fluorouracil versus fluorouracil plus cisplatin in the treatment of metastatic colorectal cancer: a Hoosier oncology group trial. *J. Clin. Oncol.* **6**, 642–648.

Lokich JJ (1985) Optimal schedule for 5-fluorouracil chemotherapy. Intermittent bolus or continuous infusion. *Am. J. Clin. Oncol.* **8**, 445–448.

Lokich JJ, Skarin AT, Mayer RJ & Frei E (1977) Lack of effectiveness of combined 5-fluorouracil and methyl-CCNU therapy in advanced colorectal cancer. *Cancer* **40**, 2792–2796.

Lokich JJ, Bothe A, Fine N *et al.* (1981) Phase I study of protracted venous infusion of 5-fluorouracil. *Cancer 48*, 2565–2568.

Lokich JJ, Ahlgren JD, Gullo JJ, Philips JA & Fryer JG (1989) A prospective randomized comparison of continuous infusion fluorouracil with a conventional bolus schedule in metastatic colorectal carcinoma: a mid-Atlantic oncology program study. *J. Clin. Oncol.* **7**, 425–432.

McDonald JS (1989) Editorial. Continuous low-dose infusion of fluorouracil: is the benefit worth the cost? *J. Clin. Oncol.* **7**, 412–414.

Marsh JC, Bertino JR, Katz KH *et al.* (1991) The influence of drug interval on the effect of methotrexate and fluorouracil in the treatment of advanced colorectal cancer. *J. Clin. Oncol.* **9**, 371–380.

Martin DS & Kemeney NE (1992) Modulation of fluorouracil by *N*-(phosphonacetyl)-L-aspartate: a review. *Semin. Oncol.* **19** (suppl. 3), 49–55.

Moertel CG, Schsutt AJ, Hahn RG & Reitemeier RJ (1975) Brief communication: therapy of advanced colorectal cancer with a combination of 5-fluorouracil, methyl-1,3-*cis*(2-chlorethyl)-1-nitrosourea, and vincristine. *J. Natl. Cancer Inst.* **54**, 69–71.

Nordic Gastrointestinal Tumor Adjuvant Therapy Group (1989) Superiority of sequential methotrexate, fluorouracil and leucovorin to fluorouracil alone in advanced symptomatic colorectal carcinoma: a randomized trial. *J. Clin. Oncol.* **7**, 1437–1446.

Nordic Gastrointestinal Tumor Adjuvant Therapy Group (1992) Expectancy of primary chemotherapy in patients with advanced asymptomatic colorectal cancer: a randomized trial. *J. Clin. Oncol.* **10**, 904–911.

O'Dwyer PJ, Paul AR, Walczak J. Weiner LM, Litwin S & Comis RL (1990) Phase II study of biochemical modulation of fluorouracil by low-dose PALA in patients with colorectal cancer. *J. Clin. Oncol.* **8**, 1497–1503.

Ogawa M, Rozencweig M & Staquet MJ (ed) (1981) Mitomycin C current impact on cancer chemotherapy. In: *Proceedings of a Symposium on Mitomycin C presented during the Third NCI-EORTC Symposium on New Drugs in Cancer Therapy*. Brussels, Belgium.

Pazdur R, Ajani JA, Patt YZ *et al.* (1990) Phase II study of fluorouracil and recombinant interferon alfa-2a in previously untreated advanced colorectal carcinoma. *J. Clin. Oncol.* **18**, 2027–2031.

Petrelli N, Douglass HO, Herrera L *et al.* (1989) The modulation of fluorouracil with leucovorin in metastatic colorectal carcinoma: a prospective randomized phase III trial. *J. Clin. Oncol.* **7**, 1419–1426.

Pinedo HM & Peter GFD (1988) Fluorouracil: biochemistry and pharmacology. *J. Clin. Oncol.* **6**, 1653–1664.

Poon MA, O'Connell MJ, Moertel CG *et al.* (1989) Biochemical modulation of fluorouracil: evidence of significant improvemnt of survival and quality of life in patients with advanced colorectal carcinoma. *J. Clin. Oncol.* **7**, 1407–1418.

Rezkalla S, Kloner RA, Ensley J *et al.* (1989) Continuous ambulatory ECG monitoring during fluorouracil therapy: a prospective study. *J. Clin. Oncol.* **7**, 509–514.

Saenz NC, Cady B, McDermott WV Jr & Steele GD Jr (1989) Experience with colorectal carcinoma metastatic to the liver. *Surg. Clin. North Am.* **69**, 361–370.

Scott NA & Beart RW Jr (1988) Colorectal cancer: flow cytometric DNA analysis. *Aust. N.Z. J. Surg.* **58**, 189–191.

Seifert P, Baker LH, Reed ML & Vaitkevicius VK (1975) Comparison of continuously infused 5-fluorouracil with bolus injection in treatment of patients with colorectal adenocarcinoma. *Cancer* **36**, 123–128.

Sobrero A, Nobile MT, Vidili MG *et al.* (1989) Randomized trial of the maximum tolerated dose of weekly bolus 5-fluorouracil alone or combined with high dose leucovorin in advanced, measurable colorectal cancer. In: Pinedo HM, Rostum YM (eds) *Leucovorin Modulation of Fluoropyrimidines: A New Frontier in Cancer Chemotherapy*, pp. 47–51. London: Royal Society of Medicine Services.

Stehlin JS Jr, de Ipolyi PD, Greeff PJ, McGaff CJ Jr, Davis BR & McNary L (1988) Treatment of cancer of the liver. Twenty years' experience with infusion and resection in 414 patients. *Ann. Surg.* **208**, 23–37.

Tannock IF (1987) Tumour growth and cell kinetics. In: Tannock IF & Hill RP (eds) *The Basic Science of Oncology*, pp. 140–159. New York: Pergamon Books. 140–159.

Trump DL, Egorin MJ, Forrest A, Willson JKV, Remick S & Tutsch KD (1991) Pharmacokinetics and pharmacodynamic analysis of fluorouracil during 72-hour continuous infusion with and without dipyridamole. *J. Clin. Oncology* **9(11)**, 2027–2035.

Valone FH, Friedman MA, Wittlinger PS *et al.* (1989) Treatment of patients with advanced colorectal carcinoma with fluorouracil alone, high-dose leucovorin plus fluorouracil, or sequential methotrexate, fluorouracil, and leucovorin: a randomized trial of the northern California oncology group. *J. Clin. Oncol.* **7**, 1427–1436.

Van De Velde CJH and De Brauw LM (1989) Developments in the management of metastasis of colorectal tumours in the liver. Management of liver metastases. *Scand. J. Gastroenterol.* **24** (suppl. 171), 91–98.

Van der Wilt CL, Pinedo HM, Smid K, Cloos J, Noordhuis P & Peters GJ (1992) Effect of folinic acid on fluorouracil activity and expression of thymidylate synthase. *Semin. Oncol.* **19** (suppl. 3), 16–25.

Wadler S & Wiernik PH (1990) Clinical update on the role of flourouracil and recombinant interferon alfa-2a in the treatment of colorectal carcinoma. *Semin. Oncol.* **17**, 16–21.

Wadler S, Schwartz EL, Goldman M *et al.* (1989) Fluorouracil and recombinant alfa-2a-interferon: an active regimen against advanced colorectal carcinoma. *J. Clin. Oncol.* **7**, 1769–1775.

Wirth A, Green M, Penfold C *et al.* (1992) Recent advances in the treatment of colorectal cancer. *Aust. N.Z. J. Med.* **22**, 61–68.

Zhang Z-G, Harstrick A & Rustum YM (1992) Modulation of fluoropyrimidines: role of dose and schedule of leucovorin administration. *Semin. Oncol.* **19** (suppl. 3), 10–15.

8

Regional cytotoxic therapy in patients with colorectal liver metastases

Colin S. McArdle and D.J. Kerr

The results of systemic chemotherapy for patients with multiple liver metastases secondary to colorectal cancer are disappointing. For example, single-agent 5-fluorouracil (5-FU) has a response rate of approximately 10–15%. Most cytotoxic drugs have a steep dose–response curve and it is therefore a basic pharmacokinetic principle that if one can increase drug delivery to a tumour, one can increase response rate (Frei & Canellos, 1980). However attempts to increase the response rate to systemic chemotherapy further by escalating the dose have been limited by unacceptable toxicity. In an attempt to enhance tumour exposure to cytotoxic agents and reduce systemic toxicity, many workers have therefore turned to the use of targeted therapy.

Targeting of cytotoxic drugs can occur at three levels, as described by Widder *et al.* (1979):

1. The drug is selectively distributed to the organ harbouring tumour – in this case, the liver (Fig. 8.1).
2. The drug is directed to tumour rather than normal tissue within the target organ.
3. The drug is taken up preferentially by tumour cells.

It has long been recognized that colorectal liver metastases (>1 cm in diameter) receive their blood supply predominantly from the hepatic artery (Ridge *et al.*, 1987) and the first-level targeting can therefore be achieved by the administration of drugs via a hepatic artery catheter.

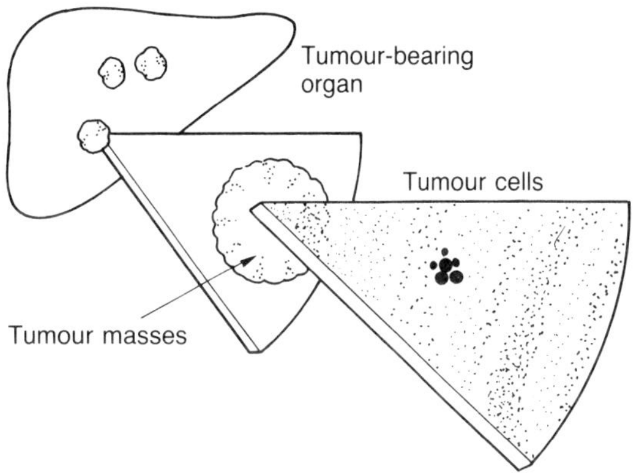

Figure 8.1 Theory of targeting.

In patients with a classical vascular anatomy, the common hepatic artery arises from the coeliac axis and gives off the gastroduodenal branch before dividing into right and left hepatic arteries. Access to the hepatic artery can be achieved by inserting a catheter into the gastroduodenal artery so that the tip of the catheter lies at its origin (see chapter 6).

The choice of an appropriate chemotherapy regimen thereafter is critical. Because bolus 5-FU administered via the hapatic artery catheter is rapidly washed out from the liver, rapid administration of 5-FU through the hepatic artery catheter confers no regional advantage when compared with the same drug given

Table 8.1 Comparison of systemic clearance of 5-fluorouracil (5-FU) from plasma after bolus injection, 2-h and 24-h infusion intravenously and intra-arterially

	n	Clearance of 5-FU (bolus injection) (1/min)	*n*	Clearance of 5-FU (2 h infusion; 1/min)	*n*	Clearance of 5-FU (24-h infusion; 1/min)
Intravenous	9	0.94±0.3	7	1.75±0.2*	6	18.4±6.5*
Intra-arterial	9	0.81±0.2	7	2.66±0.4*	6	42.0±27.1*

*$p<0.05$.

Table 8.2 Randomized trial of regional compared with systemic therapy

Study	Route	No.	Response (%)	*P* value	Survival	*P* value
MSKCC	i.a.	48	52	0.001	17 months (median)	NS
(Kemeny *et al.*, 1987)	i.v.	51	20		12 months	
NCOG	i.a.	58	42	0.001	17 months (median)	NS
(Hohn *et al.*, 1987)	i.v.	59	10		16 months	
National Cancer Institute	i.a.	21	62	0.003	22% (2 years)	NS
(Chang *et al.*, 1987)	i.v.	29	17		15%	
MAYO	i.a.	36	48	0.02	12.6 months (median)	NS
(Martin *et al.*, 1990)	i.v.	33	21		10.5 months	
France	i.a.	81	43	0.001	15 months (median)	0.02
(Rougier *et al.*, 1992)	i.v.	82	9		11	

i.a. = intra-arterial; i.v. = intravenous; NS = Not significant.
MSKCC = Memorial Sloan Kettering Cancer Center
NCOG = Northern California Oncology Group

intravenously (Goldberg *et al.*, 1988). This is probably because the extraction mechanism of the liver is saturated. It is clear, however, that hepatic arterial infusion of 5-FU significantly reduces systemic exposure, as manifested by lower peak plasma concentrations and area under the curve and higher rates of clearance, compared with intravenous infusion (Goldberg *et al.*, 1990). This effect becomes more obvious as the duration of infusion is increased (Table 8.1).

It is therefore essential to improve drug uptake by enhancing second- and third-level targeting. Methods of doing so include:

1. The prolonged administration of 5-fluorodeoxyuridine (FUDR) using an Infusaid pump. Based on the encouraging results obtained in early non-randomized studies (Balch *et al.*, 1983; Niederhuber *et al.*, 1984; Cohen *et al.*, 1985), Infusaid pumps were widely used in the USA.

Kemeny (1992) has recently reviewed the results of those studies where regional therapy using FUDR was compared with systemic therapy. Although response rates were consistently higher with regionally administered therapy, this did not consistently translate into a survival advantage (Table 8.2). This may have been due in part to the small numbers in some studies and the cross-over design employed in others. For example, in the Memorial Sloan Kettering Cancer Center study, 99 patients were randomized to a 14-day infusion of FUDR administered by Infusaid pump regionally or systemically. In the 45 evaluable patients receiving intrahepatic arterial therapy, there were 2 complete and 23 partial reponses (53%) and in the 48 evaluable patients receiving systemic therapy there were no complete responses and 10 partial responses (21%). Median survival for the intra-arterial and systemic treatment groups was 17 and 12 months respectively. However, interpret-

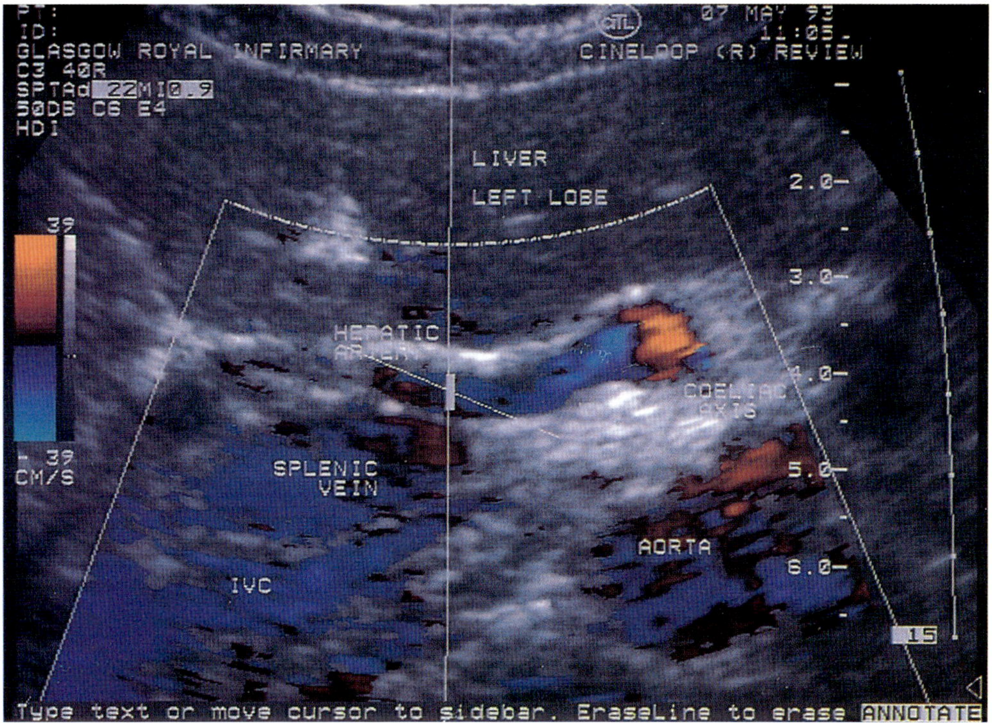

Plate 1 Transverse sonographic scan of the epigastrium showing the longitudinal section of the common hepatic artery with the Doppler cursor overlying the lumen.

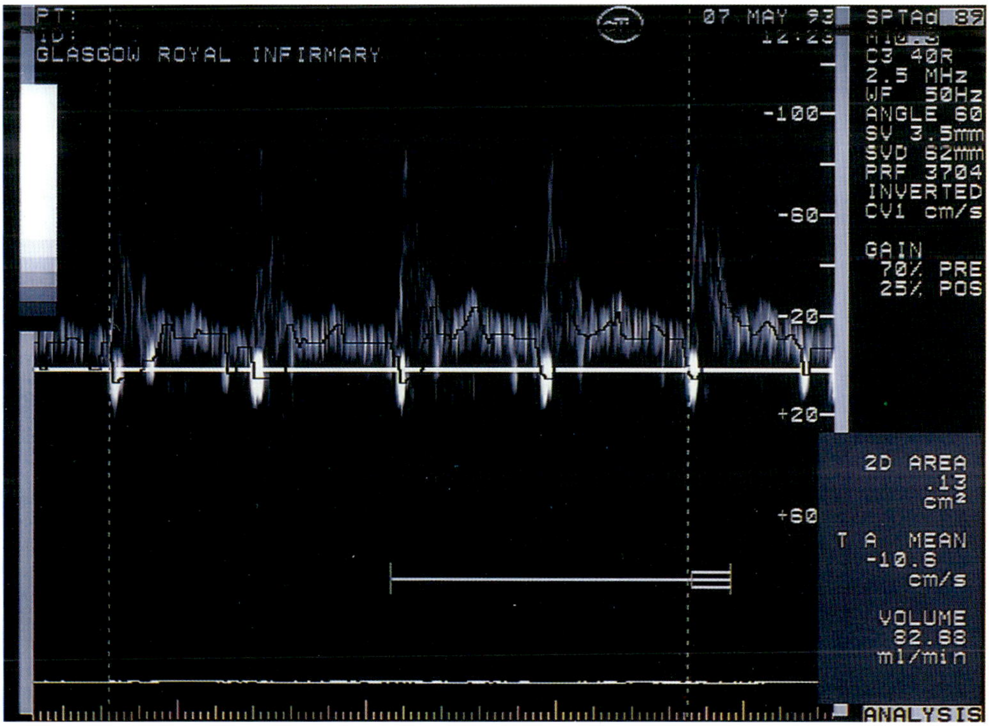

Plate 2 Measurement of time-averaged velocity (TAV) of the hepatic arterial flow from the velocity waveform, over four cardiac cycles.

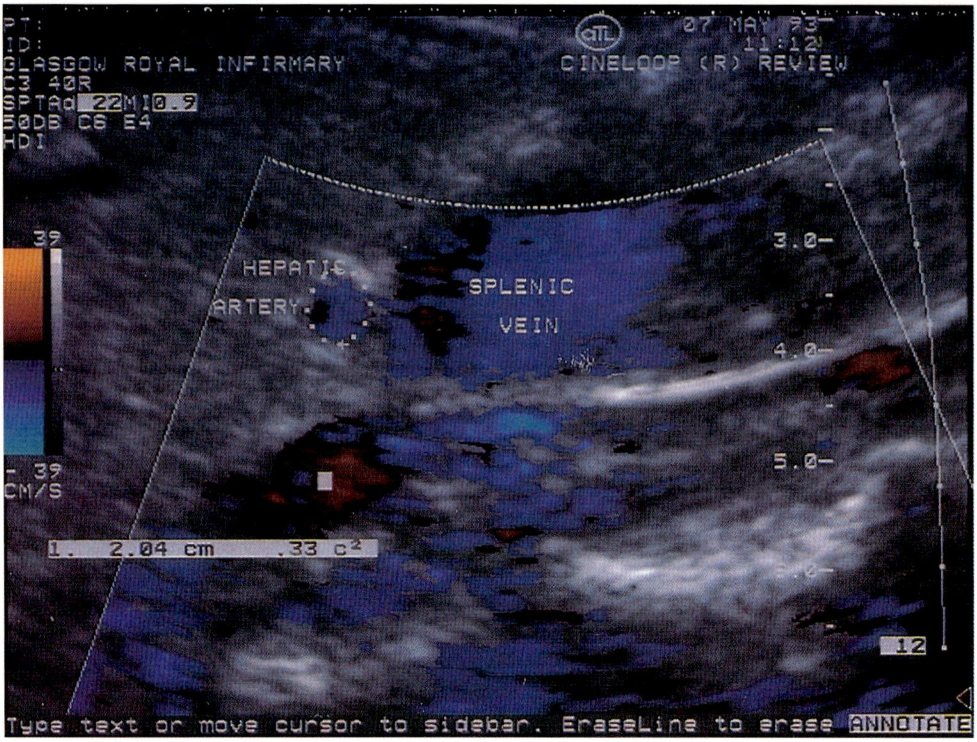

Plate 3 Measurement of the cross-sectional area of the hepatic artery.

(a)

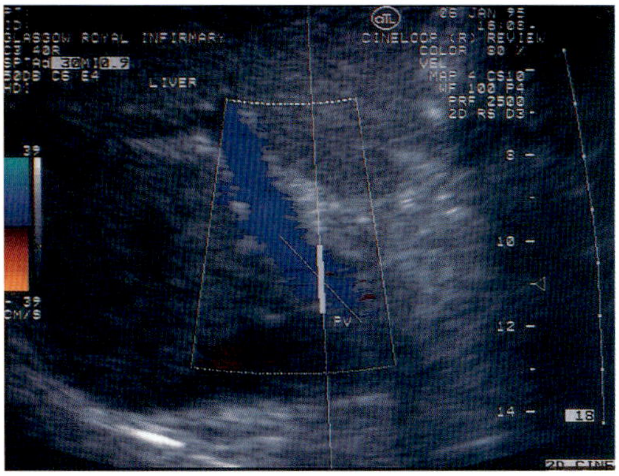

Plate 4 (a) Longitudinal section of the portal vein with the Doppler cursor overlying the lumen.
(b) Measurement of the cross-sectional area of the portal vein.

(b)

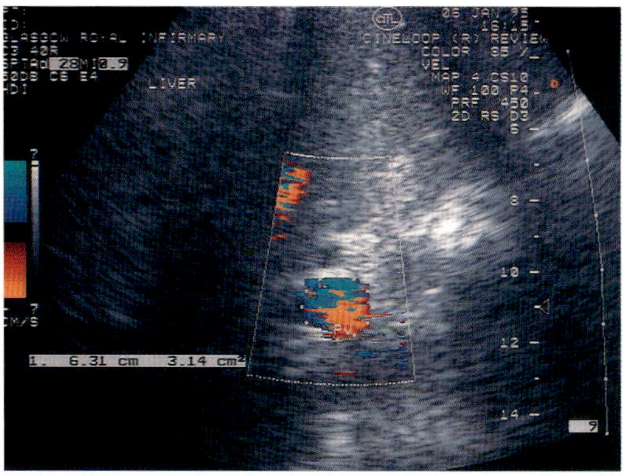

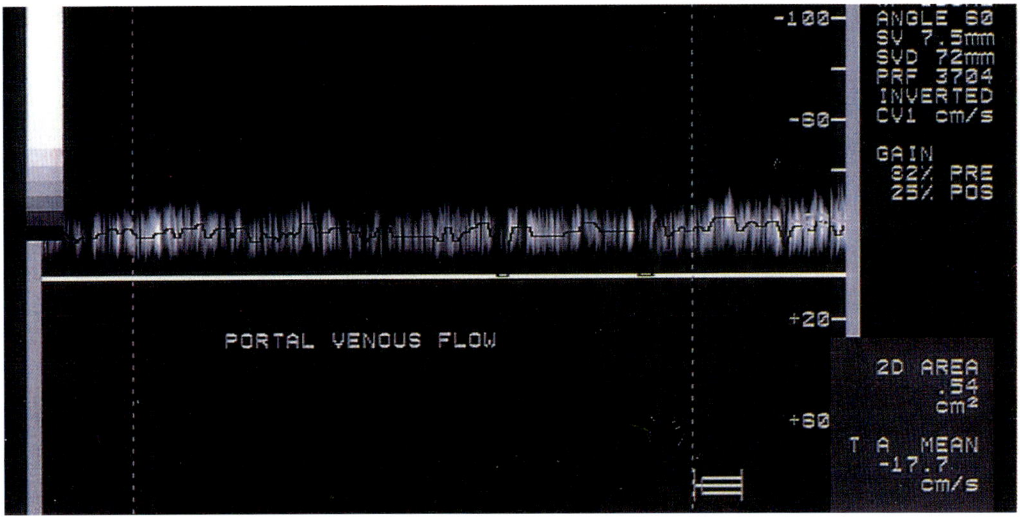

Plate 5 Measurement of time-averaged velocity (TAV) of portal venous flow.

Plate 6 (a) Biodegradable human albumin microspheres (15-40 μm diameter) on screening electron microscopy. (b) Adriamycin-loaded albumin microspheres (15-50 μm) on dark ground illumination. (c) Mitomycin-C ethylcellulose microcapsules (200 μm diameter). (d) Glass yttrium-90 microspheres (40 μm diameter).

(a) (b)

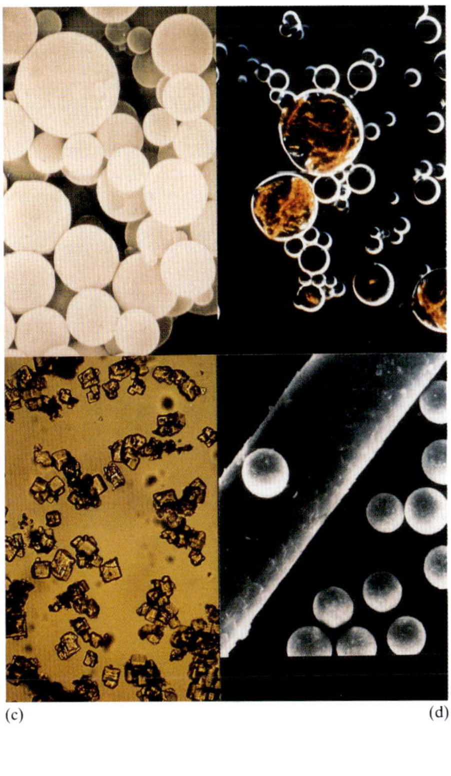

(c) (d)

Plate 7 (a) Adriamycin-loaded albumin microspheres trapped in pulmonary capillary bed following intravenous injection in rat. (b) Biodegradation of the microsphere occurring after 48 hours. (c) The presence of microspheres within tumour in animal tumour model. (d) Fluorescent micrograph showing leakage of Adriamycin from microsphere into surrounding tissue. (McArdle *et al.*, 1988)

(a) (b)

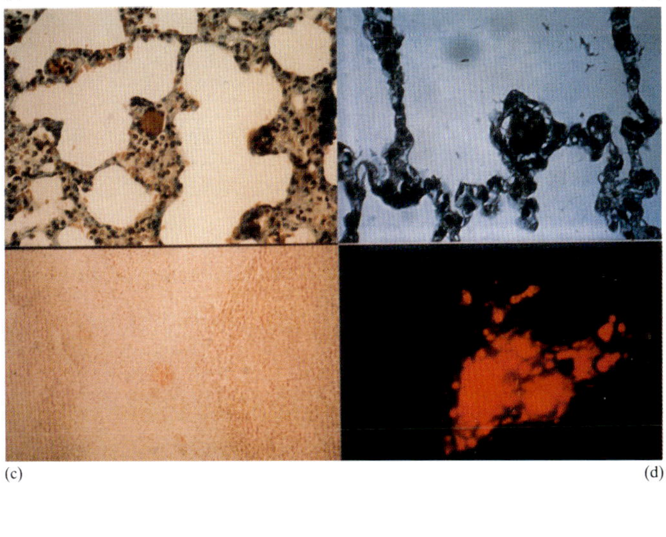

(c) (d)

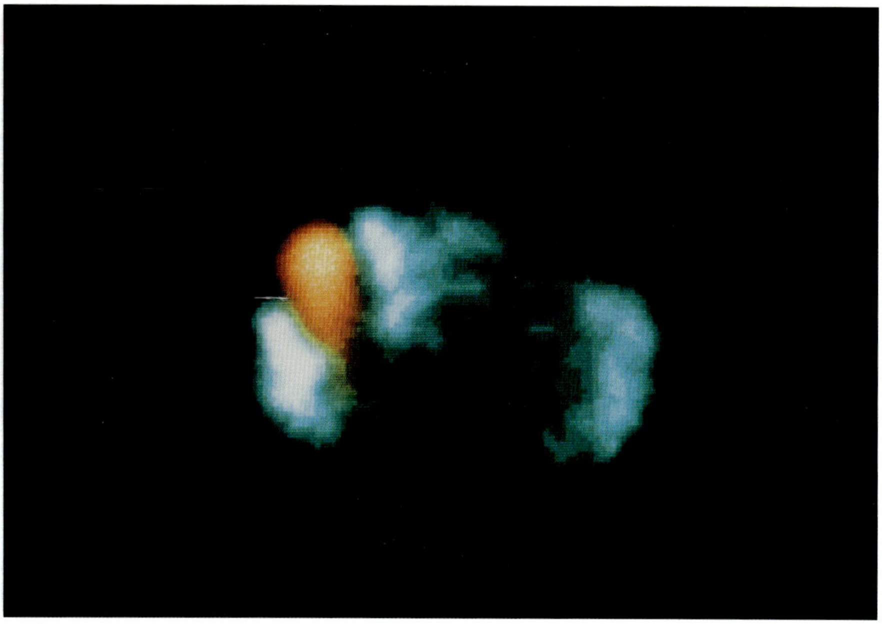

Plate 8 Microspheres trapped in tumour bed (orange). Normal liver and spleen are shown in green (Goldberg *et al.*, 1991b)

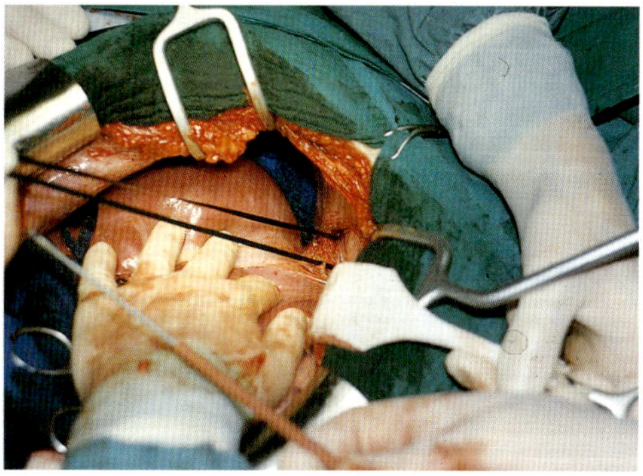

Plate 9 Exposure of vena cava intrapericardially

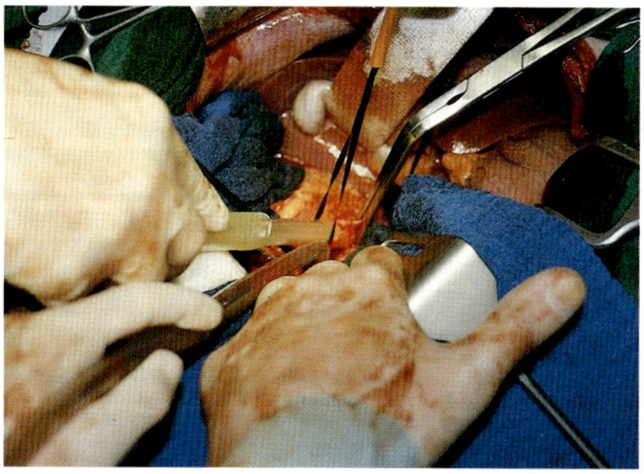

Plate 10 Cannulation of vena cava infrarenally with the double-lumen catheter

ation of the survival data was complicated by the fact that 60% of the patients in the systemic treatment group received intra-arterial therapy after failing to respond to systemic therapy. The patients who crossed over had a median survival of 18 months compared to 8 months for those who received only systemic therapy. In the most recent study reported (Rougier *et al.*, 1992), the response rate in 81 patients receiving intra-arterial therapy was 43% compared to 9% in the 82 patients receiving systemic therapy ($P<0.001$); 1-year survival was also higher in the regional therapy group (64 versus 44%; $P<0.02$). However, this study could be criticized on the basis that half the patients allocated to the systemic limb did not receive chemotherapy and the remaining patients received a regimen generally regarded as inadequate.

2. The coadministration of biodegradable microemboli to 'dam back' hepatic blood flow and hence improve drug uptake. The use of biodegradable starch microspheres has been extensively investigated in this context. However, a prospective randomized controlled trial to evaluate the use of biodegradable starch microspheres failed to show a significant overall survival benefit in patients receiving chemotherapy with 5-FU and biodegradable starch microspheres, although those with low-volume disease did appear to fare better (Hunt *et al.*, 1990).
3. The use of biodegradable or non-biodegradable drug-loaded or radioactive microspheres that are trapped in the microcirculation of the tumour and therefore release the cytotoxic agent locally. These microspheres may be coadministered with vasoactive agents, for example angiotensin II, to improve targeting further.

Over the last 5 years we have developed or tested a variety of biodegradable and non-biodegradable, blank, cytotoxic-loaded or radioactive microspheres (Plate 6). For example, Adriamycin-loaded albumin microspheres (15–40 μm in diameter) incorporating 1% by weight of Adriamycin were prepared by cross-linking albumin with glutaraldehyde (McArdle *et al.*, 1988). After systemic administration in rats the microspheres were trapped in the pulmonary capillary bed (Plate 7). The albumin matrix then degraded, releasing the Adriamycin locally. Following selective injection via the hepatic artery approximately 95% of injected microspheres were trapped in the liver; less than 1% were found in blood (Table 8.3). Parallel pharmacokinetic studies (Kerr *et al.*, 1988) showed that when equivalent doses of cytotoxic drug were administered as free solution or in the form of cytotoxic-loaded microspheres, serum levels after microsphere injection were significantly lower than following the administration of free drug (Fig. 8.2). In this manner, high drug levels can be achieved within the target organ with minimal systemic exposure. Subsequent studies in a rat liver tumour model (Goldberg *et al.*, 1992) showed that cytotoxic-loaded microspheres had a significantly greater inhibitory effect on tumour

Table 8.3 Distribution of radiolabelled microspheres after selective intrahepatic arterial injection (%)

Liver	Kidney	Lung	Blood (per litre)
93±5	1.2±0.4	5.2±4.9	0.3±0.2

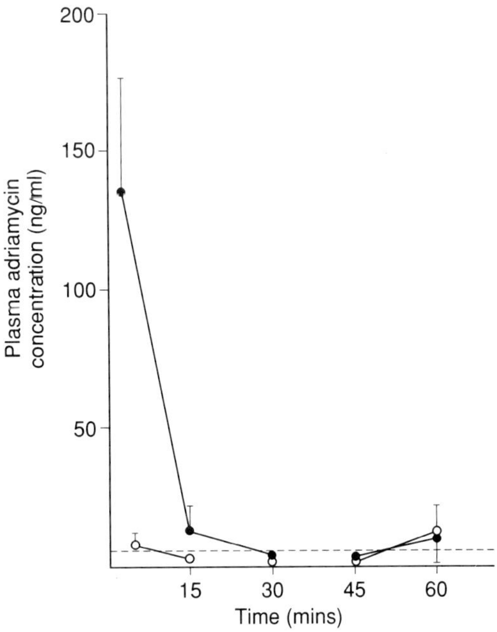

Figure 8.2 Plasma concentrations following administration of the same dose of Adriamycin either as free drug or as Adriamycin-loaded albumin microspheres. The dashed line represents the lower level of detection. (Kerr *et al.*, 1988)

Table 8.4 Mean weight of tumour following treatment

Group	*n*	Mean tumour weight (g)	s.d.
Intra-arterial Adriamycin in solution	6	0.74*	0.12
Intra-arterial Adriamycin-loaded albumin microspheres	6	0.45*	0.08

*$p<0.05$

growth compared to free cytotoxic drug administered regionally or systemically (Table 8.4).

Furthermore, it is well-established that tumours are supplied by relatively immature blood vessels that are deficient in smooth muscle and have an attenuated response to vasoactive agents such as noradrenaline and angiotensin II (Sasaki *et al.*, 1985). This property provides a potential method of diverting organ blood flows to the tumour, thereby increasing the delivery of cytotoxic agents to the tumour (Fig. 8.3).

Using a double-isotope technique at the time of surgery, we measured the distribution of radiolabelled microspheres in tumour and normal liver tissue before and after angiotensin II infusion (Goldberg *et al.*, 1991a). The median increase in tumour : normal ratio following angiotensin II was almost threefold. These results were subsequently confirmed in the conscious patient using scintigraphic planar and tomographic imaging (Plate 8; Fig. 6 Goldberg *et al.*, 1991b).

The temporal changes in hepatic arterial blood flow have also been assessed using duplex colour Doppler sonography (Leen *et al.*, 1993a, 1993b). In patients with less than 30% hepatic replacement, hepatic arterial flow falls by 75–80% within 30 s of commencing an angiotensin II infusion. After cessation of the infusion, there was a rebound phenomenon, flow increasing by up to 20% above normal (Fig. 8.4). In patients with more extensive hepatic replacement, hepatic arterial blood flow showed no reduction but rose continuously from the start of the infusion. These observations are clearly relevant to the optimal timing of microsphere administration.

By administering the cytotoxic-loaded or radioactive microspheres during an angiotensin

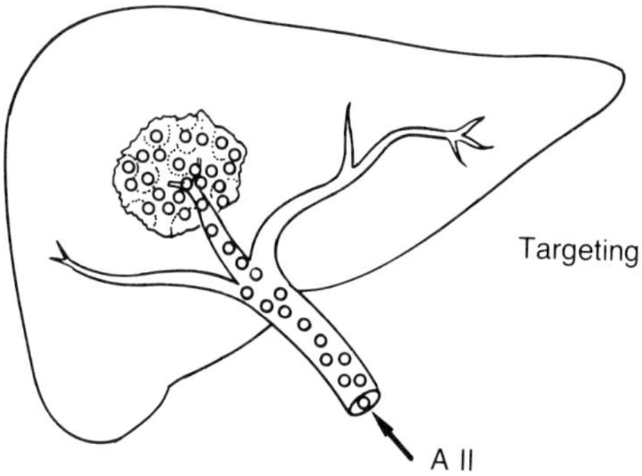

Figure 8.3 Effect of angiotensin II (AII). Microspheres injected during an angiotensin II infusion are directed preferentially towards tumour.

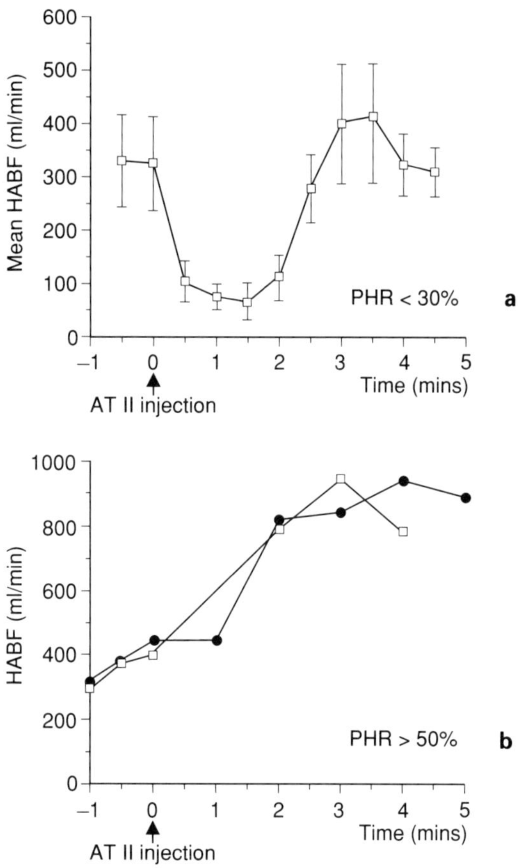

Figure 8.4 The effects of intra-arterial angiotensin II (AT II) infusion on hepatic arterial blood flow in patients (a) with less than 3% hepatic replacement and (b) with greater than 50% hepatic replacement. HABF = Hepatic arterial blood flow; PHR = Percentage hepatic replacement. (Leen *et al.*, 1993b)

II infusion, it was therefore anticipated that a significant proportion of the administered dose would be directed selectively towards the tumour, where the microspheres would lodge in the tumour circulation and produce high levels of cytotoxic agent locally.

In our initial clinical study we used biodegradable albumin microspheres (diameter 40 μm) to reduce local blood flow and hence increase drug uptake (Goldberg *et al.*, 1990). Responses were seen in one-third of patients. Median survival was 9 months. Half the deaths were from progressive liver metastases but one-quarter died of extrahepatic disease and a further quarter from non-cancer-related causes, suggesting that we had altered the natural history of the disease.

We subsequently produced ethylcellulose microencapsulated Mitomycin C (200 μm diameter), as described by Kato and his colleagues (1981). Patients received up to 40 mg Mitomycin C intra-arterially at the time of laparotomy without evidence of systemic toxicity (Anderson *et al.*, 1991a). The value of these Mitomycin C/ethylcellulose microcapsules was limited by the non-biodegradable nature of the polymer coating and the large particle size, which precluded easy administration via an indwelling catheter. We therefore looked for other alternatives.

Studies of radioactive resin microspheres were undertaken in the early 1970s. Unfortunately, the radioactive isotope leached from these microspheres, causing pancytopenia in some patients. Since then a number of potential carriers have been investigated, including ceramics and glass.

We assessed the use of glass yttrium-90 microspheres (40–50 μm) coadministered with angiotensin II (Anderson *et al.*, 1992a). Yttrium-90 is a β-emitter with a half-life of approximately 64 h. Up to 150 Gy was delivered to the liver without local or systemic toxicity. Six of the 7 patients developed extrahepatic disease, mainly lung metastases. Median survival was 11 months.

In each of the above studies, designed to deliver high doses of cytotoxic drug or radiotherapy to the liver, some patients appeared to benefit from a reduction in the rate of growth of their liver metastases (Fig. 8.5). Median survival appeared to be prolonged compared to historical controls. It is not clear, however, to what extent this simply represents an element of selection. A feature common to each of the studies was that the majority of patients, in whom stable hepatic disease or regression was obtained, developed extrahepatic progression, predominantly lung metastases.

Survival was clearly limited by the development of extrahepatic disseminated disease and it would therefore seem reasonable that future therapy should be designed not only to achieve high therapeutic levels within the liver but also in the systemic circulation.

This might be achieved in two ways:

1. By combining regional and systemic therapy.
2. By allowing high-dose regional chemotherapy to spill over into lung and generate systemic drug levels which would be effective against microsopic pulmonary disease (Fig. 8.6).

Recent studies suggest that the addition of folinic acid significantly improves response rate and may increase survival in advanced colorectal cancer patients receiving systemic 5-FU (Machover *et al.*, 1986; Petrelli *et al.*, 1987; Erlichman, 1988; Poon *et al.*, 1989; Advanced Colorectal Cancer Meta-Analysis Project, 1992). In essence, 5-FU is metabolized to fluorodeoxyuridylate (FdUMP), which binds to and inhibits the enzyme thymidylate synthetase. The addition of folinic acid enhances 5-FU activity by stabilizing the binding of the FdUMP to thymidylate synthetase, thus increasing the degree of enzyme inhibition and promoting further thymidine depletion. While the use of 5-FU/folinic acid combinations may represent an important therapeutic advance, a significant proportion of patients experience severe systemic toxic side-effects. The use of a regional approach might circumvent these problems and at the same time enhance response rates to 5-FU administered via the hepatic artery.

We therefore compared the pharmacokinetic profiles of folinic acid when administered regionally and systemically in patients receiving regional 5-FU (Anderson *et al.*, 1991b). A small but statistically significant therapeutic advantage was demonstrated for the regional route of administration (Fig. 8.7). However, 3 of 6 patients receiving regional folinic acid developed hepatic artery catheter occlusion, suggesting that the possible risk to catheter patency outweighed the pharmacokinetic advantage. We therefore reverted to the use of

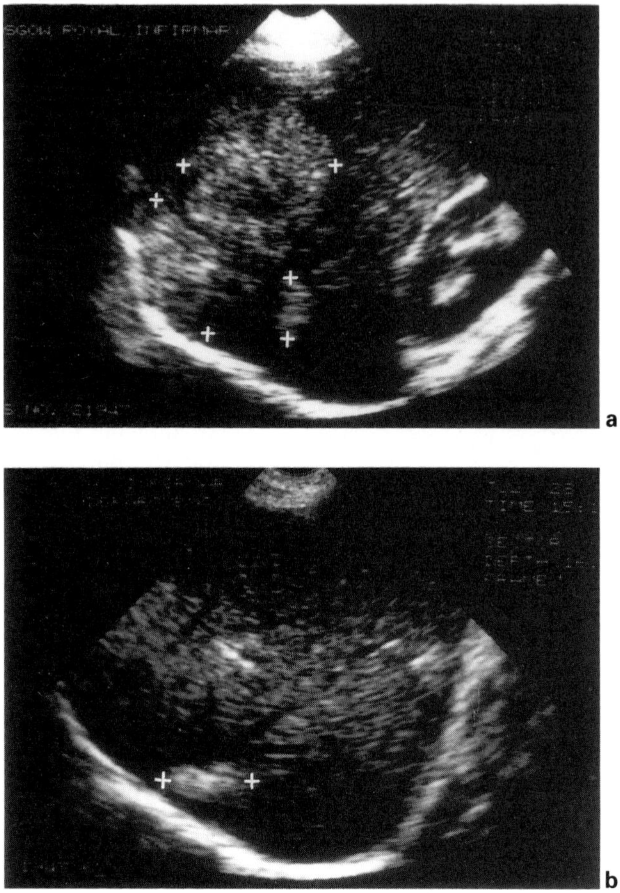

Figure 8.5 Ultrasound showing (a) extensive liver replacement by tumour prior to regional chemotherapy and (b) substantial tumour reduction 18 months later. (Reproduced with permission from the *European Journal of Surgical Oncology*)

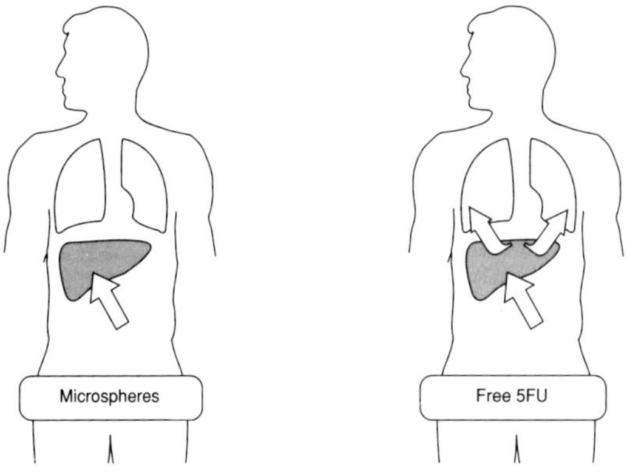

Figure 8.6 Concept of regional therapy with systemic overspill. 5FU = 5-Fluorouracil.

the intravenous route for the administration of folinic acid.

In a phase I study (Anderson *et al.*, 1992b) patients received weekly 24-h infusions of 5-FU, while folinic acid was administered intravenously at a fixed total dose of 400 mg/m^2 per week over the first, second, 23rd and 24th hours of the 5-FU infusion (Fig. 8.8). *In vitro* studies have suggested that a minimum extracellular L-folate concentration of 10 μmol/l is required to maximize 5-FU-induced thymidylate synthetase inhibition. A 2-h intravenous infusion of 200 mg/m^2 would be expected to achieve this level. We therefore elected to deliver a loading dose of folinic acid during the initial 2 h of the 5-FU infusion with a further dose during the final 2 h of the infusion when peak intracellular

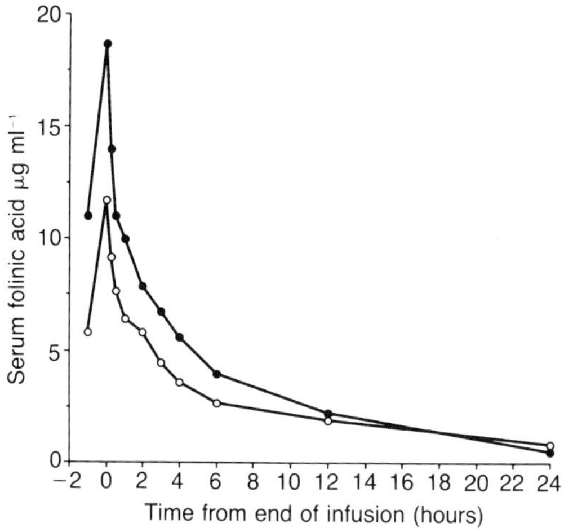

Figure 8.7 Plasma levels of folinic acid (100 mg/ m^2) following intrahepatic arterial and intravenous administration over 2 h. (Anderson *et al.*, 1991b.)

0.6–2.0g 5FU / m^2 / week

IA 0 ———————————————— 24

IV 0 —— 2 400mg FA / m^2 / week 22 —— 24

Figure 8.8 Design of phase I study. IA = Intra-arterial; IV = intravenous; 5FU = 5-fluorouracil; FA folinic acid.

5-FU levels would be present. We chose to use a 24-h infusion of 5-FU, because previous studies had shown a significant advantage over bolus (Goldberg *et al.*, 1990). The initial dose of 5-FU was 0.6 g/m^2 per week, the dose at which Petrelli *et al.* (1987) reported a 27% incidence of life-threatening toxicity. The dose of 5-FU was subsequently escalated to 2.0 g/m^2 per week.

Only 1 of 7 patients who received 1.5 g/m^2 per week experienced moderate side-effects. In contrast, 4 of 8 patients treated at 2.0 g/m^2 per week required hospital admission for treatment-related side-effects, the predominant symptoms being vomiting and diarrhoea (Fig. 8.9). Weekly full blood count and liver function tests showed no evidence of myelosuppression or hepatotoxicity in any patient.

Based on these data, a phase II study using this regimen was established. Patients with histologically proven metastases confined to the liver and an indwelling hepatic arterial catheter received a weekly 24-h infusion of 5-FU (1.5 g/

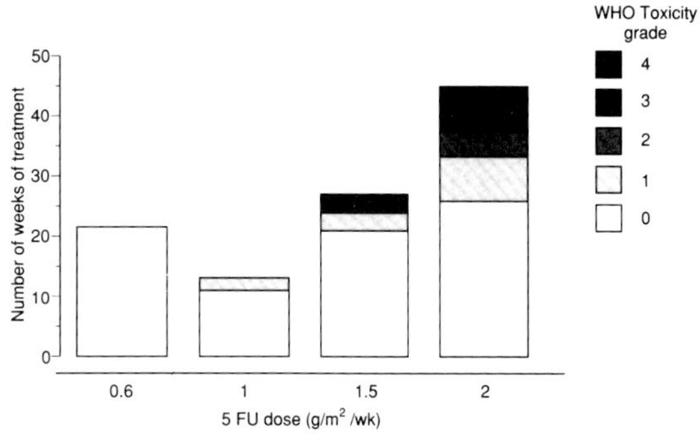

Figure 8.9 Toxicity. WHO = World Health Organization; 5FU = 5-fluorouracil.

1.5g 5FU / m^2 / week

IA 0 ———————————————— 24

IV 0 —— 2 400mg FA / m^2 / week 22 —— 24

Figure 8.10 Design of phase II study. IA = Intra-arterial; IV = intravenous; 5FU = 5-fluorouracil; FA = folinic acid.

m^2 per week) through the hepatic artery catheter, while folinic acid (400 mg/m^2 per week) was administered intravenously during the first, second, 23rd and 24th hours of 5-FU infusion (Fig. 8.10). Treatment pulses were given weekly for 6 weeks followed by a 2-week respite prior to the next cycle.

Thirty patients have been included in the study, of whom 27 are evaluable. The physical characteristics are shown in Table 8.5. The mean age was 58 years; most patients had less than 25% of liver replaced by tumour. Six

Table 8.5 Physical characteristics of patients (n = 30)

Mean age	
years	58
range	36–77
M : F	21:9
Hepatic replacement (%)	
25	21
25–50	6
>50	1
Pretreatment	
5-FU	1
5-FU/FA	3
M/S	2

5-FU = 5-Fluorouracil; FA = folinic acid; M/S = cytotoxic-loaded microspheres.

Table 8.6 Response rates

CR	1
PR	11
MR	2
SD	10
PD	3

CR = complete response; PR = partial response; MR = minimal response; SD = stable disease; PD = progressive disease.

Table 8.7 Toxicity (66 cycles)

	WHO grade	No. of patients
Nausea	I	5
	II	1
Vomiting	II	5
	III	2
Diarrhoea	I	3
	II	2
	III	1
Stomatitis	I	1
Hepatitis	I	1

WHO = World Health Organization.

Table 8.8 Recurrence (n = 17)

Locoregional	4
Intra-abdominal	3
Lung	8
Bone	4
Liver	6
Soft tissue	2

Table 8.9 Deaths (n = 12)

Locoregional	2
Intra-abdominal	2
Lung	3
Bone	1
Liver	3
Intercurrent disease	3

patients had been pretreated with systemic 5-FU, systemic 5-FU and folinic acid or cytotoxic-loaded microspheres.

The median follow-up is 16 months. At the initial assessment (2 months) 14 of the 27 patients had responded and 10 had stable disease (Table 8.6). Toxicity was mild. Two

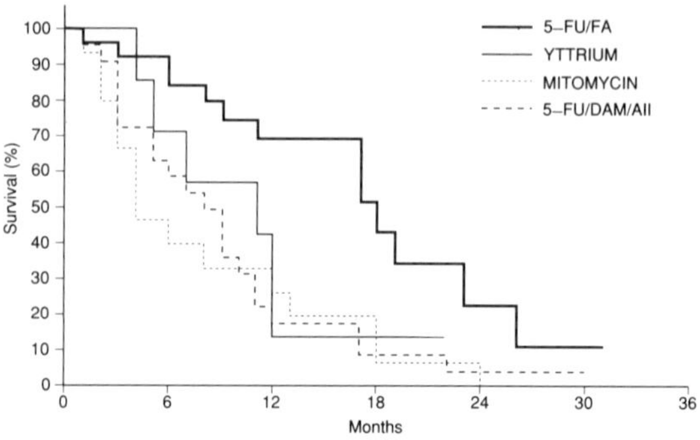

Figure 8.11 Predicted survival of patients receiving regional 5-fluorouracil (5-FU)/systemic folinic acid (FA) compared with outcome in patients receiving microsphere-based therapy. DAM = degradable albumin microspheres; AII = angiotensin II.

patients had grade III vomiting or diarrhoea (Table 8.7); this was readily controlled by antiemetics and/or dose modification.

Seventeen patients have recurred (Table 8.8), the median time to progression being 7 months. The majority of patients developed extrahepatic disease, particularly lung metastases. Twelve patients have died (Table 8.9); the majority of these had developed extrahepatic disease and in only 3 was liver progression the main cause of death. Three patients died of non-cancer-associated conditions.

Median survival was 18 months (Fig. 8.11). This appears to be significantly prolonged compared with historical controls and previous studies undertaken in this unit using microsphere-based therapy.

Clearly these results are of interest. They suggest that a combination of regionally administered 5-FU plus systemic folinic acid may offer a significant advance in the management of patients with colorectal liver metastases.

A phase III study comparing the above regimen with conventional systemic therapy is now planned.

References

Advanced Colorectal Cancer Meta-Analysis Project (1992) Modulation of fluorouracil by leucovorin in patients with advanced colorectal cancer: evidence in terms of response rate. *J. Clin. Oncol.* **10**, 896–903.

Anderson JH, Goldberg JA, Eley JG *et al.* (1991a) A phase I study of regionally administered mitomycin microcapsules for patients with colorectal liver metastases. *Eur. J. Cancer* **27**, 1189–1190.

Anderson JH, Kerr DJ, Setanoians A, Cooke TG & McArdle CS (1991b) A pharmacokinetic comparison of intravenous versus intra-arterial folinic acid. *Br. J. Cancer* **65**, 133–135.

Anderson JH, Goldberg JA, Bessent RG *et al.* (1992a) Glass yttrium-90 microspheres for patients with colorectal liver metastases. *Radiother. Oncol.* **25**, 137–139.

Anderson JH, Kerr DJ, Coke TG & McArdle CS (1992b) A phase I study of regional 5-fluorouracil and systemic folinic acid for patients with colorectal liver metastases. *Br. J. Cancer* **65**, 913–915.

Balch CM, Urist MM & McGregor ML (1983) Continuous regional chemotherapy for metastic colorectal cancer using a totally implantable infusion pump. *Am. J. Surg.* **14**, 285–290.

Chang AE, Schneider PD & Sugarbaker PH (1987) A prospective randomized trial of regional versus systemic continuous 5-fluorodeoxyuridine chemotherapy in the treatment of colorectal liver metastases. *Ann. Surg.* **206**, 685–693.

Cohen AM, Kaufman SD & Wood WC (1985) Treatment of colorectal cancer hepatic metastases by hepatic artery chemotherapy. *Dis. Colon Rectum* **28**, 389–393.

Erlichman F (1988) 5-Fluorouracil (fUra) and folinic acid (FA) therapy in patients with colorectal cancer. *Adv. Exp. Med. Biol.* **244**, 185–192.

Frei E III & Canellos GP (1980) Dose: a critical factor in cancer chemotherapy. *Am. J. Med.* **69**, 585–594.

Goldberg JA, Kerr DJ, Willmott N, McKillop JH & McArdle CS (1988) Pharmacokinetics and pharmacodynamics of locoregional 5-fluorouracil (5FU) in advanced colorectal liver metastases. *Br. J. Cancer* **57**, 186–189.

Goldberg JA, Kerr DJ, Watson DG *et al.* (1990a) The pharmacokinetics of 5-fluorouracil administered by arterial infusion in advanced colorectal hepatic metastases. *Br. J. Cancer* **61**, 913–915.

Goldberg JA, Kerr DJ, Willmott N, McKillop JH & McArdle CS (1990b) Regional chemotherapy for colorectal liver metastases: a phase II evaluation of targeted hepatic arterial 5-fluorouracil for colorectal liver metastases. *Br. J. Surg.* **77**, 1238–1240.

Goldberg JA, Murray T, Kerr DJ *et al.* (1991a) The use of angiotensin II as a potential method of targeting cytotoxic microspheres in patients with intrahepatic tumour. *Br. J. Cancer* **63**, 308–310.

Goldberg JA, Thomson JAK, Bradnam MS *et al.* (1991b) Angiotensin II as a potential method of targeting cytotoxic-loaded microspheres in patients with colorectal liver metastases. *Br. J. Cancer* **64**, 114–119.

Goldberg JA, Willmott N, Kerr DJ, Sutherland C & McArdle CS (1992) An *in vivo* assessment of Adriamycin-loaded albumin microspheres. *Br. J. Cancer* **65**, 393–395.

Hohn D, Stagg R, Friedman M *et al.* (1987) The NCOG randomized trial of intravenous (IV) vs hepatic arterial (IA) FUDR for colorectal cancer metastatic to the liver. *Proc. Am. Soc. Oncol.* **6**, 85.

Hunt TM, Flowerdew ADS, Birch SJ, Williams JD, Mullee MA & Taylor I (1990) Prospective randomised controlled trial of hepatic arterial embolization or infusion chemotherapy with 5-fluorouracil and degradable starch microspheres for colorectal liver metastases. *Br. J. Surg.* **77**, 779–782.

Kato T, Nemoto R, Mori H, Takahashi M & Harada M (1981) Arterial chemoembolisation with mitomycin C microcapsules in the treatment of primary or secondary carcinoma of the kidney, liver, bone and intrapelvic organs. *Cancer* **48**, 674–680.

Kemeny N (1992) Review of regional therapy of liver metastases in colorectal cancer. *Semin. Oncol.* **19**, 155–162.

Kemeny N, Daly J, Reichman B *et al.* (1987) Intrahepatic or systemic infusion of fluorodeoxyuridine in patients with liver metastases from colorectal carcinoma. *Ann. Intern. Med.* **107**, 459–465.

Kerr DJ, Willmott N, Lewi H & McArdle CS (1988) The pharmacokinetics and distribution of Adriamycin-loaded albumin microspheres following intra-arterial administration. *Cancer* **62**, 878–882.

Leen E, Angerson WJ, Warren H *et al.* (1993a) Hepatic arterial haemodynamics changes following intra-arterial angiotensin II infusion: duplex/colour Doppler sonography. *Clin. Radiol.* **47**, 321–324.

Leen E, Angerson WJ, Warren H *et al.* (1993b) Duplex/colour Doppler sonography: measurement of changes in hepatic arterial haemodynamics following intra-arterial angiotensin II infusion. *Br. J. Cancer* **67**, 1381–1384.

McArdle CS, Lewi H, Hansell D, Kerr DJ, McKillop J & Willmott N (1988) Cytotoxic-loaded albumin microspheres: a novel approach to regional chemotherapy. *Br. J. Cancer* **75**, 132–134.

Machover D, Goldschmidt E, Chollet P *et al.* (1986) Treatment of advanced colorectal and gastric adenocarcinomas with 5-fluorouracil and high dose folinic acid. *J. Clin. Oncol.* **4**, 685–696.

Martin JK Jr, O'Connell MJ, Wieand HS *et al.* (1990) Intra-arterial floxuridine vs systemic fluorouracil for hepatic metastases from colorectal cancer. A randomized trial. *Arch. Surg.* **125**, 1022.

Niederhuber J, Ensminger W, Gyves J, Thrall J, Walker S & Cozzi E (1984) Regional chemotherapy of colorectal cancer metastatic to the liver. *Cancer* **53**, 1336–1343.

Petrelli N, Herrera L, Rustum Y *et al.* (1987) A prospective randomised trial of 5-fluorouracil vs 5-fluorouracil and high dose leucovorin + 5-fluorouracil and methotrexate in previously untreated patients with advanced colorectal carcinoma. *J. Clin. Oncol.* **5**, 1559–1565.

Poon MA, O'Connell MJ, Moertel CG *et al.* (1989) Biochemical modulation of fluorouracil: evidence of significant improvement of survival and quality of life in patients with advanced colorectal carcinoma. *J. Clin. Oncol.* **7**, 1407–1417.

Ridge JA, Bading JR, Gelbard AS, Benua RS & Daly JM (1987) Perfusion of colorectal hepatic metastases. Relevant distribution of flow from the hepatic artery and portal vein. *Cancer* **59**, 1547–1553.

Rougier P, Laplanche A, Huguier M *et al.* (1992) Hepatic

arterial infusion of floxuridine in patients with liver metastases from colorectal carcinoma: long-term results of a prospective randomized trial. *J. Clin. Oncol.* **10**, 1112–1118.

Sasaki Y, Shingi I, Yoshihisa H *et al.* (1985) Changes in distribution of hepatic blood flow induced by intra-arterial infusion of angiotensin II in human hepatic cancer. *Cancer* **55**, 311–316.

Widder KJ, Senyei AE & Ranney DF (1979) Magnetically responsive microspheres and other carriers for the physical targeting of antitumour agents. *Adv. Pharmacol. Chemother.* **16**, 213–271.

Editors' note

Subsequent to the submission of this chapter, another prospective controlled trial of hepatic artery chemotherapy has reported a significant (P=0.03) prolongation in survival in patients with colorectal liver metastases (median 405 vs. 226 days) (Allen/Mersh *et al.*, 1994). Importantly, this study also measured quality of life and showed that this was maintained in treated patients.

Reference

Allen/Mersh TG, Earlen S, Efordy C, Abrams K, Houghton J (1994) Quality of life and survival with continuous hepatic artery floxuridine infusion for colorectal liver metastases. *Lancet*. **344**, 1255/60.

9

Aspects of portal vein chemotherapy in the management of colorectal liver metastases

I. Taylor

The development of colorectal liver metastases remains a major problem in management. In most series 15–20% of patients with primary colorectal cancer have multiple liver metastases at the time of initial surgery, although this figure could be much higher depending upon the techniques used to determine diagnostic accuracy. In addition to this, as many as 50% of patients will eventually develop liver metastases, often in the absence of recurrence elsewhere (Cedermark *et al.*, 1977).

Much is now known about the mechanisms for the development of liver metastases but simplistically it is thought that tumour cells invade the mesenteric venous radicles and enter the liver as tumour emboli via the portal veins. While the majority of these cells will be destroyed, some undoubtedly survive and may subsequently develop into micrometastases. These then enter a period of dormancy, although some 'awaken' and develop into macroscopic metastases. This chapter will deal with mechanisms by which knowledge of portal venous dissemination might be used in the possible prevention of liver metastases as well as for aspects of treatment of established metastases.

Circulating tumour cells

In order for malignant cells to disseminate they must gain access to the circulation and for this to occur the tumour must grow and develop a functional microcirculation from the surrounding host tissues. There is now extensive evidence to suggest that intravasation is most likely to occur at the tumour periphery where new vessel formation is pronounced and the vessels susceptible to penetration. The mechanisms for penetration are complex and depend upon a balance between angiogenic polypeptides, angiogenesis inhibitors, proteolytic enzymes and the matrix proteins of the tumour stroma rather than a single angiogenesis factor. This multiplicity of requirements undoubtedly explains the heterogeneity observed in the vascular composition of individual tumours which in turn would undoubtedly influence their metastatic potential.

If it is assumed that hepatic metastases from colorectal cancer arise as a result of embolization of tumour cells into the portal circulation, then clearly the tumour must invade tributaries of this system. Many studies have dealt with the question of venous invasion in colorectal cancer. However, the incidence reported depends very much upon histological techniques and different definitions of blood vessel invasion (Table 9.1). There is, however, general agreement that the incidence of blood vessel invasion increases as tumour differentiation deteriorates and the depth of infiltration of the bowel wall increases (Minsky & Mies, 1989). In addition, Shirouzu *et al.* (1991) have demonstrated that, as the frequency of venous invasion increases, so too does the incidence of metachronous liver metastases.

Table 9.1 Incidence of venous invasion

Authors	Study	Incidence
Brown and Warren (1938)	Postmortem	38%
Dukes and Bussey (1958)	Operative specimens (1800)	11%
Talbot *et al.* (1980)	Operative specimens (703)	52%
Chapuis *et al.* (1985)	Operative specimens (709)	19%

In addition, survival in Dukes stage B and C carcinoma is related to the degree of venous invasion. So much so, that survival of patients with Dukes B tumours showing vascular invasion is less than that of Dukes C tumours without vascular invasion (Krasna *et al.*, 1988). There is, however, inconsistency in relating vascular invasion to the incidence of circulating tumour cells and the subsequent development of hepatic metastases. Some studies have demonstrated that patients with infiltration of extramural veins do not inevitably develop hepatic metastases (Shirouzu *et al.*, 1991). It is possible, however, that patients recorded as having no overt evidence of liver metastases actually harbour microscopic foci of tumour (Finlay & McArdle, 1986). These will subsequently develop into liver metastases and are undoubtedly associated with a poorer prognosis. However, the metastatic process is relatively inefficient and other variables enter into the equation. These include:

1. Operative manipulation (Fisher & Turnbull, 1955). As a result, a no-touch technique was introduced. A recent randomized trial by Wiggers *et al.* (1988) has shown that application of this technique results in a reduction in the number of metastases, although not necessarily an improvement in survival.
2. Site selectivity (Murphy *et al.*, 1988). This takes account of 'trapping' in the organ of first encounter and local factors determining the growth of malignant cells.

Dormant liver metastases

There is clinical and experimental evidence to suggest that not all micrometastases within the liver eventually develop into overt clinical metastases. Malignant cells entering the liver may remain dormant for a period of time. However, it is known that various stimuli can disrupt this mechanism and malignant cells will subsequently grow. A recent study in an animal model has shown that undetectable liver metastases can be stimulated both by cyclosporin A and by posthepatectomy liver regeneration (Panis *et al.*, 1992). Finlay and McArdle (1986) have provided evidence in patients that the presence of occult metastases results in a much worse prognosis.

Portal blood supply of colorectal liver metastases

It is generally accepted that the majority of the blood supply to established liver metastases is derived from the hepatic artery. The original evidence for this was based on postmortem studies (Breedis & Young, 1954). Recently more sophisticated methods have been used to distinguish portal vein and hepatic arterial distribution. Using coloured silicone rubber injected into the portal vein and hepatic artery, Lin *et al.* (1984) showed that 71 out of 83 metastases had a blood supply from both vessels. Importantly, many arterioportal anastomoses were demonstrated and colorectal metastases are, in general, hypovascular, compared to normal liver tissue, whatever their blood supply.

Isotope imaging and particularly hepatic perfusion index (HPI) (discussed in Chapter 3) have emphasized the importance of the arterial blood supply to developing liver metastases. Other techniques have included xenon clearance where, interestingly, following hepatic artery ligation there appeared to be an increased portal vein perfusion into established liver metastases, suggesting a collateral circulation (Taylor *et al.*, 1979; Taylor, 1981).

There is therefore extensive evidence demonstrating the predominance of arterial blood supply to the growth of established liver metastases. However, the portal vein does play a part in the development of liver metastases, particularly in colorectal cancer. The malignant cells from the primary tumour invade the portal venous circulation and it is via this route that the malignant cells enter the liver. Dormancy undoubtedly occurs and not all metastases develop into overt tumours. The initial phase of tumour development depends upon a blood supply from the portal vein; however, eventually an arterial supply develops. This seems rather simplistic and it is likely that the tumour itself secretes vasoactive substances which determine arterial blood flow. Can this information be utilized in any way to prevent the development of colorectal liver metastases?

Portal vein infusion as prophylaxis

Accepting that there is a risk of tumour embolization in patients with colorectal cancer, it would seem logical to try and prevent its sequelae. The risk for this developing appears maximal both during and immediately following colorectal resectional surgery. Measures available for the prevention of liver metastases include:

1. Early ligation of the vascular pedicle.
2. Adjuvant chemotherapy.

Early ligation of the vascular pedicle

A purely mechanical approach to prevention of liver metastases consequent on manipulation of tumour at operation is the 'no-touch isolation' technique of Turnbull. He described a method of resecting colonic tumour which involved early ligation of lymphovascular pedicles, whilst the tumour-bearing area of the colon remained untouched until this time. In a series of 471 patients operated on for colon cancer, the age-corrected 5-year survival rate was 81.6%, almost doubling the expected survival rates (Turnbull, 1970). As previously mentioned, Wiggers *et al.* (1990) have investigated this technique in a prospective randomized trial. The incidence of liver metastases was reduced in those patients treated by the no-touch technique; overall survival was only minimally affected.

Adjuvant chemotherapy

There have now been numerous studies looking at the effect of systemic chemotherapy in colorectal cancer. Initial studies utilized systemic 5-fluorouracil (5-FU) alone, with little improvement in overall survival. However, more recent studies have combined 5-FU with additional agents and some encouraging data are beginning to emerge. This is particularly true for the combination of 5-FU with levamisole (Moertel *et al.*, 1990).

An additional adjuvant approach is to deliver the chemotherapy in the perioperative period via the portal venous system. Cruz *et al.* (1956) demonstrated in an animal model that the incidence of liver metastases could be reduced by giving nitrogen mustard directly to the portal vein after the injection of a cancer cell suspension. The importance of the route of administration and the timing of chemotherapy have been emphasized over a number of years. Sutanto-Ward *et al.* (1992) demonstrated this in an animal model. Immediate portal vein infusion of a chemotherapeutic agent was able to delay the appearance of hepatic tumour and changed the cause of death from hepatic to extrahepatic disease with associated prolonged survival. However, if the infusion was given into the portal vein 72 h later, it did not have any effect on delaying the appearance of hepatic tumour or on prolonging survival.

Clinical trials of portal vein infusion

In an attempt to reduce the incidence of metachronous colorectal liver metastases, and hopefully improve survival, a randomized prospective trial of perioperative portal vein infusion of 5-FU was initiated in 1975 (Taylor *et al.*, 1985). Patients with colorectal cancer but without evidence of established liver metastases were randomized to receive no further treatment following surgical resection, or a 7-day continuous portal vein infusion of 5-fluorouracil (1 g/day with 5000 units of heparin). In this original study 22 patients in the control group and 5 patients in the treated group developed liver metastases ($P = 0.002$). The incidence of local recurrences was not affected and a survival benefit was limited to patients with Dukes B colon cancer. The incidence of cytotoxicity using this technique was minimal.

Direct access to the portal vein can be difficult but there are alternative means of cannulating the portal venous system. These include:

1. The obliterated umbilical vein. This vein lies in the free edge of the falciform ligament

Table 9.2 Randomized trials comparing portal vein infusion of 5-fluorouracil (5-FU) to control arm

Group/institution	Authors	No. of patients	Treament arms versus control
Liverpool	Taylor *et al.* (1985)	257	5-FU + heparin
Rotterdam	Wereldsma *et al.* (1990)	304	5-FU + heparin urokinase
NSABP	Wolmark *et al.* (1990)	1158	5-FU + heparin
Mayo/NCCTG	Beart *et al.* (1990)	224	5-FU + heparin
Australia/New Zealand	Gray *et al.* (1987)	372	5-FU + heparin Systemic 5-FU
Virginia Mason	Ryan *et al.* (1988)	154	5-FU + heparin + Mitomycin C Heparin
St Mary's	Fielding *et al.* (1992)	451	5-FU + heparin
SAKK	Metzger *et al.* (1989)	533	5-FU + heparin + Mitomycin C

SAKK = Swiss Group for Clinical Cancer Research.

and can be dissected free. Following dilatation of the vein a cannula is passed into the portal vein and infusion commenced.

2. Access via the gastroepiploic or gastroduodenal veins which lie on the greater curvature of the stomach.
3. Cannulation of a small bowel mesenteric vein.
4. Direct cannulation of the inferior mesenteric vein.

As a result of the initial report of portal vein infusion, several prospective randomized trials have been initiated (Table 9.2). Some comment on a number of them is warranted.

The Swiss Group for Clinical Cancer Research (SAKK) reported the results of a large randomized trial in which surgery alone was compared with immediate postoperative portal vein 5-FU and mitomycin C (Metzger *et al.*, 1989). In the 469 patients randomized, an operative mortality of 1.85% was noted. After a median follow-up of some 4 years an actuarial survival of 70% in the treatment arm and 57% in the observation arm was obtained. In the Australia and New Zealand trial (Gray *et al.*, 1987), only patients with colon cancer were included and 372 were randomized either to observation or to portal vein infusion of 5-FU, or to systemic 5-FU. An improved survival accrued for portal vein infusion in patients with Dukes C colon cancer.

The trial reported from the Mayo Clinic randomized 224 patients with B2 or C colorectal cancer to either no therapy or to 7 days of 5-FU via the portal vein (Beart *et al.*, 1990). This is the only study in which treatment was delayed for up to 5 days postoperatively. It should be noted that in this study no improvement in survival was noted at a median follow-up of 5.5 years. In addition, the number of patients developing liver metastases were the same in both arms of the study. It should be noted, however, that in this trial portal vein 5-FU was not necessarily given in the perioperative period, but was delayed. In the Rotterdam study (Wereldsma *et al.*, 1990) patients were randomized to observation alone, portal vein infusion of 5-FU and heparin, or portal vein infusion of urokinase. However, the urokinase offered no benefit in preventing liver metastases. 5-FU infusion, on the other hand, decreased the number of liver metastases to one-third of the control group ($P = 0.001$). The average death rate in the 5-FU arm was 75% of the death rate in the control arm but did not quite reach statistical significance.

The largest study so far reported in the NSABP report of 1158 patients randomized to portal vein infusion with 5-FU and heparin or observation alone (Wolmark *et al.*, 1990). A disease-free survival of 74 versus 64% and an overall survival of 81 versus 73% ($P = 0.07$) in favour of the treated group was reported. The incidence, however, of liver metastases was not statistically significantly different.

A meta-analysis incorporating the results of all the reported trials does show a benefit in terms of overall survival and a reduction in the incidence of liver metastases. However, because each of the trials is relatively too small to demonstrate a convincing moderate improvement in overall survival, a much larger trial has been organized (the Adjuvant X-ray and

Infusion Study, known as the AXIS study). This trial is intended to randomize up to 4000 patients into either portal vein infusion or surgery only, with rectal carcinoma patients also randomized to radiotherapy. It is only in a trial of this size and magnitude that small differences in survival and reductions in liver metastases will be demonstrated.

Portal vein infusion for the treatment of established liver metastases

Adjuvant chemotherapy following liver resection for colorectal liver metastases has not been extensively investigated, although such patients might benefit. A phase II study of intraportal 5-FU chemotherapy following liver resection in 12 patients with colorectal liver metastases has been reported (Elias *et al.*, 1987). Only 40% of the patients were able to tolerate five courses of 14 days of 5-FU infusion, mostly due to catheter-related complications. However, no significant haematological complications were noted.

In view of the blood supply characteristics of liver tumours, it is unlikely that portal infusion alone will deliver sufficient drug to the tumour to be of benefit. However, because of the compensatory haemodynamic changes which occur following hepatic artery ligation, resulting in increased portal vein infusion of liver metastases (Taylor *et al.*, 1979; Ackerman, 1986), the combination of hepatic artery ligation and portal vein cytotoxic infusion could, theoretically, be beneficial. Murray-Lyon *et al.* (1970) describe 5 patients in whom this was performed. All 5 derived symptomatic benefit and survived between 10 and 20 months. Laufman *et al.* (1984) described 19 patients treated with hepatic artery ligation and portal vein infusion of 5-FU with Mitomycin C. A 63% response rate was recorded, with a median survival of 13 months from the start of treatment and 14 months from the date of diagnosis.

A larger series of 35 patients with synchronous multiple colorectal liver metastases has been reported with strict selection criteria and categorization depending upon the extent of liver involvement (Taylor, 1981). Hepatic artery ligation was performed with portal vein infusion of 5-FU early in the postoperative period. Patients with less than 20% tumour had a median survival of 15 months, patients with 20–70% tumour involvement 10.5 months, and patients with greater than 70% tumour involvement only 5.5 months. The overall median survival was 10 months. Gerard *et al.* (1991) carried out a multicentre prospective randomized trial to study the efficacy of hepatic artery ligation with and without portal vein infusion of 5-FU in patients with colorectal liver matastases. Thirty-five patients were eligible in the hepatic artery ligation + portal vein infusion group and 32 in the hepatic artery ligation alone group. Complications of hepatic artery ligation were relatively high, including 4 hepatic failures. Five patients had a partial response and 1 patient had a complete response in the hepatic artery ligation + portal vein infusion group. Only 1 patient had a partial response in the hepatic artery ligation alone group. Median survival for both groups was 12 months. This study does not show any great advantage for portal vein infusion in addition to hepatic artery ligation in terms of progression of disease. It would be surprising if this locoregional approach is as effective as long-term hepatic arterial infusion considering the relative blood supply of liver metastases.

Conclusions

A great deal is now understood about the development of metastases, and in particular about the blood supply of the liver. There are many mechanisms involved in invasion of the venous blood supply and the establishment of micrometastases within the liver itself. Nevertheless, by manipulating our knowledge with regard to blood supply, a greater understanding of the mechanisms has been achieved. Undoubtedly a desirable aim would be to prevent the establishment of metachronous liver metastases and ongoing trials of portal vein infusion are awaited with interest. With regard to the treatment of established liver metastases, it is unlikely that portal vein infusion will have a major role to play. A further promising approach is adjuvant portal vein infusion following resection of liver metastases and this avenue requires further investigation by randomized controlled trials.

References

Ackerman NB (1986) Experimental studies on the role of portal circulation in hepatic tumour vascularity. *Cancer* 58, 1653–1657.

Beart RW, Moertel CG, Wieand HS *et al.* (1990) Adjuvant therapy of resectable colorectal carcinoma with 4-fluorouracil administrated by portal infusion. *Arch. Surg.* **125**, 897–901.

Breedis C & Young G (1954) The blood supply of neoplasms in the liver. *Am. J. Pathol.* **30**, 969–977.

Brown CE & Warren S (1938) Visceral metastases from rectal carcinoma. *Surg. Gynecol. Obstet.* **66**, 611–621.

Cedermark BJ, Blumenson LE, Pickren JW *et al.* (1977) The significance of metastases in adenocarcinomas of the colon and rectum. *Surg. Gynecol. Obstet.* **144**, 537–546.

Chapuis PH, Dent OF & Fisher R (1985) A multi-variate analysis of clinical and pathological variables in prognosis after resection of large bowel cancer. *Br. J. Surg.* **72**, 698–702.

Cruz EP, McDonald GO & Cole WH (1956) Prophylactic treatment of cancer. The use of chemotherapeutic agents to prevent tumour metastases. *Surgery* **40**, 291–296.

Dukes CE & Bussey HJR (1958) The spread of rectal cancer and its effect on prognosis. *Br. J. Cancer* **12**, 309–320.

Elias D, Lasser P, Rougier P *et al.* (1987) Early adjuvant intraportal chemotherapy after curative hepatectomy for colorectal liver metastases. *Eur. J. Surg. Oncol.* **13**, 247–250.

Fielding LP, Hiltinger R, Grace RH *et al.* (1992) Randomized controlled trial of adjuvant chemotherapy by portal-vein perfusion after curative resection for colorectal adenocarcinoma. *Lancet* **340**, 502–506.

Finlay IG & McArdle CS (1986) Occult hepatic metastases in colorectal cancer. *Br. J. Surg.* **73**, 732–735.

Fisher ER & Turnbull RB (1955) The cytological demonstration and significance of tumour cells in the mesenteric venous blood in patients with colorectal carcinoma. *Surg. Gynecol. Obstet.* **100**, 102–108.

Gerarde A, Buyse M & Pector JC (1991) Hepatic artery ligation with and without portal infusion of 5-FU. A randomized study in patients with unresectable liver metastases from colorectal carcinoma. *Eur. J. Surg. Oncol.* **17**, 289–294.

Gray BN, de Zwart J, Fisher R *et al.* (1987) The Australia and New Zealand trial of adjuvant chemotherapy in colon cancer. In: Jones SE and Salmon (eds) *Adjuvant Therapy of Cancer V*. New York: Grune & Stratton, p. 537.

Krasna MJ, Flancbaum L, Cody RP *et al.* (1988) Vascular and neural invasion in colorectal carcinoma: incidence and prognostic significance. *Cancer* **61**, 1018–1023.

Laufman LR, Nims TA, Guy JT *et al.* (1984) Hepatic artery ligation and portal vein infusion for liver metastases from colon cancer. *J. Clin. Oncol.* **2**, 1382–1389.

Lin G, Lunderquist A, Hagerstrand I *et al.* (1984) Post mortem examination of the blood supply and vascular pattern of small liver metastases in man. *Surgery* **96**, 517–526.

Metzger U, Laffer U, Castiglione M *et al.* (1989) Adjuvant intraportal chemotherapy for colorectal cancer – 4 year results of the randomized Swiss study. *Proc. ASCO* **8**, 407.

Minsky B & Meis C (1989) The clinical significance of vascular invasion in colorectal cancer. *Dis. Colon Rectum* **32**, 794–803.

Moertel CG, Fleming TR & McDonald JS (1990) Levamisole and fluorouracil for adjuvant therapy of resected colon cancer. *N. Engl. J. Med.* **322**, 352–358.

Murphy P, Alexander P, Senior PV *et al.* (1988) Mechanisms of organ selective tumour growth by blood-borne cancer cells. *Br. J. Cancer* **57**, 19–31.

Murray-Lyon FM, Parsons VA, Blendis LM *et al.* (1970) Treatment of secondary hepatic tumours by ligation of hepatic artery and infusion of cytotoxic drugs. *Lancet* **2**, 172–175.

Panis Y, Ribeiro J & Chretien Y (1992) Dormant liver metastases: an experimental study. *Br. J. Surg.* **79**, 221–223.

Ryan J, Heiden P, Crowly J *et al.* (1988) Adjuvant portal vein infusion for colorectal cancer: a 3-arm randomized trial. *Proc. ASCO* **7**, 361.

Shirouzu K, Isomoto H, Kakegawa T *et al.* (1991) A prospective clinico-pathological study of venous invasion in colorectal cancer. *Am. J. Surg.* **162**, 216–222.

Sutanto-Ward E, Sigurdson ER, Tremiterra S *et al.* (1992) Adjuvant chemotherapy for colorectal hepatic metastases: role of route of administration and timing. *Surg. Oncol.* **1**, 87–95.

Taylor I (1981) Studies on the treatment and prevention of colorectal liver metastases. *Ann. R. Coll. Surg. Engl.* **63**, 270–276.

Taylor I, Bennett R & Sherriff S (1979) The blood supply of colorectal liver metastases. *Br. J. Cancer* **39**, 749–756.

Taylor I, Machin D, Mullee M *et al.* (1985) A randomized controlled trial of adjuvant portal vein cytotoxic perfusion in colorectal cancer. *Br. J. Surg.* **72**, 359–363.

Turnbull RB (1970) Cancer of the colon. The 5 and 10 year survival rates following resection utilizing the isolation technique. *Ann. R. Coll. Surg.* **46**, 243–250.

Wereldsma JCJ, Bruggink EDM, Meijer WS *et al.* (1990) Adjuvant portal liver infusion in colorectal cancer with 5-fluorouracil/heparin versus urokinase versus control. *Cancer* **65**, 425–432.

Wiggers T, Jeekel J, Arends JW *et al.* (1990) No-touch isolation technique in colon cancer: a controlled prospective trial. *Br. J. Surg.* **75**, 709–715.

Wolmark N, Rockette H, Wickerham DL *et al.* (1990) Adjuvant therapy of Dukes' A, B and C adenocarcinoma of the colon with portal-vein fluorouracil hepatic infusion: preliminary results of national surgical adjuvant breast and bowel project protocol C-02. *J. Clin. Oncol.* **8**, 1466–1475.

10

Isolated liver perfusion

K. R. Aigner

The principle of isolation perfusion for locoregional chemotherapy was first described by Creech *et al.* in 1958 for treatment of disseminated melanoma of a limb. The concept behind this strategy is to supply extremely high drug exposure to the tumour-invaded organ while systemic toxicity is prevented or at least extremely reduced (Creech *et al.*, 1958; Stephens, 1988). The technique of isolated liver perfusion (ILP), as described herein, was first performed in 1981 (Aigner *et al.*, 1982). Due to the poor chemosensitivity of colorectal liver metastases (Link *et al.*, 1986, 1988; De Bruijn *et al.*, 1988), there seemed to be a need for an isolated procedure as a means of increasing the total dose and concentration of cytotoxic drugs to an extent that is only limited by local tissue tolerance. Complete isolation of the perfused system avoids systemic side-effects. Modifications, according to the type of tumour to be treated, technical improvements and new drugs, have been continuously incorporated into the method by our group (Aigner, 1988, 1993a) as well as other investigators (De Brauw *et al.*, 1988; Schalhorn *et al.*, 1988; Hafstroem *et al.*, 1990; Naredi *et al.*, 1992).

Perfusion technique

Complete isolation of the liver is accomplished with a special double-lumen liver perfusion catheter (Perfufix, Braun Melsungen, Germany), introduced into the vena cava, and shunting the caval blood from the lower hemibody to the right atrium (Fig. 10.1).

First the liver is exposed via a midline incision and costal retractors, and mobilized away from the diaphragm. The hepatoduodenal ligament is then exposed and tourniquet tapes are placed around the common hepatic artery, gastroduodenal artery and two around the portal vein for cannulation in both directions. The gastroduodenal artery is then distally ligated. Collateral hepatic arterial branches are dissected. In case of anatomical variations, replaced right or left hepatic arteries are ligated.

Through a transverse incision in the diaphragm the vena cava is exposed intrapericardially and secured with a tourniquet tape. Further tourniquets are placed around the vena cava above and (two) below the renal veins. The lumbar veins entering the vena cava in this area are divided and ligated. Then the patient is heparinized with 150 u/kg.

For cannulation of the vena cava through a longitudinal incision between two vascular clamps, the perfusion catheter is introduced while temporarily blocked with a central guide tube in order to avoid blood loss through the side openings. For complete introduction into the vena cava the guide is removed and the end of the catheter occluded with a strong clamp. When it is in its proper position all tourniquets are fixed.

Cannulation of the portal vein in both directions is performed through a transverse incision. The distal cannula towards the gastrointestinal tract is immediately connected with the portocaval shunt tube of the perfusion catheter. The proximal tube, directed towards

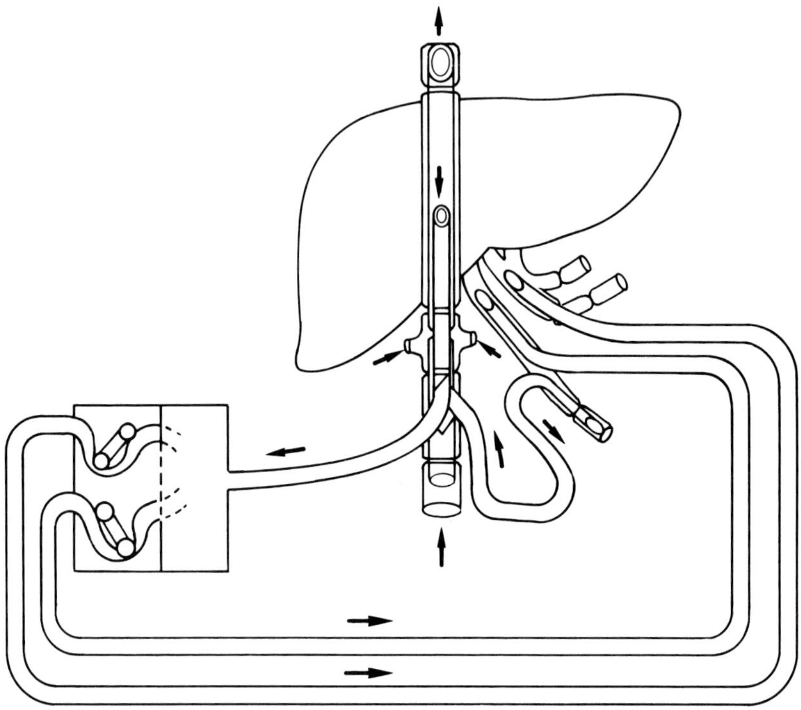

Figure 10.1 The isolated liver perfusion circuit.

the liver, is connected with the portal perfusion line of the heart–lung machine, and the venous hepatic return line of the perfusion catheter is connected to the venous line of the heart–lung machine. At this time the common hepatic artery must be clamped in order to prevent systemic blood loss into the isolated perfusion circuit. Once the suprarenal and intrapericardial vena cava tourniquets are narrowed too, the so-called portal isolation is established and the heart–lung machine can be turned on. The flow rate is adapted to the hepatic venous return.

The hepatic artery is usually cannulated through the gastroduodenal artery. At this time the portal flow rate for immediate oxygenation of the liver is adapted to about 300–400 ml/min. During infusion of drugs into the hepatic arterial line over 15–30 min, depending on the drug used and its total dose, the blood flow in this line is kept low, at about 100 ml/min, in order to reach a high local drug concentration. The volume level in the oxygenator is maintained at a steady state, mainly regulated through the venous return and the portal flow. In cases of hyperthermic perfusion, before application of drugs, high flow rates are aimed at in both lines for heating up the liver parenchyma to 39.5–40°C. The temperature is measured with thermistor probes in both liver lobes. At this temperature, blood supply to the metastases is at its optimum. Blood temperature in the oxygenator has to be kept at 41.5–42°C.

After 60 min of isolated cytotoxic perfusion, the venous line is cut through and the perfusate washed out. The hepatic vascular system is refilled with plasma expander and 1 unit of blood that is usually obtained by preoperative haemodilution. After decannulation the vena cava is repaired with a running suture while the bulldog clamp is already removed from the common hepatic artery. The portal vein, too, is repaired with a running Prolene suture. After removal of the hepatic arterial tube a port catheter is inserted into the gastroduodenal artery for subsequent infusion chemotherapy.

Prerequisites for optimal drug exposure and response

Quality of response is basically dependent on tumour vascularization, chemosensitivity and local drug exposure (concentration × time).

Blood supply is different in various histological types of tumour tissue: however, within one histological type small metastases are better vascularized than large ones. Measurements of drug levels in large versus small hepatic lesions as well as in the centre versus the periphery of metastases have confirmed this theory (Aigner *et al.*, 1988).

Chemosensitivity testing has proved to be useful for selecting drugs that are likely to be effective in the tumour to be treated, and to determine which concentration is required to induce an optimal response. In colorectal cancer, drug levels achieved with systemic chemotherapy have turned out to be not sufficiently active. As a consequence, complete remission is rarely seen. This supports the administration of high local concentrations in an isolated perfusion circuit. With reduction of the arterial blood flow via the roller pumps and infusion of cytotoxics into the arterial line, the speed of infusion regulates the drug concentration and, alone, determines the necessary infusion duration. Thus the product of concentration and time (area under the curve, AUC) is predictable and the efficacy of isolation perfusion is optimized.

An easier technique of isolation of the liver has been described recently (Aigner, 1995), where a double-balloon stopflow catheter (PfM, Cologne, Germany) with central shunts isolates the hepatic venous return. The catheter is introduced through the femoral artery. The liver is perfused selectively through the hepatic artery while the portal vein is clamped (Fig. 10.2).

Clinical cases

Overall, 57 patients with disseminated non-resectable liver metastases were submitted to ILP. Fifty-three patients had colorectal liver metastases, 1 had liver metastases from ocular melanoma and received 150 mg Cisplatinum (CDDP) and 30 mg Phenylalanine mustard (L-Pam), 2 had carcinoid and 1 had hepatoma. Fifteen colorectal cases had ILP with 1000 mg 5-fluorouracil (5-FU) alone without further therapy. Three of these patients died in the early postoperative phase when ILP was being developed. Since then, no further early post-operative deaths have occurred.

In 19 patients, which was the early group, ILP was performed with 5-FU alone. Forty patients received subsequent hepatic arterial infusion (HAI) with Mitomycin (MMC) (14 mg) and 5 × 5-FU (1000 mg). Thirty-eight of 40 had prior ILP with MMC/5-FU, 2/40 had ILP with 5-FU alone. In these 2 patients response was more impressive during subsequent HAI, which leads to the conclusion that alkylating agents should be used for perfusion. Total MMC dose was continuously increased up to 50 mg without major evidence of local toxicity. Therefore, the study has to be considered a dose-finding pilot trial, particularly since clinical stages were not uniform and consisted of 67% clearly palpable liver enlargement with elevation of the alkaline phosphatase.

Results

Response was generally estimated according to the course of tumour markers. Second-look surgery was only performed in cases where resectability of bulky lesions was to be expected while small lesions had disappeared. On these occasions it became evident that even totally necrotic colorectal metastases with normal carcinoembryonic antigen levels usually do not disappear on the computed tomographic scan – they just shrink – while histologically calcifications and connective tissue are observed. One of those patients, who had turned out to be resectable 4 weeks after ILP at second look, 5 years post-ILP had no evidence of any small lesions, but died after 6 years from myocardial infarction. Another patient presented with a second tumour metastatic to the liver (hypernephroma) 34 months post-ILP and died at 38 months due to the new disease. One patient developed local recurrence 40 months post-ILP and died after 45 months. Two patients are still alive after 9.5 and 10.5 years. The median survival of the total group of 40 patients receiving ILP/HAI was 18 months.

The advantage of ILP with increasing doses of Mitomycin is demonstrated by an increasing number of complete remissions. Although the total percentage of responses is about the same in the 5-FU group and the MMC/5-FU group, the complete response rate is higher in the latter (62%) as compared with the 5-FU group (16%). The partial response rate, however, is only 28% in the MMC/5-FU group versus 79% in the 5-FU group. This indicates a clear dose–response behaviour of Mitomycin.

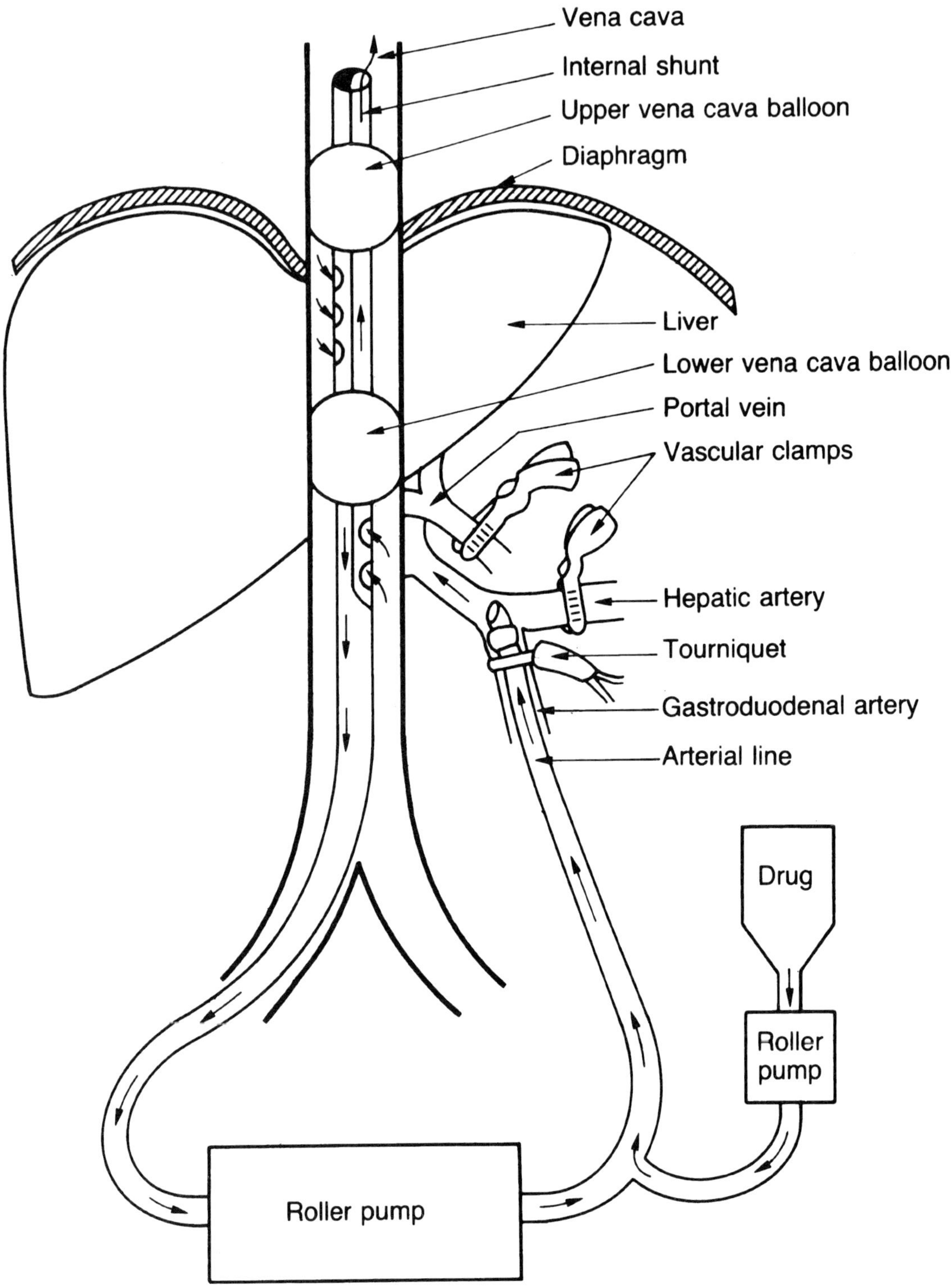

Figure 10.2 Isolated liver perfusion with a double-balloon vena cava catheter.

Table 10.1 Manifestation of extrahepatic lesions following isolated liver perfusion (ILP) or ILP/hepatic arterial infusion (HAI)

Method	Extrahepatic metastases	Postoperative peritoneal carcinosis
ILP (5-FU)	After 4 months	74%
ILP (5-FU/MMC) + HAI	After 11.5 months	20%

5-FU = 5-Fluorouracil; MMC = Mitomycin.

Side-effects

Generally, liver tissue damage is unexpectedly mild despite high-dose cytotoxic therapy. A transient increase of serum glutamic oxaloacetic and pyruvic transaminase to 100–200 u/l uusually occurs, but normalizes within 1 week. Performance after ILP does not differ from that after any other laparotomy, lasting 3–4 h. Cholinesterase decreases to 800–1200 u/l and returns to normal within 1 month. Biliary sclerosis was never observed after ILP.

Extrahepatic metastases

A total of 87% of patients developed extrahepatic lesions (peritoneum, lungs, bone, brain or a combination) after therapy at a median interval of 4 months in the ILP 5-FU group and 11.5 months following ILP with MMC/5-FU (Table 10.1). More than 70% of all patients – among them more than 90% of those in clinical stages III and IV (Khayat *et al.*, 1988) – develop peritoneal carcinomatosis, even in cases of complete response in the liver. Metastatic invasion of the porta hepatis was diagnosed in 74% of our patients after ILP with 5-FU alone and in 20% after ILP with MMC/5 FU. This indicates less metastatic spread from the liver to other areas following initial high-dose therapy. In the course of longer follow-up there is a shift towards bone and brain metastases.

Discussion

It is evident that in resistant tumour tissue like colorectal metastases, systemic chemotherapy and even HAI fail to provide sufficient local control, since the required local drug exposure due to lack of local concentration or even poor vascularization can never be achieved (Link *et al.*, 1986, 1988; Sigurdson *et al.*, 1987; De Bruijn *et al.*, 1988). Further, it remains questionable whether a high partial response rate in liver metastases really can definitely induce prolonged life expectancy. The answer is most probably no, except in those cases of central metastases adjacent to the bile ducts, where even a partial remission with slight shrinkage of the lesion may postpone the occurrence of jaundice with consecutive liver failure due to biliary occlusion. However, this is not the rule in the majority of the patients at risk, and may certainly not influence the median survival rate of all patients. Since the main criterion is the median survival rate, and not a possibly augmented number of a few more long-term survivors in the lower part of the survival curve, it seems mandatory to investigate further treatment modalities that induce an improved complete/partial response ratio and consequently prolong median survival due to long disease-free intervals. In recent years chemoembolization, performed with the suitable drugs and embolisate, appeared to bear unexpected potential (Konno *et al.*, 1992; Stagg *et al.*, 1992; Taguchi, 1992).

However, we should not forget that all new forms of cancer therapy have been controversial regarding the administered drugs, the mode of delivery, the clinical stage of the patients treated and, specifically, the tumours treated. Nevertheless, during recent years some progress has been made in the understanding of regional chemotherapy (Pettavel *et al.*, 1984; Krementz, 1986; Wile *et al.*, 1987; Van de Velde, 1988; Ishida *et al.*, 1992; Kemeny *et al.*, 1992). The basic questions arising now are: Has the best drug for the specific tumour been used (Link *et al.*, 1986, 1988; Hafstroem *et al.*, 1990; Naredi *et al.*, 1992)? Is the catheter technique optimal – does the drug get to the tumour? Is there any chemosensitivity in the high dose range that can be achieved by arterial delivery (Link *et al.*, 1986, 1988)? Is the suggested toxicity acceptable and can quality of life be improved? It should be taken into consideration that colorectal cancer, from the point of view of chemosensitivity and vascularization, is certainly not the most suitable tumour in which to investigate the benefit of regional drug application.

In the perfusion situation it became obvious that isolation techniques with flow reduction and possibly even hypoxia (Aigner, 1993) for further enhancement of the cytotoxic potential of melphalan and Mitomycin might provide – not yet overseeable – possibilities for further improvement of local control. The pitfall, however, that could be foreseen at the very beginning, was that, regarding the tremendous number of patients at risk, the relatively few number of tumour centres able to perform isolation techniques would never be able to cope with it. Furthermore, it became obvious in our study that only lower tumour stages are candidates for isolation perfusion, since distant metastases, first of all in the peritoneum, occur even in cases of local control in the liver. This is a challenge first, to simplify isolation perfusion techniques substantially and, second, to improve local control of peritoneal relapse. Therefore, the technically much easier and less time-consuming stopflow and above all vena cava double-balloon techniques (Aigner, 1993, 1995) for isolation of the hepatic venous return should be taken into consideration, since this can easily be achieved from the femoral access. In addition cannulation of the gastroduodenal artery and clamping of the portal vein are low-risk procedures. Immediate peritoneal lavage (Sugarbaker *et al.*, 1988), hyperthermic peritoneal perfusion (Fujimoto *et al.*, 1988, 1993) or abdominal stopflow or hypoxic perfusion may be useful adjuvants to prevent peritoneal progression, which up to now terminates all local therapeutic endeavours. To obtain definite information concerning the value of isolation perfusion for colorectal liver metastases, randomized trials of the ILP with and without adjuvant modalities should be carried out.

References

Aigner KR (1988) Isolated liver perfusion: 5-year results. *Reg. Cancer Treat.* **3**, 11–20.

Aigner KR (1993) Aortic stopflow infusion (ASI) and hypoxic abdominal perfusion (HAP) for disseminated bulky peritoneal carcinomatosis – rationale and technique. *Reg. Cancer Treat.* (suppl. 1), abstracts A4: 3.

Aigner KR (1995a) A simplifed technique for isolated liver perfusion using a vena cava double balloon catheter with central shunt. *Reg. Cancer Treat.* (in press).

Aigner KR, Walther H, Tonn JC *et al.* (1982) Die isolierte Leberperfusion mit 5-Fluorouracil (5-FU) beim Menschen. *Chirurg.* **53**, 571–573.

Aigner KR Müller H, Walther H & Link KH (1988) Drug filtration in high dose chemotherapy. In: Aigner KR, Patt YZ, Link KH & Kreidler J (eds) *Reg. Cancer Treat.* Vol. 29, pp. 261–280. Basel: Karger.

Creech OJ, Krementz ET, Ryan RF & Winblad JN (1958) Chemotherapy of cancer: regional perfusion utilizing an extracorporeal circuit. *Ann. Surg.* **148**, 616–632.

De Brauw LM, Van der Velde CJH, De Bruijn EA & Tjaden UR (1988) Controlled release of 5-FU ra by application of isolated liver perfusion in the treatment of hepatic metastases. *Reg. Cancer Treat.* Vol. 29, pp. 217–221. Basel: Karger.

De Bruijn EA, Slee PhThJ, Kuppen PJK *et al.* (1988) The importance of exposure time in regional chemotherapy: mitomycin C and fluoropyrimidines. *Reg. Cancer Treat.* Vol. 29, pp. 43–48. Basel: Karger.

Eggermont AMM, Van Ooijen B & Wiggers T (1992) Locoregional immunotherapy for nonresectable malignant hepatic disease. *Reg. Cancer Treat.* **4**, 227–231.

Fujimoto S, Shresta RD, Kokobun M *et al.* (1988) Intraperitoneal hyperthermic perfusion combined with surgery effective for gastric cancer patients with peritoneal seeding. *Ann. Surg.* **208**, 36–41.

Fujimoto S, Takakashi M, Kokobun M *et al.* (1993) Clinical usefulness of cimetidine treatment for prevention of scald injury on the peritoneo-serosal membrane in intraperitoneal hyperthermic perfusion for patients with advanced gastric cancer. *Reg. Cancer Treat.* **1**, 1–6.

Hafstroem L, Rudenstam CM, Holmberg SB, Schersten T & Ehrsson H (1990) The pharmacokinetics of melphalan in regional hyperthermic liver perfusion. *Reg. Cancer Treat.* **3**, 23–25.

Ishida H, Jurama T & Mishima Y (1992) Comparison between portal vein chemotherapy and hepatic artery chemotherapy on experimental liver micrometastases. *Reg. Cancer Treat.* **5**, 74–78.

Kemeny MM, Alava G, Oliver JM & Smith FB (1992) The use of circadian flow patterning to reduce toxicity in continuous infusions of recombinant interleukin-2. *Reg. Cancer Treat.* **4**, 260–264.

Khayat D, Le Cesne A, Weil M *et al.* (1988) Intraarterial treatment of hepatic metastasis using fluorouracil, adriamycin and mitomycin C (FAM) chemotherapeutic regimen. *Reg. Cancer Treat.* **1**, 62–64.

Konno T, Yamashita R, Oda T, Maeda H, Taguchi T & Nagamitsu A (1992) Targeting cancer chemotherapy used lipiodol as a carrier of anticancer agents for hepatocellular carcinoma. *Reg. Cancer Treat.* **5**, 110–116.

Krementz ET (1986) Regional perfusion – current sophistication. What next? *Cancer* **57**, 416–432.

Link KH, Aigner KR, Kuehn W, Schwemmle K & Kern DH (1986) Prospective correlative chemosensitivity testing in high-dose intraarterial chemotherapy for liver metastases. *Cancer Res.* **46**, 4837–4840.

Link KH, Aigner KR & Kessler D (1988) *In vitro* chemosensitivity profiles of human malignancies for high-dose (regional) chemotherapy. In: Aigner KR, Patt YZ, Link KH & Kreidler J (eds) *Reg. Cancer Treat.* Vol. 29, pp. 28–42. Basel: Karger.

Naredi P, Holmberg SB, Hafstroem L, Heath DD, Shalinsky DR & Howell SB (1992) Pharmacokinetics of cisplatin in an isolated liver perfusion system in humans. *Reg. Cancer Treat.* **4**, 254–257.

Pettavel J, Leyvraz S & Douglas P (1984) The necessity for staging liver metastases and standardizing treatment-response criteria. The case of secondaries of colo-rectal origin. In: Van de Velde CJH & Sugarbaker PH (eds) *Liver Metastasis*. pp. 154–168. Dordrecht: Nijhoff.

Schalhorn A, Peyerl G & Denecke H (1988) Pharmacokinetics of 5-fluorouracil during isolated liver perfusion. *Reg. Cancer Treat.* **1**, 21–27.

Sigurdson ER, Ridge JA, Kemeny N & Daly JM (1987) Tumor and liver drug uptake following hepatic artery and portal vein infusion. *Clin. Oncol.* **5**, 1836–1840.

Stagg RJ, Venook AP, Chase JL, Frye JW, Ring EJ & Hohn DC (1992) Chemoembolization of primary and metastatic liver tumors. *Reg. Cancer Treat.* **5**, 53–57.

Stephens FO (1988) Why use regional chemotherapy? Principles and pharmacokinetics. *Reg. Cancer Treat.* **1**, 4–10.

Sugarbaker PH, Cunliffe W, Belliveau JF *et al.* (1988) Rationale for perioperative intraperitoneal chemotherapy as a surgical adjuvant for gastrointestinal malignancy. *Reg. Cancer Treat.* **1**, 66–79.

Taguchi T (1992) A comparative randomized study on the treatment of primary and secondary liver tumors with intraarterial chemotherapy with or without degradable starch microspheres (DSM) (Spherex). *Reg. Cancer Treat.* **5**, 117–120.

Van de Velde CJH, de Brauw LM, Sugarbaker PH & Tranberg K (1988) Hepatic artery infusion chemotherapy: rationale, results, credits and debits. *Reg. Cancer Treat.* **1**, 93–101.

Wile AG, Kar R, Cohen RA, Jakowatz JG & Opfell RW (1987) The pharmacokinetics of cisplatin in experimental regional chemotherapy. *Cancer* **59**, 695–700.

11

Radiotherapy

Bruce N. Gray and Mark A. Burton

The development of liver metastases is a common outcome for many patients with cancer, but particularly for those with primary tumours originating in the gastrointestinal tract. For some forms of cancer, liver metastases can be treated with either chemotherapy or hormonal therapy, resulting in effective palliation, and occasionally even cure. However, for the great majority of patients, surgery, systemic chemotherapy or hormonal treatment will not be of value.

In clinical practice it is common to find that primary tumours of the gastrointestinal tract metastasize to the liver without spreading to other organs. It is this subgroup of patients who may be considered for some form of localized treatment, be it hepatic perfusion chemotherapy, surgery or radiotherapy. This contrasts with many other forms of cancer spread such as from melanoma, breast or prostate, where the liver metastases are merely one manifestation of the metastatic process.

Radiotherapy is a widely used modality for treating localized cancer. However, in the case of liver metastases, radiotherapy has not gained wide acceptance as a viable treatment option, and has until now played a small part in the overall patient management. The reasons for this are several. First, any consideration of treating secondary cancer in the liver with radiotherapy has to be positioned against the need to treat other sites of malignancy as well. As radiotherapy is purely a localized form of treatment, patients with widespread disease are not candidates for any form of localized treatment. Second, the upper limit of radiation that can be applied to the normal liver parenchyma limits its effectiveness.

In 1965 Ingold *et al.* showed that up to 30 Gy of radiation could be delivered without inducing significant radiation hepatitis, but that the risk rose sharply with increasing doses. The recommended tolerance limits of the liver with conventional fractionation techniques indicate that a whole-liver dose of 35 Gy will have a 50% incidence of radiation hepatitis (Rubin, 1975). These and other studies indicate that as radiation doses exceed 30 Gy the risk of developing radiation hepatitis rapidly increases, although there have been isolated reports of using higher doses up to 50 Gy (Lightdale *et al.*, 1979).

The distribution of liver metastases also limits the ability to treat them from externally applied radiation beams. Whereas it is possible to direct an external beam on to single tumours within the liver, multiple metastases usually spread widely throughout the liver parenchyma, thereby rendering it necessary to apply the radiation to the whole of the liver, which in turn limits the dose that can be applied.

Despite these limitations, radiotherapy has been evaluated as treatment for liver metastases and some of the newer and more novel techniques of applying radiotherapy appear to have great promise. In fact, some recent reports are encouraging enough to require that all patients who are not considered candidates for surgical resection should be considered for radiation therapy. The criteria that might be applied for selecting patients as potential candidates for treatment are:

1. Patients whose metastatic disease is largely limited to the liver.
2. Patients in whom the liver metastases cannot be treated by other techniques such as surgical removal.
3. Patients in whom control of the liver metastases is likely to result in either a quantitative or qualitative improvement in survival.
4. Patients without clinically apparent metastatic cancer, but who are at high risk of developing liver metastases (adjuvant radiotherapy).

Radiotherapy can be classified as external or internal, depending on the route of administration.

External-beam radiotherapy

Case and Warthin first demonstrated the potential of external-beam therapy for treating liver metastases in 1924, and this has been the traditional technique used since then. Since that time there have been many anecdotal reports in the literature of small series of patients with liver metastases treated with external-beam radiotherapy, and this subject has been reviewed many times (Gray, 1980; Minsky & Leibel, 1989).

Objective response rates have varied, but in some reports there has been evidence of tumour regression in the majority of patients (Gray, 1980). Despite the objective evidence that confirms that externally applied radiation will cause tumours to regress in about half the patients, there is no real evidence that this translates into a survival advantage. Furthermore, there has been considerable variation in technique, dose, tumour type, patient selection and methods for reporting results that makes it difficult to recommend standard radiation techniques as proven effective therapy.

Hyperfractionation

Several variations in standard techniques have been explored in order to increase effectiveness of treatment. Hyperfractionation techniques have theoretical advantages and have been assessed in the treatment of liver malignancy. The Radiation Therapy Oncology Group study evaluated the use of hyperfractionation radiation in combination with chemotherapy in a series of 59 patients with hepatocellular cancer and compared these results to 131 patients treated with conventional radiation schedules. Although radiation doses were only of the order of 21–24 Gy, the response rate of approximately 20% was the same for both groups (Stillwagon *et al.*, 1989). They concluded that the low response rate could not be improved with hyperfractionation, although the acute toxicity was increased. It is unlikely that hyperfractionation techniques can offer much improvement over conventional techniques for metastatic disease as well as primary liver tumours.

In order to try and increase effective doses delivered to tumours within the liver, attempts have been made to develop three-dimensional treatment planning, with higher doses being applied to tumour when it was possible to exclude more of the normal liver parenchyma from the treatment field (Lawrence *et al.*, 1991). This technique deserves further evaluation, as it does allow high radiation doses to be delivered when dose prescription is guided by dose–volume histograms. This technique has been used to treat liver metastases with much higher radiation doses than would otherwise be tolerated and in combination with chemotherapy, although an objective response can only be detected in about half the patients treated (Lawrence *et al.*, 1991).

Radiation plus chemotherapy

Because of the difficulty in using high radiation doses to the liver, most studies have combined radiation with other forms of treatment such as chemotherapy. Indeed, there is ample evidence that shows that these two treatment modalities are complementary and the biological basis for interaction of radiation and chemotherapy has been well described (Fu, 1985). There is also evidence that radiation and chemotherapy should be administered either sequentially or in an alternating manner to get the optimal effect (Fu, 1985).

Response rates using the combination of radiation and chemotherapy have varied widely, with some reports claiming high response rates of up to 70% (Barone *et al.*, 1979), whereas others have failed to demonstrate any improvement over that of either conventional radiation therapy or chemotherapy alone. For instance, a small study of 25 patients with liver metastases treated with a combination of whole-liver radiation plus razoxane produced a response rate of 65% (Hellman *et al.*, 1992).

There have been many attempts to increase response rates by administering the chemotherapy directly into the hepatic artery. This has the potential of not only increasing the direct cytotoxic effect of the chemotherapy, but is also more likely to potentiate the radiation effect. Several reports have suggested that a combination of radiation and hepatic artery chemotherapy can prolong survival. In a study of 33 patients with colorectal metastases in the liver, Webber *et al.* (1978) compared hepatic perfusion chemotherapy, hepatic radiation or a combination of the two, with a median survival of 9, 5 and 13 months respectively. Herbsman *et al.* (1978) also produced an encouraging report using a combination of hepatic artery perfusion chemotherapy and external radiotherapy of up to 30 Gy with a mean survival of 16 months from the start of treatment and 20 months from diagnosis.

However, other reports suggest that the combination of hepatic perfusion chemotherapy and radiotherapy has little to offer over that of chemotherapy alone. In another randomized trial comparing hepatic perfusion chemotherapy alone or in combination with 25.5 Gy liver radiation in 37 patients with colorectal liver metastases, there was no improvement in either response or survival by adding the radiotherapy to chemotherapy, with only a third of patients showing a response to the combination treatment (Wiley *et al.*, 1989). A further similarly designed study produced a comparable result. In this trial of 27 patients with liver metastases from the colorectum, Miller *et al.* (1988) found that the addition of liver radiation added nothing to hepatic arterial chemotherapy, with only 5 of 23 patients showing a response to treatment. In this latter study the radiotherapy was added after the chemotherapy, and hence the effect of the radiation could be measured over and above that of chemotherapy.

Perhaps the most convincing study to assess the combination of radiation and hepatic perfusion chemotherapy was that of the North California Oncology Group, in which 166 patients were randomized between liver irradiation alone or in combination with either intra-arterial or systemic chemotherapy. Although there was no significant difference between the rate of tumour regression or survival in each of the three groups, there did appear to be a longer period of tumour control when chemotherapy was added to the radiotherapy (Friedman *et al.*, 1988) but this does not, of course, demonstrate an advantage over chemotherapy alone.

Adjuvant radiotherapy in high-risk patients

There is another area in which liver radiation may have a role to play. As certain subgroups of patients who are at high risk of developing liver metastases can be identified prior to clinical appearance of the metastases, it would be rational to administer radiotherapy to the liver as an adjuvant in these high-risk patients and before the metastases become obvious. This concept of adjuvant therapy using chemotherapy has recently been shown to be of benefit to patients undergoing resection of primary tumours in the large bowel, and hence there may be a role for radiotherapy to the liver as well.

The Gastrointestinal Tumour Study Group (GITSG) (1991) investigated this concept in a clinical trial in which 300 patients undergoing resection for stage B or C colon cancer were randomized to observation or treatment with liver radiation plus systemic chemotherapy with 5-fluorouracil. Although the study failed to show any advantage from this adjuvant protocol, the concept certainly needs further evaluation. The GITSG protocol used a relatively low radiation dose of 21 Gy, and systemic chemotherapy at best is associated with a low response of the order of 20%. Targeted internal radiotherapy techniques using higher doses, either with or without hepatic perfusion chemotherapy, certainly deserve further study.

As liver metastases are a very common sequel to primary tumours of the pancreas, the concept of prophylactic liver irradiation has been assessed in this patient group also. There are at least two phase 2 trials that indicate that prophylactic hepatic irradiation can result in fewer patients developing liver metastases than would otherwise have been expected (Komaki *et al.*, 1988; Wiley *et al.*, 1988). In order to study the concept of prophylactic liver irradiation further, the Radiation Therapy Oncology Group irradiated the liver with 23.4 Gy of radiation plus chemotherapy as a prophylactic measure as one facet of therapy for patients with non-resectable carcinoma of the pancreas.

The results of this multi-institutional study of 81 patients suggested that the liver irradiation could decrease the incidence of subsequent liver metastases, but this did not translate into benefit for the patients, as failure to control either the primary tumour and intra-abdominal spread overwhelmed any potential benefit from the liver radiation (Komaki *et al.*, 1992). These results highlight the need to control liver metastases, which is only part of overall patient management.

Radiotherapy for control of symptoms

Improvements in quality of life are an important aim of cancer treatment and to this end liver irradiation has been used to control symptoms. In one study, 79 patients with symptomatic liver metastases were evaluated. Although symptomatic control in this patient group was good, the short median survival in this group of patients of only 4 months meant that liver irradiation was not the optimal treatment for symptomatic patients (Heimdal *et al.*, 1988).

Radiotherapy plus hyperthermia

The biological interaction of hyperthermia and radiotherapy has been described elsewhere in this book. There are numerous studies that show that these two modalities are complementary and result in improvements in response. This subject has been summarized under the heading of hyperthermia (Chapter 15).

Internal radiotherapy

As the inherent problems of external radiation limit its use in the treatment of liver metastases, a number of novel techniques have been developed in order to localize the radiation into the immediate tumour environment. All of these techniques attempt to increase the radiation dose to the metastases, while maintaining that to the normal liver parenchyma to a tolerable level. These targeted forms of internal radiotherapy include:

1. Selective internal radiation therapy by embolizing the tumour vasculature with radioactive particles.
2. Direct implantation of radioactive materials.
3. Sludging of the tumour vasculature with lipiodol-containing radionuclides.
4. Specific targeting of tumours with antibodies containing radionuclide.

Selective internal radiation therapy

Liver metastases are fed almost exclusively from the hepatic artery, as opposed to normal liver parenchyma, which receives blood from both the artery and portal vein (Stribley *et al.*, 1982; Archer & Gray, 1989). This provides an opportunity not only to perfuse cytotoxic drugs directly into tumour metastases, but also selectively to embolize particulate material by injecting it into the hepatic artery. This selective embolization of liver metastases can be further enhanced by the use of vasoactive drugs which cause normal liver vessels to constrict, but not those supplying tumours (Burton *et al.*, 1985; Burton & Gray, 1987). In 1951, Muller and Rossier first used this concept of selectively irradiating metastases by embolizing radioactive material into the liver via the vascular tree. The original technique used by these authors was relatively crude and until recently has not shown much promise.

However, the basic technique of selectively targeting high local radiation doses into the vascular compartment of metastases has been intensively studied in recent years. Although the earliest attempts to use this technique met with only moderate success, the technique has now been refined with the use of better microspheres, higher radiation doses, intraoperative radiation dosimetry, and an understanding of dose distribution within the liver and metastases (Burton & Gray, 1989; Burton *et al.*, 1989; Gray *et al.*, 1989). The main isotope now used in this technique is yttrium 90, which is incorporated into either ceramic or plastic microspheres. The ability to target the radiation therapy to tumours has overcome the major stumbling block of externally applied beams and allowed high radiation doses to be delivered to tumours. The dosimetric distribution for selective internal radiation therapy is complex, and conventional understanding of liver tolerance has to be recalculated (Gray *et al.*, 1990; Fox *et al.*, 1991).

At Royal Perth Hospital, we have now treated over 100 patients with various modifications of this technique. The most recent report on this technique of selective internal radiation therapy has combined the use of internally delivered radiotherapy with hepatic perfusion chemotherapy, with virtually all patients showing some evidence of tumour regression (Gray *et al.*, 1992). These response rates are certainly higher than other forms of treatment for liver metastases and require further evaluation. Selective internal radiation therapy is currently being evaluated in a randomized trial that is assessing whether this high rate of tumour regression will translate into improved survival.

Direct implantation of radioactive seeds

This technique involves directly implanting seeds or wires containing either radioactive iodine or iridium into the tumour. Donath *et al.* (1990) reported the results in 6 patients in whom radioactive seeds containing iodine 125 were directly implanted into unresectable metastases at the time of surgery. They reported a fall in carcinoembryonic antigen levels and concluded that there was good local control of tumour growth at the sites treated with the seeds.

Direct implantation of iridium 192 was similarly used to treat 6 patients with liver metastases that were found at laparotomy to be not resectable. This treatment seemed to result in good local control of tumour, although there are significant logistic problems associated with this form of interstitial intraoperative treatment and it is unlikely that the technique would have wide application (Holt *et al.*, 1988).

Lipiodol iodine 131

It has been known for some time that lipiodol sludges in the vascular network of tumours when injected into the hepatic artery. Lipiodol has therefore been used as a carrier for cytotoxic drugs, and more recently also for transport and localization of radionuclides. Most work in this area has been with the use of iodine 131-labelled lipiodol. This technique has been used mainly for the treatment of primary hepatocellular carcinomas, but also for liver metastases. In both situations there is a relatively greater concentration of the isotope in tumour, as opposed to normal parenchyma, and this should result in enhanced irradiation of tumour tissue (Raoul *et al.*, 1988). The therapeutic response however, appears much better for primary tumours than for metastases, with no response occurring in 8 patients treated in one study (Bretagne *et al.*, 1988).

Highly selective subsegmental embolization with intra-arterial iodine 131-labelled lipiodol has been used to irradiate selectively isolated tumours in the liver. The response rates for small hepatomas is high, but the technique is limited to isolated tumours and hence is of little value in metastatic disease, when multiple metastases require treatment (Yoo *et al.*, 1991).

Antibody targeting

Another novel isotopic approach has been to couple a radionuclide to an antibody that can then be injected into patients so that it targets the tumour. This approach has been tried in patients with colorectal liver metastases using iodine 131-labelled anti-carcinoembryonic antigen antibody, but the radiation dose delivered to the tumour is below that needed to get a good response and the targeting ability of the antibody is poor (Order *et al.*, 1986). Higher radionuclide labelling and more specific antibodies need to be developed if this technique is to have a future.

Summary

Radiation therapy has now been used for more than 60 years for treating patients with both primary and metastatic liver cancer. Despite numerous clinical trials and improvements in external-beam therapy, there is no clearly defined role for the use of external beams for this group of patients, and there seems little scope for any major new development in this area. The primary obstacle remains the inability to target high radiation doses into the various parts of the liver that harbour the metastatic disease.

By far the most promising new development comes from the various attempts to target selectively the tumour with high cytocidal doses of radiation, while sparing the normal liver parenchyma. Certainly the objective response rates for some of these techniques, such as selective internal radiation therapy, is much higher than with the use of externally applied beams, but it remains to be shown whether this will translate into patient benefit. Several of these techniques are currently being evaluated in clinical trials.

References

Archer S & Gray B (1989) The vascularisation of small liver metastases. *Br. J. Surg.* **76**, 545–548.

Barone R, Byfield J & Frankel S (1979) *Dis. Colon Rectum* **22**, 376.

Bretagne J, Raoul J, Bourguet P *et al.* (1988) Hepatic artery injection of I-131-labelled lipiodol. Part 2. Preliminary results of therapeutic use in patients with hepatocellular carcinoma and liver metastases. *Radiology* **168**, 547–550.

Burton MA & Gray BN (1987) Redistribution of blood flow in experimental hepatic tumours with nor-adrenaline and propranolol. *Br. J. Cancer* **56**, 585–588.

Burton MA & Gray BN (1989) Intra-operative dosimetry of yttrium-90 in liver tissue. *Nucl. Med. Biol.* **16**, 495–498.

Burton MA, Gray BN, Self GW, Heggie JC & Townsend PS (1985) Manipulation of experimental rat and rabbit liver tumour blood flow with angiotensin-2. *Cancer Res.* **45**, 5390–5393.

Burton MA, Gray BN, Klemp P, Kelleher D & Hardy N (1989) Selective internal radiation therapy; distribution of radiation in the liver. *Eur. J. Cancer Clin. Oncol.* **25**, 1487–1491.

Case J & Warthin A (1924) *AJR* **12**, 27.

Donath D, Nori D, Turnbull A, Kaufman N & Fortner J (1990) Brachytherapy in the treatment of solitary colorectal metastases to the liver. *J. Surg. Oncol.* **44**, 55–61.

Fox RA, Klemp PFB, Egan G, Mina LL, Burton MA & Gray BN (1991) Dose distribution following selective internal radiation therapy. *Int. J. Radiat. Oncol. Biol. Phys.* **21**, 463–467.

Friedman M, Phillips T, Hannigan J & Carter S (1988) Phase 3 trial of irradiation plus chemotherapy for patients with hepatic metastases and hepatoma; experience of the north California oncology group. *Natl Cancer Inst. Monog.* **6**, 259–264.

Fu K (1985) Biological basis for interaction of chemotherapeutic agents and radiation therapy. *Cancer* **55**, 2123–2130.

Gastrointestinal Tumour Study Group (1991) Adjuvant therapy with hepatic irradiation plus fluorouracil in colon cancer. *Int. J. Radiat. Oncol. Biol. Phys.* **21**, 1151–1156.

Gray BN (1980) Colorectal cancer; modern treatment of disseminated disease. *Aust. N.Z. J. Surg.* **50**, 647–658.

Gray BN, Burton MA, Kelleher D, Anderson J & Klemp P (1989) Selective internal radiation (SIR) therapy for treatment of liver metastases; measurement of response rate. *J. Surg. Oncol.* **42**, 192–196.

Gray BN, Matz L, Burton MA, Kelleher D & Klemp P (1990) Tolerance of the liver to yttrium-90 irradiation. *Int. J. Radiat. Oncol. Biol. Phys.* **18**, 619–623.

Gray BN, Anderson JE, Burton MA, Codde JP, Morgan C & Klemp P (1992) Regression of liver metastases following treatment with yttrium 90 microspheres. *Aust. N.Z. J. Surg.* **62**, 105–110.

Heimdal K, Hannisdal E & Fossa S (1988) Survival after palliative radiotherapy of liver metastases. A search for prognostic factors. *Acta Oncol.* **28**, 63–65.

Hellman K, Goold M, Higgins N & Phillips R (1992) Responses of liver metastases to radiotherapy and razoxane. *J.R. Soc. Med.* **85**, 136–138.

Herbsman H, Hassan A & Gardner B (1978) *Surg. Gynecol. Obstet.* **147**, 13.

Holt R, Nauta R, Lee T *et al.* (1988) Intraoperative interstitial radiation therapy for hepatic metastases from colorectal carcinoma. *Am. Surg.* **54**, 231–233.

Ingold J, Reed G, Kaplan H & Bagshaw M (1965) Radiation hepatitis. *AJR* **93**, 200–208.

Komaki R, Hansen R, Cox J & Wilson J (1988) Phase 1–2 study of prophylactic hepatic irradiation with local irradiation and systemic chemotherapy for adenocarcinoma of the pancreas. *Int. J. Radiat. Oncol. Biol. Phys.* **15**, 1447–1452.

Komaki R, Wadler S, Peters T *et al.* (1992) High dose local irradiation plus prophylactic hepatic irradiation and chemotherapy for inoperable adenocarcinoma of the pancreas. A preliminary report of a multiinstitutional trial (radiation therapy oncology group protocol 8801) *Cancer* **69**, 2807–2812.

Lawrence T, Tesser R & ten Haken R (1990) An application of dose volume histograms to the treatment of intrahepatic malignancies with radiation therapy. *Int. J. Radiat. Oncol. Biol. Phys.* **19**, 1041–1047.

Lawrence T, Dworzanin L, Walkers-Andrews S *et al.* (1991) Treatment of cancers involving the liver and porta hepatis with external beam irradiation and intraarterial hepatic fluorodeoxyuridine. *Int. J. Radiat. Oncol. Biol. Phys.* **20**, 555–561.

Lightdale C, Wasser J & Coleman M (1979) *Cancer* **43**, 174.

Miller R, Bukowski R, Andresen S & Gahbauer R (1988) Phase 3 evaluation of sequential hepatic artery infusion of 5-fluorouracil and hepatic irradiation in metastatic colorectal carcinoma. *J. Surg. Oncol.* **37**, 1–4.

Minsky B & Leibel S (1989) The treatment of hepatic metastases from colorectal cancer with radiation therapy alone or combined with chemotherapy or misonidazole. *Cancer Treat. Rev.* **16**, 213–216.

Muller J & Rossier D (1951) *Acta Radiol. (Stockh.)* **35**, 449.

Order S, Klein J, Leicher P *et al.* (1986) Radiolabelled antibody treatment of primary and metastatic liver malignancies. *Rec. Adv. Cancer Res.* **100**, 307–314.

Raoul J, Bourguet P, Bretagne J *et al.* (1988) Hepatic artery injection of I-131-labelled lipiodol. Part 1. Biodistribution study results in patients with hepatocellular carcinoma and liver metastases. *Radiology* **168**, 541–545.

Rubin P (ed) (1975) In: *Radiation Biology and Radiation Pathology Syllabus*. pp. 59–75. Chicago: Waverly Press.

Stillwagon G, Order S, Guse C *et al.* (1989) 194 hepatocellular cancers treated by radiation and chemotherapy combinations; toxicity and response; a radiation therapy oncology group study. *Int. J. Radiat. Oncol. Biol. Phys.* **17**, 1223–1229.

Stribley KV, Gray BN,. Chmiel R, Heggie JCP & Bennett RC (1982) Internal radiotherapy for hepatic metastases; the blood supply of hepatic metastases. *J. Surg. Res.* **33**, 25–32.

Webber B, Solderberg C & Leone L (1978) *Cancer* **42**, 1087.

Wiley A, Wirtanen G, Mehta M, Ramirez G & Shahabi S (1988) Treatment of probable subclinical liver metastases and gross pancreatic carcinoma with hepatic artery 5-fluorouracil and radiation therapy. *Acta Oncol.* **27**, 377–381.

Wiley A, Wirtanen G, Stephensen A, Ramirez G, Demets D & Lee J (1989) Combined hepatic artery 5-flouorouracil and irradiation of liver metastases. A randomised study. *Cancer* **64**, 1783–1789.

Yoo H, Lee J, Kim K *et al.* (1991) Nodular hepatocellular carcinoma. Treatment with subsegmental intraarterial injection of iodine 131-labelled iodised oil. *Cancer* **68**, 1878–1884.

12

Cryotherapy

I Hepatic cryosurgery: technical considerations

Gary M. Onik

In the USA alone, 150 000 cases of colorectal carcinoma are diagnosed each year. Over 60 000 patients per year will die of this disease, approximately half from hepatic metastatic disease. While it is still controversial whether systemic chemotherapy affects survival, only surgical resection has been shown to offer long-term disease-free survival in up to 30% of patients (Scheele, 1993). Unfortunately, since surgical techniques are limited in dealing with multiple metastases involving both lobes or metastases adjacent to major vascular structures, there is only a small group of patients with hepatic metatases who are candidates for resection (Foster, 1984).

Cryosurgery, a treatment in which tumours are frozen and then left *in situ* to be resorbed, has an advantage in that it is a focal treatment which can spare more normal liver tissue than resection. This allows multiple lesions affecting both lobes of the liver to be treated. In addition, because major vessels with flowing blood in them protect themselves from cryosurgery, tumours adjacent to these vessels can be treated without sacrificing this vasculature.

Although the possible advantages of hepatic cryosurgery were recognized very early, the application of this procedure was limited due to the poor monitoring of the freezing process. Recent advances in the intraoperative ultrasound (IOUS) monitoring of hepatic cryosurgery have now made the wider application of this modality feasible. IOUS has solved the major problems associated with monitoring hepatic cryosurgery – identifying the tumour, even deep within the hepatic parenchyma, and its relationship to vascular structures; guiding placement of the cryosurgical probes exactly into the lesions; and documenting the cryosurgical margin by visualizing the freezing. With the aid of this new technical advance, it has been shown that by applying cryosurgery, long-term survival in both primary and metastatic hepatic malignances can be achieved in previously unresectable tumours (Onik *et al.*, 1991a, 1991b; Cady *et al.*, 1992; Zhou *et al.*, 1992). In this section we will review the technical considerations associated with hepatic cryosurgery.

Patient selection

While patient selection for hepatic cryosurgery is dealt with later in this chapter, two areas of patient selection that have a direct effect on technique, the number of lesions treated and the treatment of lesions adjacent to major vessels, will be discussed here.

Based on data that are available from surgical series showing a decreased efficacy of resection in patients with more than three lesions, some authors limit to three or fewer the number of lesions they will treat with hepatic cryosurgery (Ravikumar *et al.*, 1991). At this time, we differ in this view in that these data may not hold the same validity for hepatic cryosurgery due to the inherent difference between resection and cryosurgery and the way the body must deal with the healing process of both.

Since cryosurgery does not denature cellular proteins that are then left *in situ* to be resorbed, hepatic cryosurgery may have immunological implications different from a simple resection.

Enough immunological evidence exists justifying the development of a surgical series to see if the data for cryosurgery differ from that for resection regarding lesion number and its effect on survival.

Animal studies by Jacob *et al.* (1984) have shown that animals treated with cryosurgery had increased survival due to appearance of less metastatic disease then those animals treated with resection. Also a recent study by Bayjoo *et al.* (1991) demonstrated increased natural killer (NK) cell activity in those animals exposed to hepatic cryosurgery. If valid in the human patient population, it is possible that patients with larger numbers of lesions could possibly gain some benefit from cryosurgery due to an additional immunological effect.

For this reason we have treated patients with more than three hepatic lesions to determine the feasibility of the procedure in this patient population. At this point our initial data indicate that the number of lesions treated has no effect on the outcome of hepatic cryosurgery. Of 68 patients with greater than 6 months follow-up who fell within our protocol, 20 patients have no evidence for disease at this time and are in complete remission. Of these patients, 10 had more than three lesions treated (mean 7.4 lesions) with a mean follow-up of 18.7 months, and 10 had three or fewer lesions treated (mean 1.6 lesions) with a follow-up of 12.3 months. When the 22 patients who died were examined, 11 had more than three lesions (mean lesions 5.7) with a mean survival of 21.6 months, and an identical 11 patients had three lesions or fewer (mean 1.9 lesions) with a mean survival of 20.9 months (Table 12.1).

Table 12.1 Effects of number of lesions treated on outcome of hepatic cryosurgery

	Number of lesions treated	
	Three or less	Four or more
No evidence of disease	10	10
Mean follow-up (months)	12.3	18.7
Mean number of lesions	1.6	7.4
Patients dead	11	11
Mean survival (months)	21.6	20.9
Mean number of lesions	1.9	5.7

Until further follow-up statistics are obtained, we would have to conclude that the number of lesions treated has virtually no effect on the results of hepatic cryosurgery. The decision on whether multiple lesions are treated therefore lies with the technical factors concerning the feasibility in freezing multiple lesions. Following this philosophy, we have done as many as 12 lesions in certain patients.

The location of lesions has no effect on our decision as to whether or not to treat a patient. We have found that with improved placement techniques that will be described later in this chapter, and the development of small 3 mm cryoprobes with significant freezing capacity, lesions virtually anywhere in the liver can be safely approached and treated. It has been written by some investigators that patients with lesions adjacent to major vessels should be excluded from having cryosurgery due to the heating effect of the vessel protecting the adjacent tumour. We have evidence, however, that

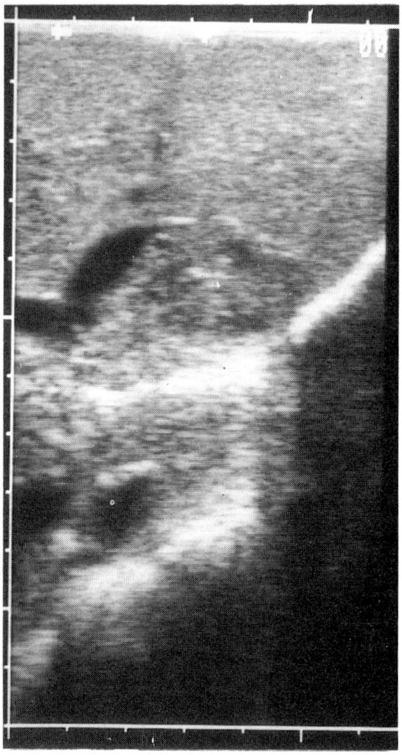

Figure 12.1(a) Intraoperative ultrasound showing a 1 cm lesion adjacent to the confluence of the middle and left hepatic veins. It was felt that this vein would be sacrificed at operation; since the patient had had a previous right lobectomy, he would be placed at significant risk of hepatic insufficiency. The lesion was sandwiched in between two flat cryoprobes and frozen.

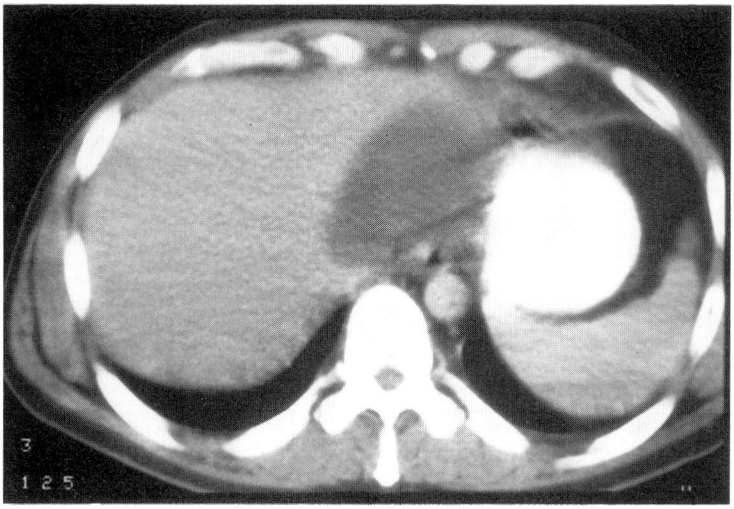

Figure 12.1(b) Postoperative computed tomographic scan shows a large hypodense lesion with sharp margins and no evidence for contrast infiltration into the area, indicating a complete lack of blood flow to the cryolesion.

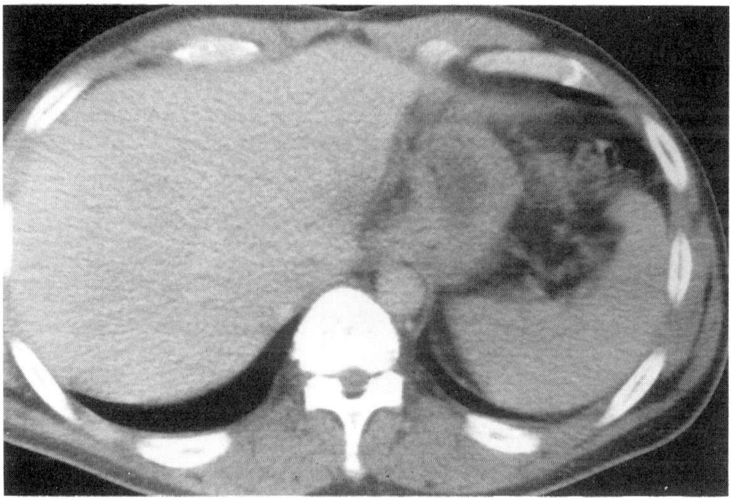

Figure 12.1(c) One year later, the lesion has resolved. Computed tomographic guided biopsy of the region showed residual fibrosis.

patients with lesions on major vascular structures, such as the inferior vena cava, can be successfully treated and are excellent candidates for cryosurgery (Fig. 12.1). These patients often have favourable tumour biology (a solitary lesion), but in a difficult location, making them unresectable.

We have found that successful cryosurgical treatment of tumours on vessels, however, requires that certain technical factors be addressed. First, the cryoprobes should be placed as close to the vessel as possible, preferably no more than 5 mm from the vessel in order to obtain as steep a cooling gradient as possible. Our animal data indicate that, when this is done, temperatures can reach as low as −65°C adjacent to the wall of the vessel, clearly consistent with tumoricidal temperatures. Second, near the vessel wall larger probes (8 mm in diameter) when possible should be

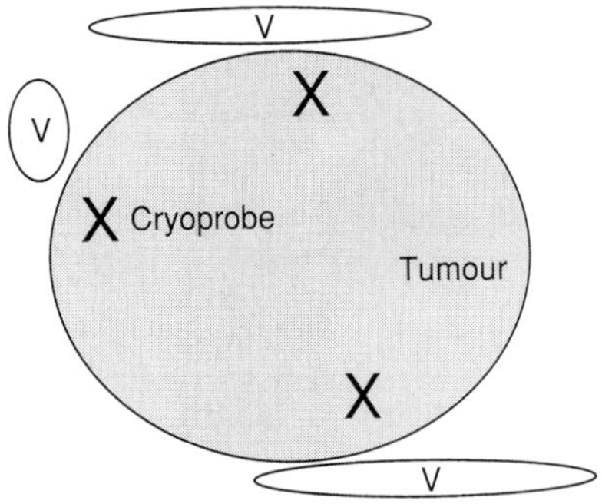

Figure 12.2 Probe placements for a tumour surrounded by multiple vessels (V). Since a very steep cooling gradient is needed near vessels to overcome the heating effect of blood within the vessel, at times multiple probes need to be placed, even though the size of the tumour might dictate fewer probes.

placed due to their greater cooling surface area and capacity. Last, multiple probes should be placed in an array through the tumour volume to compensate for the greater blood flow in the area adjacent to a vessel (Fig. 12.2). By following these principles and using improved placement techniques and cryosurgical systems with multiple probes and greater freezing capacity, excellent results can be obtained in these patients.

Technique of hepatic cryosurgery

Hepatic cryosurgery is generally done through a right subcostal incision that can be extended across the midline, adding a left subcostal incision if needed. This incision gives access to all areas of the liver, including the posterolateral aspect of the right lobe. The dome of the liver should be cleared of all adhesions so that the ultrasound probe can be placed over the dome. The ligamentous attachments of the liver should be taken down if necessary to rotate the liver to gain access to lesions in the lateral and posterior aspect of the right lobe. Access and control of the hepatic artery and portal vein should be obtained to facilitate in-flow occlusion needed to increase the efficacy of freezing. After the abdomen has been assessed for any evidence of extrahepatic tumour spread, an IOUS of the liver is obtained. Since intraoperative hepatic ultrasound and its considerations are so integral to the procedure of hepatic cryosurgery, they will be considered here.

Intraoperative ultrasound

IOUS has been shown to be a very valuable adjunct to hepatic surgery. Ultrasound's portability and real-time capabilities have brought modern cross-sectional imaging capabilities to the operating room. While external ultrasound has been found to be an insensitive modality for finding hepatic lesions, IOUS has been shown to be the most sensitive imaging modality for finding the extent of hepatic malignant disease. This difference is due to the fact that IOUS does not have to penetrate the marked sound-attenuating characteristics of skin and subcutaneous fat, allowing higher-frequency transducers to be used, which leads to finding smaller lesions. IOUS is a valuable adjunct to the surgeon by:

1. Allowing him or her to find non-palpable lesions (Fig. 12.3) not indicated by previous imaging studies; the surgeon can then map the relationship of these tumours to the hepatic vasculature. IOUS has been found to be 20% more sensitive than computed

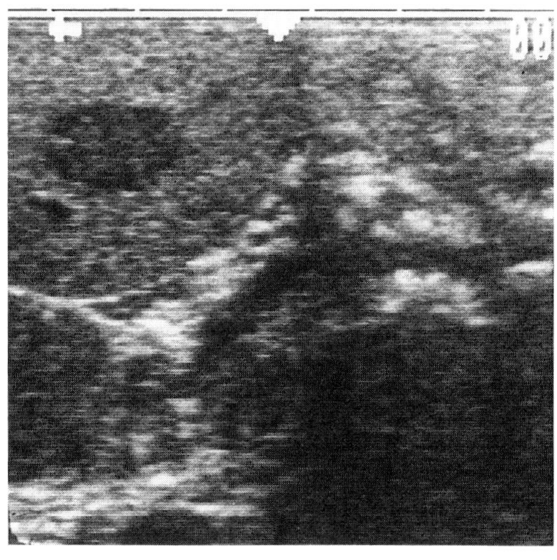

Figure 12.3 A hypoechoic hepatic metastasis is noted in the very centre of the lateral segment of the left lobe of the liver. This lesion was not seen by preoperative imaging (which is notoriously inaccurate in the lateral segment of the left lobe because of motion artefact caused by the heart). This lesion was also non-palpable.

tomographic (CT) portography in finding tumours (Clark *et al.*, 1989).
2. IOUS allows us a complete characterization of lesions at operation; for example, differentiating a cyst from a solid lesion too small to be fully characterized by CT portography or external ultrasound.
3. As with other cross-section imaging modalities, IOUS allows exact stereotaxic placement of needles for intraoperative biopsies. This is particularly important when IOUS indicates that the lesion appears atypical.
4. Ultrasound allows guidance of specific therapies intraoperatively, including resection, by better characterizing the operability of lesions, guiding ETOH injections and now guiding cryosurgical probe placement. In this chapter we will discuss the technical considerations of IOUS.

Technical considerations/IOUS

Ultrasound equipment/machine

The type of ultrasound machine used for IOUS is dictated by a number of factors. One of the most important is cost. Sophisticated ultrasound units with colour Doppler capabilities can be as expensive as a quarter of a million dollars, and such a machine is usually not feasible for dedicated operating room use. There are, however, now excellent quality machines with sophisticated processing capabilities designed specifically for operating room use. In general, because of the added flexibility, the instrument used should have electronic probe capabilities rather than mechanical probes. We prefer the Aloka 650 unit, which is relatively inexpensive, has the ability to change focal zones, and has a feature in which all the frequencies of a given probe are listened for and processed, enhancing the imaging characteristics of the probe.

Unfortunately, no single ultrasound transducer fits all the characteristics needed to do an adequate IOUS examination of the liver; therefore the machine you use is determined in part by what probes are available with it. One of the most basic relationships concerning ultrasound physics that must be understood is how the frequency of the ultrasound transducer relates to the resolution and the depth of penetration of the sound beam. The lower the frequency of the transducer, the greater the depth of penetration of the transducer; the lower the resolution of the transducer, however. As the frequency of the transducer increases, the resolution increases; conversely, the ability of the sound to penetrate the liver decreases. For this reason, no ultrasound transducer fits all situations within the liver. We suggest the following transducers for an adequate IOUS visualization:

1. A 3.5 or 5 MHz convex array probe. This visualizes lesions over 1 cm well, while giving an excellent overview of the lesion's relationship to intrahepatic structures. This type of view is important in planning probe placement routes to tumours as well as the approach to resections (Fig. 12.4).
2. A 5 MHz linear array transducer arranged in a T configuration with the cable perpendicular to the transducer head. This allows visualization of lesions over the dome of the liver and has better resolution in the far field than the convex array transducers. This, however, gives a more limited view of the liver and is less advantageous in gaining an overall feel for the anatomy in relationship to the pathology. This transducer is also the best for monitoring the freezing process during cryosurgery, since it gives the most accurate depiction of the ice ball.
3. A biplane transrectal probe with a 7.5 MHz linear array transducer and a 5 MHz sector

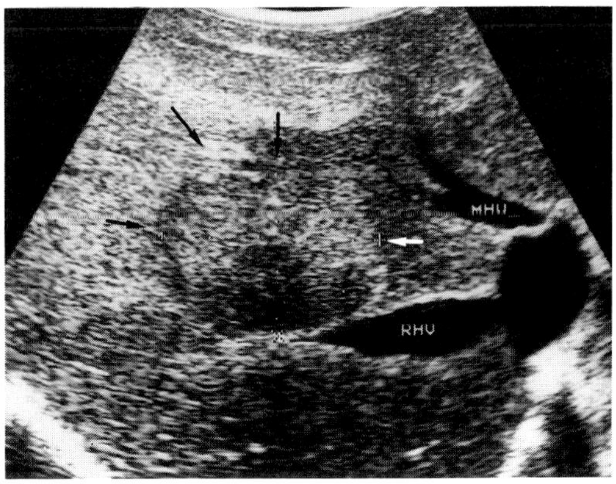

Figure 12.4 An intraoperative ultrasound generated by a 3.5 MHz convex array ultrasound probe shows a wide-angle view of the liver, giving an excellent representation of a lesion's placement within the liver (arrow), especially in relationship to hepatic vascular anatomy. MHV = middle hepatic vein; RHV = right hepatic vein.

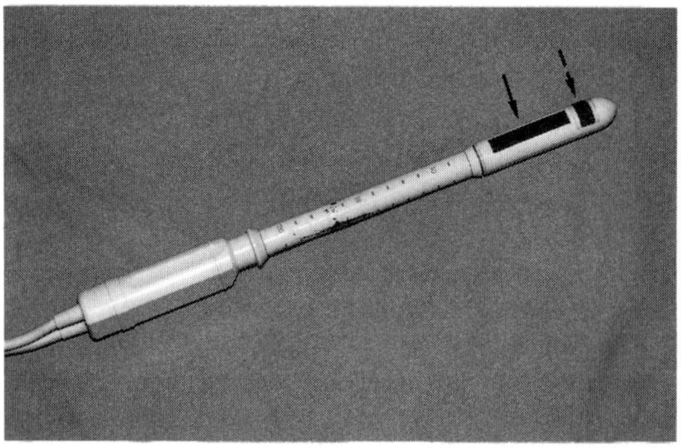

Figure 12.5 A biplane transrectal ultrasound probe that is excellent for use with hepatic cryosurgery. A linear array gives a longitudinal view of the liver (black arrow). The sector transducer built into the probe gives a right-angle axial view to the linear array probe (broken arrow).

scanner. This transducer, using the 7.5 MHz linear array, allows visualization of very small lesions not visible with either of the other two transducers. Since this transducer has limited depth penetration, however, the liver must be viewed from both above and below. Because of its biplane arrangement, this is an excellent transducer for guiding placement of needles for biopsy and cryoprobe placement (Fig. 12.5).

Technique

One of the most important factors in accomplishing a good IOUS is to orient the image correctly on the screen. The convention used with ultrasound is the same as that used for CT and magnetic resonance imaging (MRI) scans. In an axial slice, the upper half of the slice is viewed, with the right being to the left of the screen. The image should be such that if the undersurface of the liver is being scanned, the sound beams should be oriented as coming from the bottom of the screen.

Once the screen is properly oriented, the gain should be set. The gain should be set to its highest level without producing false echoes within major vascular structures. Once the overall gain is set, the time gain compensation (TGC) curve is adjusted. This setting gives the image its uniformity, with greater listening capacity being generated in the deeper portions of the liver where the sound beam is most attenuated.

So that findings are not missed, the liver should be scanned in a consistent fashion. The scanning can start in the lateral segment of the left lobe of the liver and can progress to the right lobe of the liver. The caudate lobe should have special note taken of it since it is easy to miss lesions in this region.

It is useful at times to fill the upper abdomen with warm saline, with the patient placed in a Trendelenburg position. This allows a better viewing of surface lesion due to the stand-off of the water, placing the surface of the liver more in the focal zone of the transducer, as well as allowing the curves of the lateral aspect of the liver to be better viewed. When necessary, the focal zone of the transducer can be changed while searching for lesions in various portions of the liver. This is particularly useful when viewing areas deep within the liver.

It is important to scan both the upper surface and the undersurface of the liver with the 7.5 MHz transducer, looking for small lesions. The undersurface must also be viewed due to the limited depth penetration of the 7.5 MHz probe. Occasionally lesions will only be seen from the undersurface of the liver, particularly in the region of the falciform ligament where placement of the probe directly on the falciform ligament very often results in shadowing and an inability to see beneath that region.

It is very often useful to combine palpation of the liver with your free hand while viewing the ultrasound. This technique helps confirm a lesion in a region where something abnormal has been palpated. It can also localize the approximate position of the lesion in relationship to the surface of the liver, particularly in the posterolateral aspects of the liver. Palpation can also determine whether a lesion is separate from a vessel. This can be particularly important along the inferomedial aspect of the liver where lesions can appear to be adjacent to the inferior vena cava, but actually are separated by a cleavage plane.

Appearances of metastatic lesions on intraoperative ultrasound are variable. They may appear to be hyper-, hypo- or isoechoic. A good rule to follow, however, is that all the metastatic lesions in one patient should have the same characteristics – if one metastatic lesion is hypoechoic, all of them should be. When one lesion is different, it should raise the suspicion that perhaps the pathology of that lesion is different, prompting biopsy confirmation of the atypical lesion.

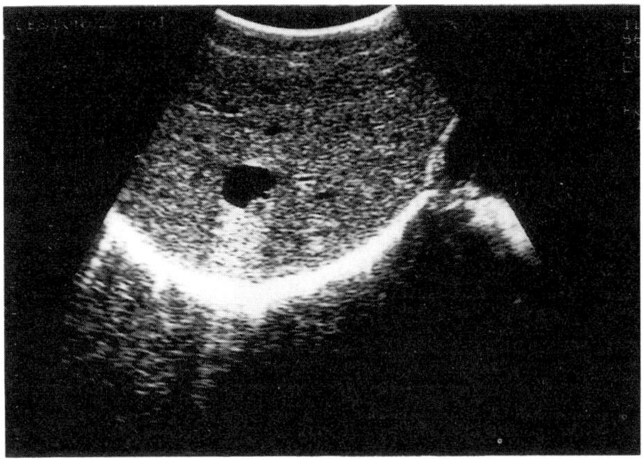

Figure 12.6 Intraoperative ultrasound showing a simple cyst. The ultrasound characteristics of a simple cyst are noted. The cyst has no internal echoes, an imperceptible wall, and increased through-sound transmission. When these characteristics are found, biopsy or aspiration of the cyst is unnecessary.

The most difficult situation encountered during an IOUS is one in which the metastatic lesion's echogenicity is isoechoic with the normal liver, making differentiation of the tumour from the normal liver extremely difficult. In these circumstances indirect signs indicating a lesion must be used, such as a disordered echogenic pattern and displacement of vessels.

Since the IOUS appearance of malignant lesions is non-specific, the only reliable differentiation of a benign lesion from a possibly malignant one is that of a simple cyst from a more complex lesion, simple cysts showing no internal echoes, an imperceptible wall, and increased through-sound transmission (Fig. 12.6). One must be careful since very small cysts can appear to have echoes within them due to the partial volume-averaging of the adjacent liver, also viewed within the thickness of the scan slice. Cystic metastases can occur but can usually be differentiated from simple cysts by their thick irregular wall.

Planning the route to the lesion

After the IOUS has identified the lesions and biopsies of suspicious lesions are obtained, the route that the cryoprobes will take to each lesion is planned. The factors that go into deciding what route to take include a number of considerations:

1. Rather than taking the shortest route possible to a lesion, in general, normal liver should be traversed by the cryoprobe on its way to the lesion, even when the lesion is easily accessible on the surface. Making a tract through normal liver to get to the lesion has two positive effects. If a vessel is injured by the cryoprobe, having a tract through normal liver allows the tract to be plugged, tamponading and controlling the bleeding. In the only case in which we have injured a vessel due to the placement of a cryoprobe (we placed a cryoprobe into the main right hepatic vein approximately 1.5 cm from its origin), the fact that we had traversed approximately 5 cm of normal liver to reach the region of the tumour enabled us to plug the tract and avoid a major catastrophe.

   Another reason not to stick surface lesions directly is that when freezing extends to the surface of the liver round the insertion site, stellate cracks occur in the liver around the cryoprobe. Placing the cryoprobes through normal liver into tumours that abut the surface of the liver prevents the need to freeze the liver surface at the cryoprobe insertion. This arkedly decreases the incidence and significance of the hepatic cracking.
2. The route to the lesion should be planned so that if the cryoprobe is inadvertently pushed too far past the lesion, other structures are

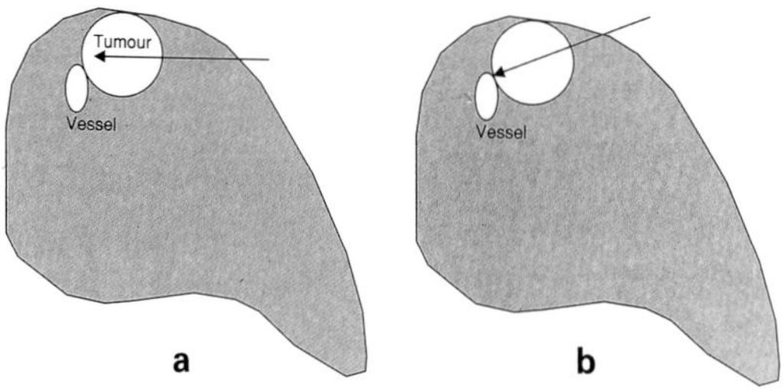

Figure 12.7 Correct path (a) through lesion to avoid having vessel in the trajectory, if the probe inadvertently extends beyond lesion. Incorrect path (b).

not injured by the cryoprobe, particularly vessels (Fig. 12.7).

3. The location of the lesion dictates the approach that must be taken as well. For instance, lesions in the dome of the liver near the origin of the hepatic veins are usually best approached through the anterior portion of the liver. If needed, even multiple probes can be placed in this way. This approach avoids a direct stick to these lesions, obviating the need to control cracking and cryoprobe lacerations in a region which is difficult to visualize.

Lesions behind the inferior vena cava are best handled by removing the posterior ligamentous attachments of the liver, rotating the right lobe of the liver anteriorly, and then placing cryoprobes along the posterior axis of the liver through normal liver into the tumour behind the inferior vena cava (Fig. 12.8).

Lesions in the caudate lobe are best handled by exposing the caudate by elevating the left lobe of the liver, working through the plane of the fissure for the ligamentum venosum and then sticking the lesions on an oblique angle so that the cryoprobe can extent slightly beyond the lesion without injuring the inferior vena cava. We found lesions in this region to be particularly difficult to deal with.

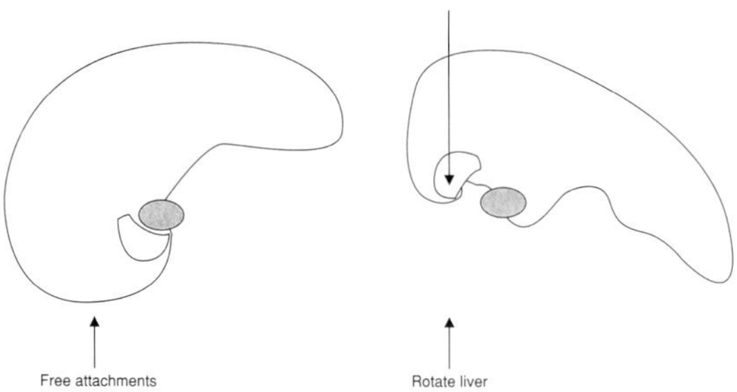

Figure 12.8 Rotation of the liver leftwards, allowing safe placement of a probe behind the inferior vena cava.

Lesions in the posterior inferior right lobe of the liver can be difficult to deal with due to main portal branches limiting anterior access to the tumour. These lesions are best handled by ultrasounding the liver from the undersurface and placing probes through the undersurface of the liver, sometimes just beneath the main portal branches.

Lesions between the hepatic veins are difficult to deal with due to the fact that the lesion is surrounded on three sides by major vascular structures. In general these lesions should be approached through a significant amount of liver to create a good tract in case a vessel is injured, but whenever possible, an approach should be taken so that if the probe is pushed too far, it will not injure a vessel. At times this is not possible in this situation (similar to caudate lesions). Great care has to be taken in the probe placement (Fig. 12.9).

Use of a biplane transrectal ultrasound probe in the placement of the cryoprobe

The results of hepatic cryosurgery are determined by the biological behaviour of the tumour as well as the technical success of the procedure, which includes the identification of the full extent of disease, the accurate placement of the cryoprobes and the confirmation of an adequate cryosurgical margin. In the past, the placement of cryoprobes has used the traditional inplane biopsy guides associated with both sector and linear array ultrasound probes. These inplane biopsy guides are known to have significant limitations in placement accuracy and needle visualization. Due to the fact that the scan thickness of ultrasound transducers is approximately 1 cm in thickness, biopsy guides that place needles parallel to the sound beam are inherently inaccurate. A needle whose length falls anywhere within the scan plane thickness can appear the same on the ultrasound picture (Fig. 12.10). Because of this phenomenon, deviations in the needle trajectory that fall inside the scan plane can cause major inaccuracies without being recognizable. It becomes necessary, therefore, to confirm

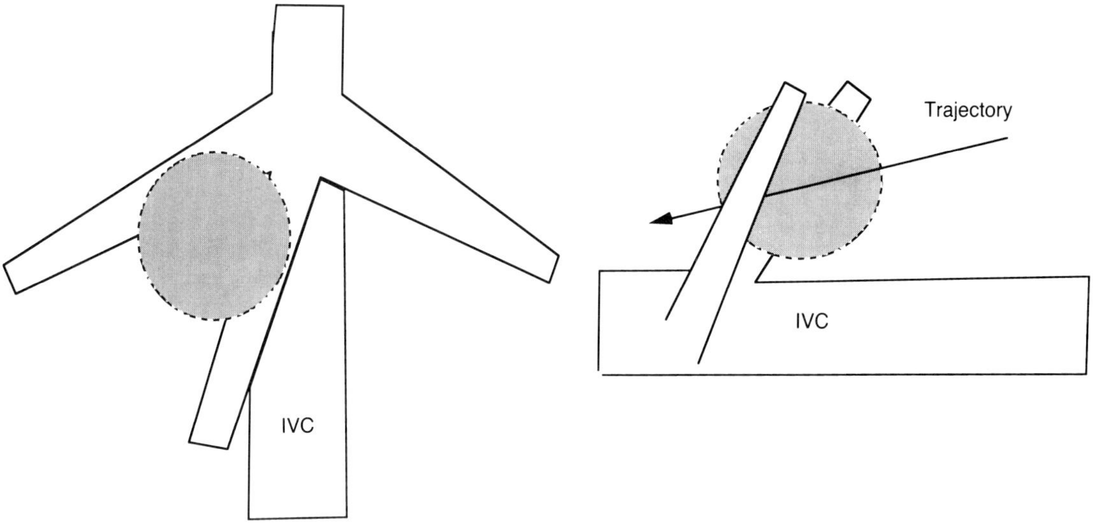

Figure 12.9 Approach to lesions between the hepatic veins. A hepatic lesion is shown between the right and middle hepatic veins. The trajectory of the needle is shown so that, if the cryoprobe extends beyond the lesion, major vascular structures are not injured. IVC = Inferior vena cava.

needle placements in a plane perpendicular to the original scan plane.

Another complicating fact in confirming needle placement is that needles are notoriously difficult to see during ultrasound placement, particularly when parallel to the sound beam. The traditional 30° angle which most biopsy guides use is suboptimal, due to the oblique angle at which the sound hits the needle (Fig. 12.11). The result of this oblique angle is that fewer echoes are reflected back directly to the transducer. This angle becomes an even greater problem when larger pointed cryoprobes are placed. Due to shadowing of the ultrasound beam when hitting metal, the position of the tip of the cryoprobe becomes obscured. Using this guidance system, this phenomenon can make deep placement of large cryoprobes near major vascular structures dangerous, particularly when depth of placement is a critical factor.

Recently the advantages of the use of a biplane *transrectal* ultrasound probe with both the longitudinal linear array and sector (axial) scanning capabilities incorporated into one probe have been noted greatly to increase accurate placement of cryoprobes. The longitudinal view with the linear transducer provides excellent depth perception of the placement due to the perpendicular arrangement of the sound beam to the needle, allowing exact recognition of the tip of the cryoprobe (Fig. 12.12a). The axial sector scan then confirms that the needle has been placed into the centre of the tumour in the xy plane (Fig. 12.12b).

This transrectal ultrasound probe has a 4 cm long linear array transducer aligned with the long axis of the probe. A separate transducer built into the tip of the probe provides an axial view of the liver at right angles to this linear array probe. The linear array is a 7.5 MHz transducer, and the sector scanner is 5 MHz.

The transrectal probe is used to guide the cryoprobes into the lesions. The 7.5 MHz linear array transducer is first used to guide the introduction needle safely through the liver, avoiding major vessels. An approximation of the correct plane of cryoprobe placement is obtained by visualizing the lesion in its greatest sagittal diameter in this longitudinal view. The needle or probe is then placed along the longitudinal plane of the transducer. The needle or cryoprobe can be guided freehand or with a biopsy guide attached to the transducer. During the needle insertion along the longitudinal plane, periodic switching to the axial view ensures that the needle is being placed correctly in the *xy* plane. Once the cryoprobe or introduction needle is placed into the lesion in the longitudinal plane, the axial view must be checked to note whether the needle is actually in the centre of the lesion. When the needle is confirmed to be in the centre of the lesion, the

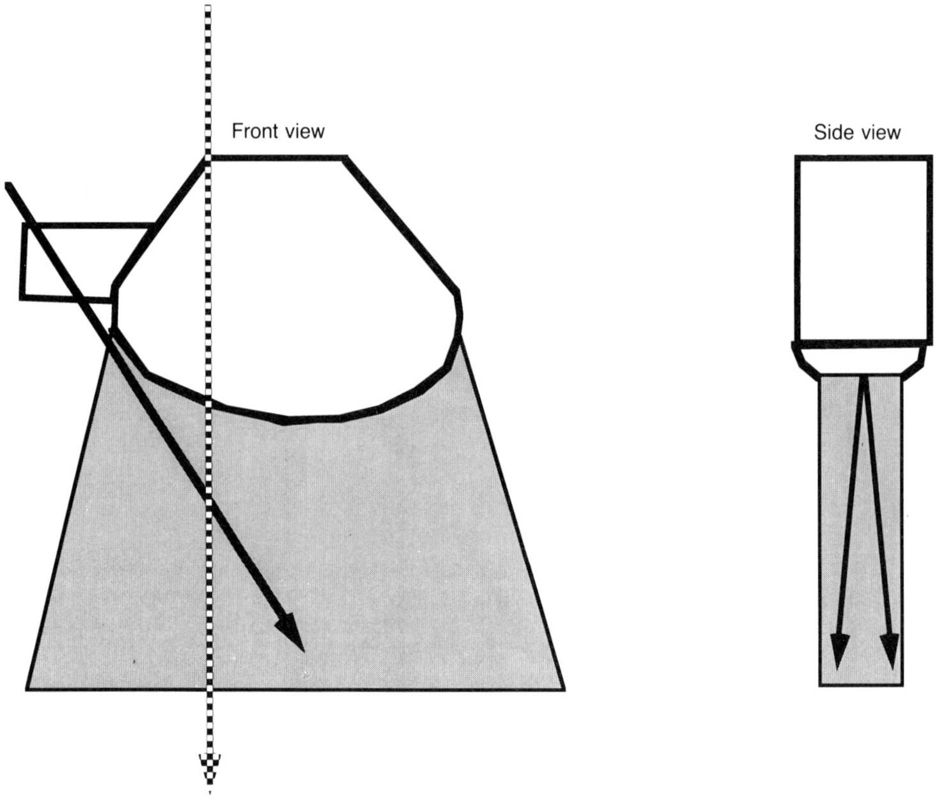

Figure 12.10 Deficiencies of an in-plane biopsy guide. Due to the fact that the scan has a certain thickness to needle trajectories in opposite directions, both within the scan plane appear exactly the same on the ultrasound. Only an ultrasound perpendicular to this scan plane can discern the difference.

longitudinal linear array transducer is used for the final depth of placement of the needle or probe.

This transrectal probe has an additional advantage in that the 7.5 MHz linear array transducer has a high resolution; and it is not unusual, due to this increased resolution, to find small lesions, 5–6 mm in diameter, that were not seen with 3.5 and 5 MHz transducers. Because of its lack of depth penetration, however, both the under- and over-surface of the liver must usually be surveyed using this transducer.

Introduction system for use in hepatic cryosurgery

The accurate placement of multiple relatively large cryoprobes deep within the hepatic parenchyma near major vascular structures has been problematic, even with the use of the biplane probe just described. The increased risk of cryoprobe placement in these situations has limited the application of the procedure. A recently developed introduction system, however, for cryoprobe placement that uses a modified Seldinger technique minimizes hepatic trauma while ensuring accurate cryoprobe placement.

The introduction system (Cook, Bloomington, Indiana) consists of an 18-gauge, 15-cm-long Teflon-coated trocar pointed needle, a 30-cm long 0.038 in, 1.5 mm J-tipped wire with a non-tapered mandril, and a one-step Teflon dilator sheath of various sizes to accommodate the appropriate cryoprobe (Fig. 12.13). The first step of the procedure involves the placement of the 18-gauge needle within the tumour (Fig. 12.14a). The needle tip is brought approximately 1 cm past the tumour's most posterior aspect. The central trocar is removed,

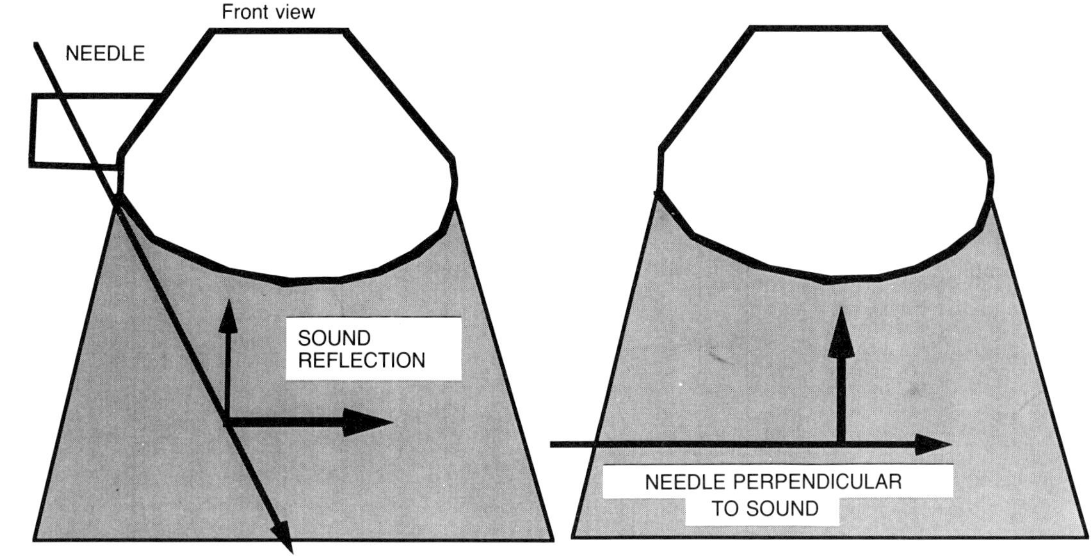

Figure 12.11 The effect of the angle of needle placement in relationship to the sound beam. When a needle is placed at an oblique angle to the sound beam, most sound is reflected in directions other than back to the transducer. This makes these needles very hard to see. A needle placed perpendicular to the sound beam, however, reflects most sound back to the transducer, making it less difficult.

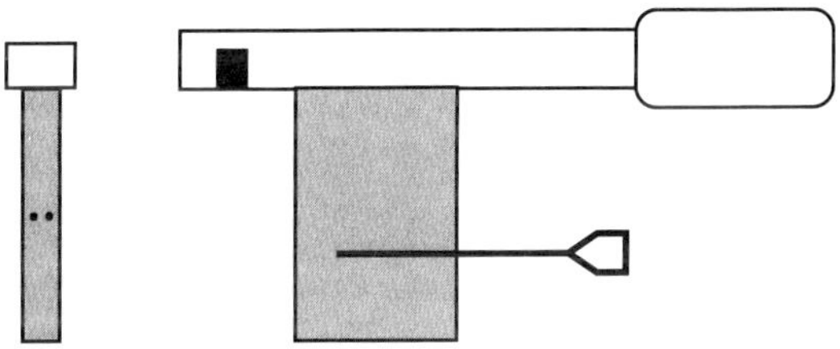

Figure 12.12(a) The longitudinal linear array transducer, when aligned parallel to the placement of the needle, shows the tip of the needle and therefore the depth of placement extremely accurately. The exact xy position of the needle when in the sound beam, however, cannot be exactly known. Both needle positions shown here give the same ultrasound appearance.

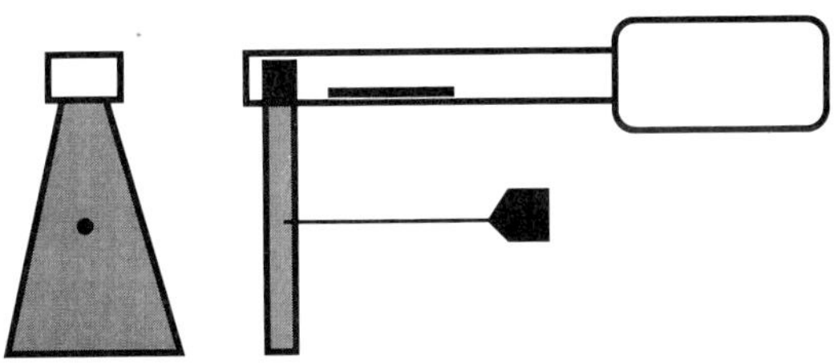

Figure 12.12(b) In order to gain the exact position in the xy plane of the tip of the needle, the axial scan needs to be used.

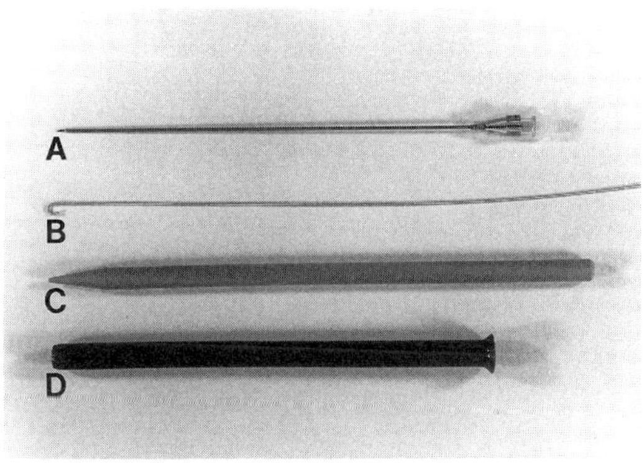

Figure 12.13 An introduction set. (A) An 18-gauge trocar pointed needle is shown. It is covered with a Teflon coating to increase its echogenicity. (B) A 30 cm long 0.038 inch wire is shown with a 1.5 mm J tip to it. The inner mandril of the wire is non-tapered and extends to the beginning of the curve of the J tip. (C) A dilator made of Teflon is shown. The dilator slips over the wire once it is in position. The sheath (D) slips over the dilator and after removing the dilator the cryoprobe is placed through the sheath.

and the 0.038 in wire is introduced into the needle until the J protrudes from the needle's end (Fig. 12.14b). The needle is then removed, leaving the wire in place (Fig. 12.14c). The cannula and dilator are then brought over the wire until the tip of the dilator is visualized at the end of the wire (Fig. 12.14d). If needed, this can be confirmed under real-time ultrasound by retracting the wire and noting the opening of the J tip. The cannula is then advanced over the dilator and through the tumour (Fig. 12.14e). The cryoprobe can then be placed through the cannula until it reaches its end (Fig. 12.14f). The cannula is then withdrawn over the cryoprobe until the complete freezing portion of the cryoprobe is exposed. The cryoprobe is activated, and the usual freeze/thaw protocol is started. The unique features of this introduction system include:

1. The echogenically coated needle to improve ultrasound visualization, the needle also having a trocar point which eliminates trajectory deviations, often seen with the use of bevelled needles.
2. The introduction wire's tight J tip minimizes – although does not eliminate – movement of the wire back and forth in the hepatic parenchyma, as the cannula and dilator are advanced over the wire.
3. The non-tapered mandril of the wire minimizes kinking of the wire, particularly when the cannula and dilator are not exactly in line with the wire placement. Our experience with the usual tapered mandril of angiographic wires showed that any error in trajectory of the cannula and dilator results in pulling the wire out of the tumour.

Technical points of note in relationship to the method include:

1. An effort to ensure that the cannula and dilator are placed in the same exact trajectory as the wire, since in soft liver, even with a non-tapered mandril, large trajectory deviations from the original wire placement can still result in bending and kinking of the wire, making passage of the cannula and dilator over the wire impossible.
2. The needle and wire complex should be placed 1 cm past the most posterior aspect of the tumour. This provides a better anchor for the system and assures a good cryosurgical margin on the posterior aspect of the lesion. In addition, it is particularly important to advance the cannula over the dilator completely through the tumour. Failure to do this will result in loss of access to the tumour, particularly in small tumours.
3. When multiple cryoprobes are to be placed through a single lesion or in separate lesions, in general we try to place all the wires first so that the bulkier cryoprobes do not limit the access to the liver and the routes that can be taken. We have found that, once cryoprobes are placed, the use of the ultrasound probe becomes much more difficult, limiting certain trajectories.
4. As opposed to most dilatation procedures that require multiple steps, a one-step dilatation of the cryoprobe tract is possible due to the soft consistency of the liver substance. This one-step dilatation is important because of the inherent instability of the wire placed within the normal liver and tumour tissue. We found that the multiple dilatations resulted in increased bleeding and frequent loss of the correct position of the wire within the tumour.

The multiple benefits of the use of this type of simple introduction system are surprising. The system solved the common problem of having a large pointed cryoprobe deflect off a relatively hard tumour, which occurs when the tumour is not approached in the exactly correct trajectory.

The system also allowed the use of cryoprobes with a much blunter point, helping to minimize potential vessel damage if a placement error occurs. Its use resulted in accurate and safe placement of large cryoprobes deep within liver parenchyma, particularly near major vascular structures, as well as accurate placement of *multiple* cryoprobes in relationship to each other. These advantages enable application of the procedure to a larger patient population. We feel that more accurate cryoprobe placements will ultimately produce superior results due to a willingness to place additional cryoprobes into a lesion to ensure more adequate freezing.

Cryoprobe selection

In general, the selection of the cryoprobes is dictated by the need to have enough freezing capacity to provide a 1 cm cryosurgical margin around the tumour. In order to understand the various determinations of freezing capacity, it is necessary to have at least a basic knowledge of cryoprobe design and cryosurgical equipment.

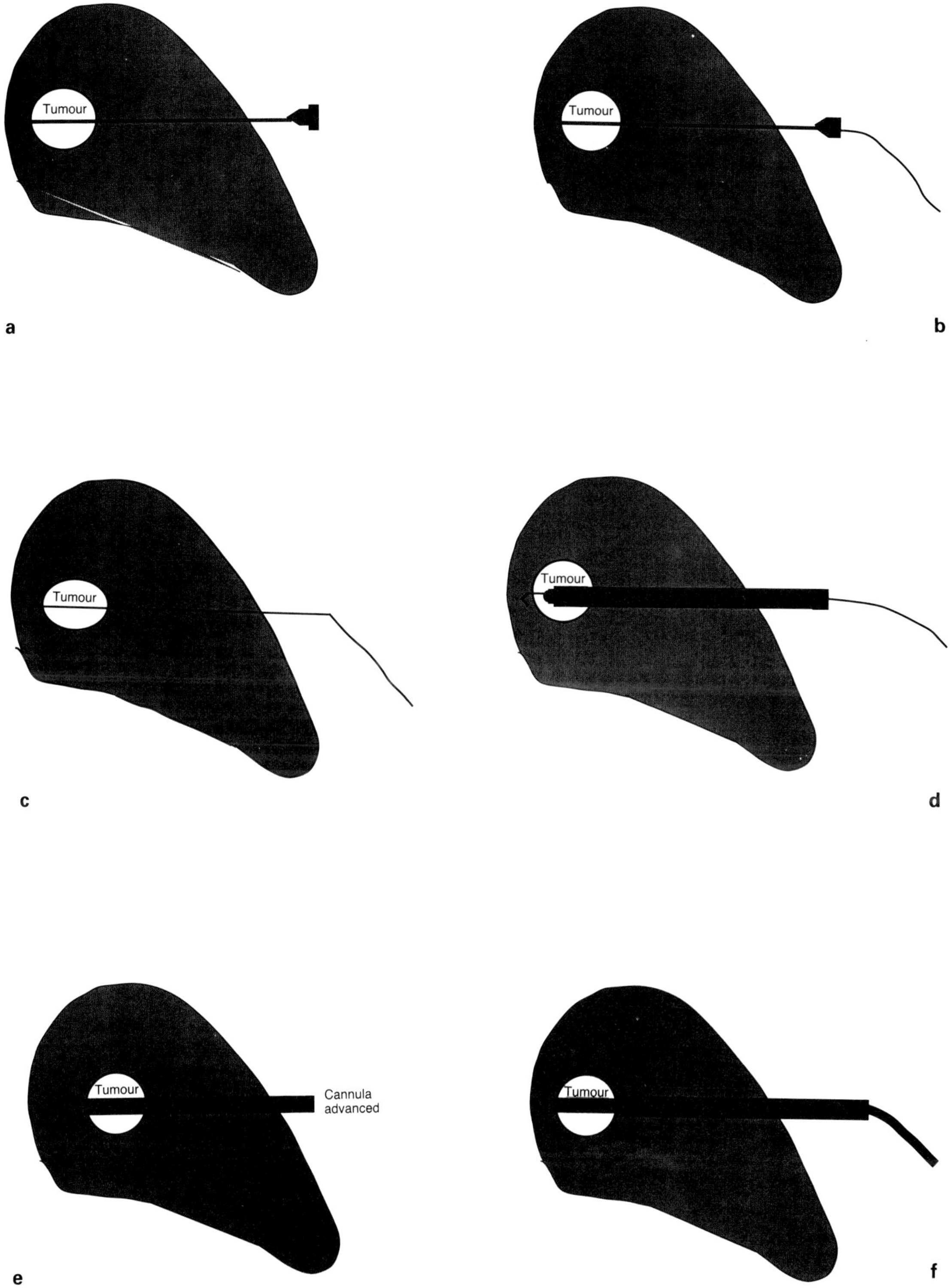

Figure 12.14 The various steps of use of the introduction system. (a) Needle placed; (b) wire placed; (c) needle removed; (d) cannula-dilator over wire; (e) wire/dilator removed; (f) cryoprobe placed.

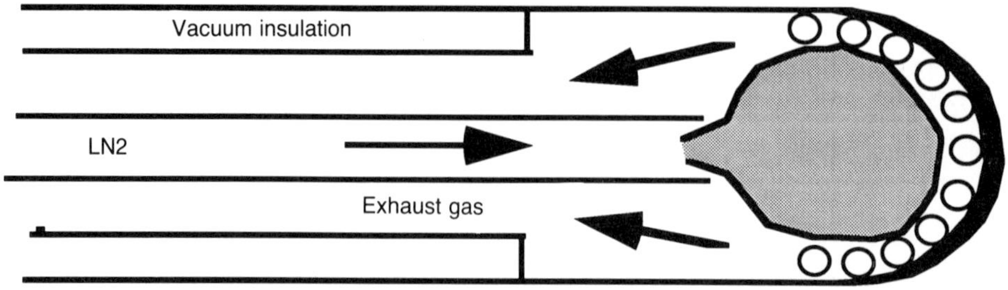

Figure 12.15 Standard cryoprobe design. A supply tube brings the cryogen down to the tip of the cryoprobe. The liquid hits the relatively warm tip metal and turns into a gas. The exhaust gas exits the space around the supply tube and exits the probe. An insulated space between the outside of the cryoprobe and the exhaust space insulates the cryoprobe and prevents freezing of that portion of the probe. Bubbles form a layer of gas between the liquid and the probe at the probe tip, essentially insulating the probe tip from the liquid nitrogen (LN_2) limiting the minimum temperature obtained by the cryoprobe to −16°C. This effect is called the Leidenfrost boiling effect.

The cryoprobe

Modern cryoprobes all have basically the same design: a vacuum-insulated shaft with a variable-sized freezing tip (Fig. 12.15). A central supply tube supplies the cryogen to the tip of the cryoprobe. When the liquid at −196°C hits the relatively warm metal of the tip, a change of phase occurs, turning the liquid into a gas. A layer of gas is then formed between the liquid and the metal of the cryoprobe, effectively insulating the metal of the cryoprobe from the −196° liquid nitrogen temperatures. This phenomen is called the Leidenfrost boiling effect. Because of this effect, the effective tip temperature of cryoprobes using liquid nitrogen at −196°C is approximately −160°. As the liquid is turned into a gas, the exhaust gas flows between the supply tube and the inner tube that creates the space for the vacuum insulation leaving the probe. It should be appreciated that, when the liquid turns into a gas, a marked expansion in volume occurs. A major limitation to the performance of a cryoprobe is the decreased flow of liquid nitrogen that occurs due to the inability of the exhaust gases to escape. For this reason there are many technical problems in developing cryoprobes of a small size. Obviously, the less cryogen that can flow through the cryoprobe, the less freezing capacity that cryoprobe will have.

In general, larger probes can freeze a greater area of tissue, in part due to the increased liquid nitrogen flow available within large probes, as well as the increased surface area in contact with the tissue.

Cryogen

The amount of freezing that can be generated from a cryoprobe is in major part determined by the cryogen used. Cryoprobes using a gas cryogen work on the principle of the Jeule Thompson effect of expanding gases removing heat from the environment. These cryoprobes using carbon dioxide or nitrous oxide are limited in their freezing capacity and will not reach temperatures below −80°C. While they can be used in ophthalmology for cryoretraction, their limited freezing capacity makes them of no value for malignant disease.

Liquid nitrogen is the standard cryogen used for tumour cryosurgery. It is relatively inexpensive and easy to handle; however, as we have discussed, due to its change of phase within the cryoprobe, it is limited in its freezing capacity and the temperature that can be achieved at the probe tip, due to the change of phase of the liquid.

A number of approaches are now being invetigated to increase the freezing capacity of traditional cryosurgical systems. One of these approaches utilizes supercooled liquid nitrogen down to −205°C. This supercooling allows the liquid nitrogen to remove heat without generating a change of phase into a gas. The result is that increased flows of liquid nitrogen through the cryoprobe can occur, and the decrease in gas generation decreases the Leidenfrost boiling effect. This allows a decrease in the size of cryoprobes while still maintaining an excellent cooling capacity. It also may allow more effective cooling from a given size cryoprobe.

Research into the use of other cryogens such as liquid helium is ongoing; this may provide advantages due to its colder temperature.

Multiple probes

Another issue to be dealt with in freezing lesions and choosing the appropriate cryoprobe is the issue of whether multiple cryoprobes need to be used for a particular lesion. It should be realized that a single cryoprobe used multiple times to cover an area is not at all equivalent to multiple cryoprobes placed in the same areas turned on all at once. Multiple applications of a single cryoprobe basically rely on overlapping circles or spheres to cover all areas of the tumour; this invariably leaves tissue between these spheres untreated. Two cryoprobes placed side by side turned on together eliminate those inpouchings of unfrozen tissue (Fig. 12.16). In addition, the temperature profile created between cryoprobes is markedly different when the two are turned on together versus separately. Therefore, when one cryoprobe does not appear to be adequate to provide the 1 cm margin around the tumour, multiple cryoprobes *must* be used simultaneously.

It should be realized that a given cryoprobe will have a maximum ice ball size that it can provide. At some point an equilibrium is established where the amount of heat removed from the ice ball by the cryoprobe is equal to the amount of heat delivered to the area by blood flow, essentially stopping ice ball growth. Therefore, more freezing cannot be obtained by simply leaving a cryoprobe on for a longer period of time. (This can be affected somewhat in in-flow hepatic occlusion.) The overwhelming majority of ice ball growth occurs in the first 15 min of the freeze cycle, and this is in general the standard time we use during our freeze cycles.

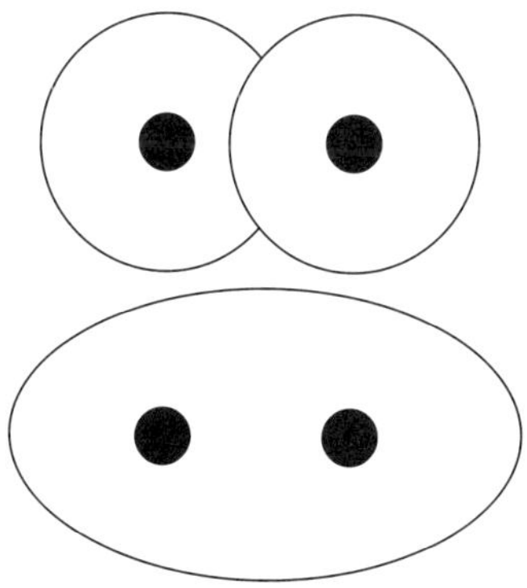

Figure 12.16 The difference between freezing when two cryoprobes that are placed in the same position are frozen together, compared with separately. The inpouching of tissue created by overlapping circles is eliminated when two cryoprobes are placed and turned on simultaneously. This allows sculpture of the ice ball to the shape of the tumour.

Blood flow

The number of cryoprobes needed to destroy a given lesion is somewhat determined by the placement of the tumour in the liver. Central lesions, particularly at the origin of hepatic veins or inferior vena cava, are in regions of extremely high blood flow and will require a greater cooling capacity, that is, larger probes or multiple probes, over lesions in peripheral areas. Some degree of extra freezing capacity for a given-size cryoprobe or cryoprobe number can be obtained by in-flow vascular occlusion to the liver. Previous work has shown that one freeze/thaw cycle with in-flow occlusion is equal to multiple freeze/thaw cycles without occlusion (Neel *et al.*, 1971a) and that approximately an additional 1 cm of lesion diameter can be achieved by in-flow occlusion (Dilley *et al.*, 1992).

Shapes of cryoprobes

Cryoprobes are manufactured in various shapes. In general, trocar probes with pointed ends are the most useful cryoprobes. Flat cryoprobes can at times be used in conjunction with a cryoprobe array when additional surface freezing is needed; however, flat cryoprobes are limited to approximately 1.5 cm depth and are usually inadequate, except for the smallest surface lesions, which are usually dealt with better by a small trocar probe placement.

The freezing protocol

Previous freezing literature emphasizes the need for multiple freeze/thaw cycles with a complete thaw between each freeze cycle. This information grew out of much of the experience learned with the cryopreservation of tissues and was derived from cell preparations *in vitro*. The cell suspensions showed that the tumour cells may survive freezing when in suspension, depending on the rate of cooling. Animal studies carried out seemed to confirm these findings, showing that control of tumour was superior when multiple freeze/thaw cycles were used (Neel *et al.*, 1971b). However, this appeared inconsistent with our own experience, in which we showed that virtually all the normal liver and frozen tumour died, even with one freeze/thaw cycle (Onik *et al.*, 1986). The difference in these findings can be explained by studies carried out by Rubinsky *et al.* (1990) showing the ultrastructural microscopic changes associated with freezing of liver within various portions of the ice ball. Close to the cryoprobe, where very high cooling rates are experienced, intracellular ice formation (which is very lethal to the cells) predominates. As the freezing rates decrease further from the cryoprobe, the ice preferentially forms within the microvasculature of the liver – the sinusoids. As water is removed from the vasculature with the formation of the ice, the surrounding cells dehydrate, trying to maintain the osmotic equilibrium. This process markedly expands and disrupts the microvasculature.

It therefore appears that there are two mechanisms at work for destruction of a tissue – the direct freezing effects on the cells, as well as the disruption of the microvasculature causing eventual ischaemic necrosis. Of interest is that these vascular effects do not appear to be immediate in the postthaw period. Continued blood flow, although decreased, continues into the cryolesion for a number of hours. This results in an interesting phenomenon of a cryolesion concentrating drugs that are within the systemic circulation. Evidence is now available that cryolesions will preferentially concentrate chemotherapeutic agents when given immediately after the thaw. The usefulness of this phenomenon remains to be explored (Gill & Long, 1971).

Other evidence appears to support the hypothesis that cellular anoxia with resultant ischaemia is a significant mechanism of the freezing injury *in vivo*. This vascular phenomenon helps to explain the survival of transplanted tissue taken from a cryolesion immediately after thawing and the almost complete destruction of surviving cells when the tissue is sampled after freeze by several hours (Gill & Long, 1971). In addition, postoperative CT scans on patients with hepatic cryosurgical lesions show complete exclusion of dye from the cryolesion, indicating complete absence of blood flow as well (Fig. 12.1).

The animal experiments which showed better control of tumour with multiple freeze/thaw cycles, however, suggested that the mechanism of freezing injury could not be one of an all-or-nothing phenomenon, as is suggested by the hypothesis of ischaemic infarction, causing complete destruction of the frozen tissue. This discrepancy may be explained by laboratory experiments which show that multiple freezing cycles result in an increased quantity of frozen tissue, with each subsequent application. With the poor monitoring of the cryolesion available in the past, it appears that the better clinical results obtained by repeated freeze/thaw cycles are probably a direct result of freezing more extensively but unknowingly.

We now have strong evidence, both clinically and experimentally, that two *complete* freeze/thaw cycles are detrimental when applied to hepatic cryosurgery. When we attempted a complete double freeze/thaw cycle in patients clinically, we found that patients developed a devastating syndrome of multisystem organ failure with evidence for diffuse damage to the patient's microscopic vasculature. Repeated freeze/thaw cycles resulted in the deaths of 3 of 4 patients in whom it was applied. Since stopping this freezing protocol, the phenomenon has not been seen again. Evidence in animals suggests that the hepatic enzyme levels increase threefold after a second freeze/thaw cycle, indicating more direct immediate cellular damage with the resultant release of greater amounts of cellular substances into the blood stream. A microscopic examination of tissue subjected to multiple complete freezes shows that the first freeze causes mainly vascular damage with the second freeze/thaw cycle causing marked cellular disruption and disorganization of the tissue.

In summary, as to freezing protocols, we feel that multiple complete freeze/thaw cycles in hepatic cryosurgery are contraindicated, with the major determinant of local tumour recurrence probably being the adequate surgical margin, as it is in traditional resection. If a 1 cm margin cannot be obtained, then *partial* thaw of the iceball can be carried out, with a second freeze to the margin of the lesion safely carried out.

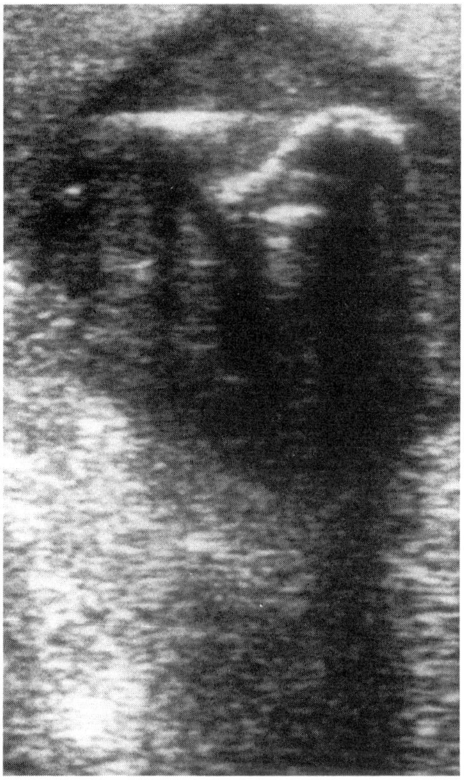

a

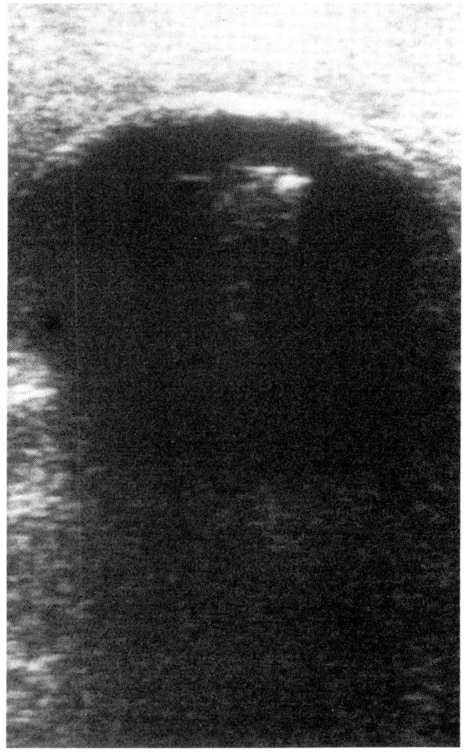

b

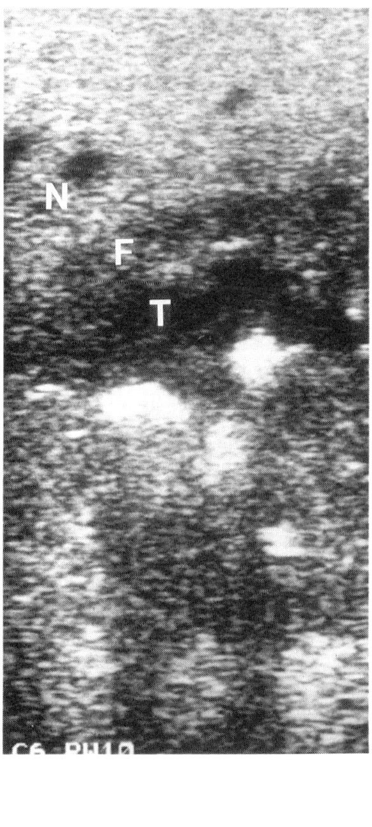

c

Figure 12.17 Four cryoprobes are placed within this lesion. (a) As the freezing is turned on, the freezing extends beyond the margins of the tumour. Note the hyperechoic rim which represents the margin of freezing and the posterior acoustic shadowing. (b) When the lesion thaws, (c) a hypoechogenicity surrounding the tumour represents the margin of the cryosurgery extending into normal liver. T = Tumour; F = frozen normal liver; N = unfrozen normal liver.

Monitoring the freezing cycle

Once again, IOUS is the key to monitoring the freezing, ensuring that an adequate cryosurgical margin has been obtained. Onik *et al.* (1984, 1985) demonstrated that the different acoustic characteristics between frozen and unfrozen tissue allow visualization of the freezing front as it emanates from the cryoprobe. It appears as a hyperechoic rim with posterior acoustic shadowing (Fig. 12.17). The rim can be observed as it encompasses the tumour and extends 1 cm beyond the tumour margin, at which point the freezing can be stopped. A few technical points have to be noted in relation to ultrasound monitoring of freezing, however:

1. The freezing margin is actually the inside surface of the hyperechoic rim as shown by ultrasound phantom studies.
2. Since frozen tissue shadows, the posterior aspect of the freezing cannot be seen and must be assumed to be adequate due to the symmetric ice ball formation. At times other ultrasound views from different aspects of the liver can be obtained to see the surface of the ice ball that was obscured by shadow.
3. Because of this shadowing effect, linear array ultrasound transducers give the most accurate depiction of the frozen area. Sector scans invariably overestimate the volume of tissue that has been frozen.
4. Once the ice ball thaws, the normal liver frozen decreases in echogenicity compared to unfrozen liver. This finding helps to document the cryosurgical margin (Fig. 12.17c).

When the freeze is completed, the cryoprobe is placed in the thaw mode; this allows the probe to be disengaged before complete thawing of the lesion. When the probe is removed, the tract can be plugged with Gelfoam or Surgicel to prevent major haemorrhage.

Conclusion

The success of hepatic cryosurgery depends on careful attention to a number of technical details, from the use of the proper-frequency ultrasound transducer to the accurate placement of cryoprobes with generation of an adequate cryosurgical margin. When properly performed, however, it provides the hepatic surgeon with a valuable adjunct in treating patients with difficult-to-resect hepatic tumours.

References

Bayjoo P, Rees RC, Goepel JR & Jacob G (1991) The effect of cryosurgery of liver tumour on natural killer cell activity in the rat. *Int. J. Immunopathol. Pharmacol.* **4**, 187–190.

Cady B, Stone MD, McDermott WV *et al.* (1992) Technical and biological factors in disease-free survival after hepatic resection for colorectal cancer metastases. *Arch. Surg.* **127**, 561–569.

Clark MP, Kane RA, Steele G *et al.* (1989) Prospective comparison of preoperative imaging and intraoperative ultrasonography in the detection of liver tumours. *Surgery* **106**, 849–855.

Dilley AV, Dy DY, Walters A *et al.* (1992) Laboratory and animal model evaluation of the Cryotech LCS2000 in hepatic cryotherapy. *Cryobiology* **30**, 74–85.

Foster JH (1984) Treatment of metastatic disease of the liver: a skeptic's view. *Semin. Liver Dis.* **4**, 170–179.

Gill W, & Long WB (1971) A critical look at cryosurgery. *Int. Surg.* **56**, 344–351.

Jacob G, Li A & Hobbs K (1984) A comparison of cryodestruction with excision or infarction of an implanted tumor in rat liver. *Cryobiology* **21**, 148–156.

Neel HB III, Ketcham AS & Hammond WG (1971a) Cryonecrosis of normal and tumor-bearing rat liver potentiated by inflow occlusion. *Cancer* **28**, 1211–1218.

Neel BH, Ketchum AJ & Hammond WG (1971b) Requisites for successful cryogenic surgery of cancer. *Arch. Surg.* **102**, 45–48.

Onik G, Cooper C, Goldberg HI, Moss AA, Rubinsky B & Christianson M (1984) Ultrasonic characteristics of frozen liver. *Cryobiology* **21**, 321–328.

Onik G, Gilbert J, Hoddick W *et al.* (1985) Sonographic monitoring of hepatic cryosurgery in an experimental animal model. *AJR* **144**, 1043–1047.

Onik G, Kane R, Steel G Jr *et al.* (1986) Monitoring hepatic cryosurgery with sonography. *AJR* **147**, 665–669.

Onik G, Rubinsky B, Zemel R & Diamond D (1991a) Cryosurgical management of hepatic malignancy. *Contemp. Oncol.* **1**, 20–24.

Onik G, Rubinsky B, Zemel R *et al.* (1991b) Ultrasound-guided hepatic cryosurgery in the treatment of metastatic colon carcinoma. Preliminary results. *Cancer* **67**, 901–907.

Ravikumar TS, Kane R, Cady B, Jenkins R, Clouse M & Steele Jr G (1991) A 5-year study of cryosurgery in the treatment of liver tumors. *Arch. Surg.* **126**, 1520–1524.

Rubinsky B, Lee CY, Bastacky J & Onik G (1990) The process of freezing and the mechanism of damage during hepatic cryosurgery. *Cryobiology* **27**, 85–97.

Scheele J (1993) Hepatectomy for liver metastases. *Br. J. Surg.* **80**, 274–276.

Zhou X-D, Yu Y-Q, Tang Z-Y, Weng J-M, Ma Z-C & Xu D-B (1992) An 18-year study of cryosurgery in the treatment of primary liver cancer. *Asian J. Surg.* **15**, 43–47.

II Cryotherapy: mechanisms of action, scientific basis for current techniques

David L. Morris and William B. Ross

Cryotherapy is currently the most advanced of the techniques of achieving imaging-controlled focal *in situ* liver destruction. At present, approximately 500 patients have been treated in the world, with good evidence of carcinoembryonic antigen reduction, as well as survival data, which are presented elsewhere in this book.

James Arnott (1851) of the Middlesex Hospital in London was probably the first person to use cryotherapy for cancer in 1851; he used a salt–ice mixture (−20°C) and described the reduction in size, pain, odour, discharge and haemorrhage. Pusey (1907) used solid sticks of carbon dioxide (−80°C) to freeze cutaneous lesions but it was not until 1961 that Dr Irving Cooper used circulating liquid nitrogen through a partially insulated probe. Dr Cooper was probably also the first to suggest that cryotherapy may be useful in the treatment of primary and secondary liver cancer. Cryotherapy is now widely used for the destruction of skin tumours, 90–97% of which will be cured at 5 years (Gage, 1982).

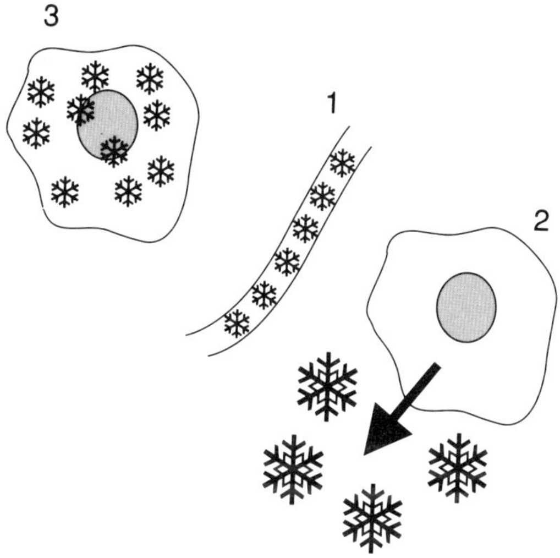

Figure 12.18 Intracellular and extracellular ice crystal formation occurs during hepatic cryotherapy. Intracellular crystals damage intracellular organelles and the cell membrane (3); extracellular crystals cause cellular dehydration (2). Intravascular crystals cause damage to vessels and secondary thrombosis (1).

Mechanisms of action

Mechanisms of tissue destruction by cryotherapy

During cryotherapy, there is formation of both extra- and intracellular ice crystals (Fig. 12.18). Slow freezing tends to be associated with more extracellular ice. Due to sequestration of extracellular water into the ice crystals, an osmotic gradient is created; the cells become dehydrated with a highly osmotic intracellular environment, causing cellular death (Fraser & Gill, 1967; Gill & Fraser, 1968).

Intracellular ice produces direct mechanical damage of cell membranes and intracellular structures. Secondary effects include denaturation of lipoprotein complexes, causing the cell membrane to leak.

Vascular effects of cryotherapy include deposition of platelet/fibrin thrombi (Whittaker, 1984) leading to reduction or cessation of blood flow, causing ischaemia. Indeed, the histological features of hepatic cryotherapy are very similar to, if not identical with, an ischaemic necrosis.

Rubinsky *et al.* (1990) very elegantly described the process of freezing a thin slice of liver on a slide with a temperature gradient. Ice was found to form and propagate within the vascular system and it is the vascular damage resulting from this process which is probably responsible for the majority of effects of at least single freeze/thaw cycles in liver.

Tumour cell viability after *in vitro* cryotherapy

In order to establish *in vitro* lethal temperature, Jacob *et al.* (1985) exposed Walker carcinoma cells to a controlled rate of freezing (16°C/min) to −10, to −40°C for 0–30 min. The cells were allowed to rewarm spontaneously. Whilst trypan blue suggested that fewer than 1% of cells were viable, significant take rates occurred when injected into animals.

The viability of cells was independent of the time held at a particular temperature. The growth of tumours from cells which did survive cryotherapy was normal – they had not been sublethally damaged. The minimal lethal temperature required was −35°C when cells were injected into skin but only −25°C when injected into liver – an interesting piece of evidence that sites are different in their ability to tolerate cancer cells.

These data, which are similar to those of Stone *et al.* (1969) and Zacarian (1977), are clearly totally incompatible with the *in vivo* experience of cryotherapy, which suggests that tissue frozen to even a few degrees below zero will undergo an apparently avascular necrosis. Gill *et al.* (1970a) reported that −2°C was sufficient. This is, in our view, clearly because the main effects of cryotherapy are *not* due to its primary effects on cancer cells but to the secondary vascular effects of cryotherapy which produce ischaemic necrosis. An alternative view of these data is that the cellular effects of cryotherapy may be much greater in the *in vivo* structural environment than in the unrealistic setting of a single-cell suspension where the formation of extracellular ice crystals would probably not occur and may have considerably less osmotic effect on a cell in a test tube than when adjacent to it in the body. Zacarian (1977) did show that an *in vitro* double freeze/thaw cycle had a considerably greater effect; 85% of cells were dead after the double cycle, compared with 55% after the single freeze/thaw.

Results of hepatic cryotherapy in animal models

The pathological evolution of hepatic cryolesions was described in rats (Fraser & Gill, 1967). By 20 h, there were grey patches and there was evidence of vascular damage and of a vascular lesion; at 24 h, there was a cellular infiltrate of polymorphs, lymphocytes and plasma cells, mainly at the margin. Together with thrombosis of vessels and disintegration of vascular walls, there was peripheral fibroblastic activity. From day 3, there was a well-demonstrated vascular lesion with irreversibly damaged cells, rapid encapsulation by the orthodox repair process, including a fibrous capsule and eventual replacement by scar tissue.

Their observations on Walker carcinosarcoma in rat liver were that there was a less well-demonstrated junction between viable and necrotic tumour.

The formation of intra- and extracellular ice crystals and irregularities in nucleus and cell membranes in mouse hepatic parenchyma was well described over 20 years ago (Trump *et al.* 1964). Large volumes of hepatic necrosis were produced by Dutta *et al.* (1979) with few post-operative problems. The pathological evolution from a swollen red area to necrosis to a fibroblastic reaction to a dense fibrous plaque was described.

Technique: physical and chemical factors

Factors affecting the speed and limiting the effect of cryotherapy

Probe diameter and temperature are clearly the most important factors. The cooling capacity of a probe could also be limited by the flow rate of the coolant, which could be increased, for example, by increasing dewar pressure. The blood flow through an organ is also important, vascular organs being harder to cool (Dilley *et al.* 1993).

Physics of cryotherapy

The steep thermal gradients achieved during cryotherapy were well understood over 20 years ago (Gill *et al.*, 1970a), with very steep fall in temperature over a small distance from the probe.

Time

There is initially a rapid growth in ice ball around a probe. After 15 min, there is usually little further growth of ice ball diameter; at this time, 80–90% of the maximum diameter is achieved (Gill *et al.*, 1970a) and eventually a steady state is achieved.

Environment

Ambient temperature has a large effect on cryotherapy – a 20% reduction produces a 60% increase in ice ball diameter and 300% increase in volume. We clamp hepatic vascular in-flow during cryotherapy of large or central hepatic tumours and have shown that, in an experimental animal model, this significantly increases speed of hepatic freezing and improves ice ball diameter (Dilley *et al.*, 1993).

Osmolality

Increased osmolality makes freezing more difficult. Methods of exploiting this phenomenon clinically have not been found. The density and specific heat of tissues also vary but this is clearly not a parameter which can be easily altered (Gill *et al.*, 1970b).

Margin and single or double freeze/thaw

We currently have little real knowledge of a safe margin for hepatic cryotherapy, and whether we need single or a double freeze/thaw cycle. Gilbert *et al.* (1986) stated that at 3 days the pathological lesion was within 1–3 mm of the diameter of the original ice ball, but the size of the original ice ball was not given and this was probably quite small because only a 5-min freeze was used. The thermal profile of an ice ball, which is an almost exponential thermal decay with distance from the probe, ensures that tissue 1 cm within the edge of small ice ball will have been exposed to a much lower temperature than in a large one. For example, 1 cm inside a 2 cm ice ball will be close to −196°C, whereas 1 cm inside a 6 cm ice ball may be only a degree or two below zero.

The thermal characteristics of refreezing tissue have been described. The second freeze is faster (or a larger ice ball achieved in the same time; Gill *et al.*, 1968) and the histological features of freezing twice are much more marked. Neel *et al.* (1971) described a fourfold increase in cellular necrosis in primate liver after a twin freeze/thaw cycle. Our group reported that twin freeze/thaw cycles achieved a higher percentage of the original ice ball, becoming necrotic in sheep liver (Dilley *et al.*, 1993) but twin freeze/thaw cycles in the liver are probably associated with excess risks. The cryoshock phenomenon experienced in Pittsburgh is of multiorgan failure and a disseminated intravascular coagulation type phenomenon. We have reported (Stewart *et al.*, 1994) much higher serum alanine transferase values after even partial double freeze/thaw cycles in humans, which we believe is a measure of hepatocellular destruction. We have also reported a close correlation between serum alanine transferase and platelet count fall post-cryotherapy (Cozzi *et al.*, 1994). At present it seems prudent to advise against a double freeze/thaw cycle in hepatic cryotherapy: our current practice is to allow the outer 1 cm of ice ball to thaw, then refreeze this. This still produces higher serum alanine transferase values than a single freeze/thaw but has not in our hands been associated with any mortality from cryoshock.

Different freeze/thaw rates

Gage *et al.* (1985) studied fast/slow freezing and thawing in the skin of dogs and assessed results by biopsy at 3 days. A slow thaw was found to be important. The speed of freezing was not important but they did suggest that the maintenance of tissue in a frozen state for several minutes was advisable; clearly, except for the very edge of a lesion, this occurs anyway.

Other authors have not found the time which the tissue is held frozen to be important.

Probe design

Open systems *must not* be used for hepatic cryosurgery. There is one reported gas embolism which was undoubtedly nearly fatal (Schlinkert & Chapman, 1990). An open system was used which was rather like a funnel. It was used on a hepatic remnant in the area of the right hepatic vein.

The design of probes which circulate liquid nitrogen varies. The simplest used, a coil of copper tubing shaped into a plate (Zhou *et al.*, 1988), whilst suitable for relatively superficial and solitary tumours, cannot readily be used for hepatic metastases where multiple lesions must be destroyed, often deep within the liver. The modern cylindrical triple-lumen probes have an active tip of varying length, an exhaust channel and the remaining probe is jacketed in a vacuum-insulated sheath. This allows the surgeon to destroy lesions deep within the liver without damaging overlying tissue.

Fatal haemorrhage due to liver surface cracking occurred in dogs where liquid nitrogen was poured directly on to the liver. This problem was avoided by putting a layer of dacron cloth soaked in KY jelly over the liver (Dutta *et al.*, 1979). We have seen surface cracking of the liver capsule when using a plate probe and the radial cracks seen with the trocar probes are described in the section on complications (p. 139).

Ultrasound-controlled cryotherapy

The demonstration that frozen tissue is very clearly seen on ultrasound was a most important step forwards in hepatic cryotherapy. Onik *et al.* (1984, 1985, 1986) showed that the ice ball was easily visible both *in vitro* and *in vivo*. Gilbert *et al.* (1986) showed that there was a very close correlation between the ultrasound image and pathology/histology at 3 days in 5 animals.

The hyperechoic border and dense black zone of the ice ball were clearly described.

IOUS is also currently the most sensitive method of detecting liver metastases (other than the micrometastases detected by HPI), which is clearly necessary before accurate staging or treatment can occur.

Large vessels and bile ducts

Proximity of a lesion to a major vascular structure is clearly a concern and may render the patient unresectable. This is not a contraindication to cryotherapy. Gage *et al.* (1967), using liquid nitrogen, subjected large arteries both with and without vascular occlusion to freezing. There was little evidence of damage to large arteries or veins and no thrombosis or aneurysm occurred. Bile duct freezing is not tolerated at all well. Inflammation, mucosal loss and stricture are seen (Gage *et al.*, 1967).

We have protected patients against biliary damage by using selectively placed bile duct warmers when freezing up to a major extrahepatic duct is required. Intrahepatic bile duct injury presumably does occur but has not been a clinical problem.

Immunological aspects of hepatic cryotherapy

Resolution of distant metastases has been described in patients after cryotherapy of primary lesions (Bayjoo & Jacob, 1992). This is a very rare observation and we have certainly not experienced this in over 100 patients. There is also, however, evidence of deleterious effects of cryotherapy on immune function. Wing *et al.* (1988) reported the generation of a population of T lymphocytes capable of suppressing lymphocyte proliferation after cryotherapy. Resistance to rechallenge by tumour was found to be lowest at around 3 weeks (Miya *et al.*, 1986). There is known to be a considerable increase in splenic weight after cryotherapy (Miya *et al.*, 1986; Wing *et al.*, 1988). Paracortical hyperplasia of lymph nodes in the area draining a tumour cryotherapy site was described and *in vitro* measures of lymphocyte function, was lowest at 3 weeks but significantly increased by 6 weeks following cryotherapy.

The use of agents which could potentially improve the immunological results of cryotherapy, for example, by suppressing T-suppressor lymphocytes with cimetidine, or stimulating lymphocyte activity with interleukin-2, has not yet been reported. The possibility that repeat cryotherapy could improve immunological response to cryotherapy has not been explored. Patients clearly can form immunological responses to their tumour and there is no doubt that there is considerable release of cancer cell antigens after cryotherapy. We have a small group of 7 patients who have had repeat hepatic cryotherapy for localized recurrence, of whom 6 are still alive, with an average follow-up from first treatment of approximately 2 years. There is at least one animal liver tumour model where cryotherapy produced better results than resection or infarction (Jacob *et al.*, 1984). We are not aware of any other data on the measurement of the effect of cryotherapy on specific antitumour response which deserves further study.

References

Arnott J (1851) *On the Treatment of Cancer by the Regulated Application of an Anaesthetic Temperature.* London: Churchill.

Bayjoo P & Jacob G (1992) Hepatic cryosurgery: biological

and clinical considerations. *J. R. Coll. Surg. Edinb.* **37**, 369–372.

Cooper IS (1963) Cryogenic surgery. A new method of destruction or extirpation of benign or malignant tumours. *N. Engl. J Med.* **268**, 743–749.

Cozzi PJ, Stewart GJ, Morris DL (1994) Thrombocytopenia after hepatic cryotherapy for colorectal metastases correlates with hepatocellular injury. *World J. Surg.* **18(5)**, 774–777.

Dilley AV, Dy DY, Warlters A *et al.* (1993) Laboratory and animal model evaluation of the Cryotech LCS 2000 in hepatic cryotherapy. *Cryobiology* **30**, 74–85.

Dutta P., Montes M and Gage AA (1979) Large volume freezing in experimental hepatic cryosurgery. *Cryobiology* **16**, 50–55.

Fraser J & Gill W (1967) Observations on ultra-frozen tissue. *Br. J. Surg.* **54**, 770–776.

Gage AA (1982) Current issues in cryosurgery. *Cryobiology* **19**, 219–222.

Gage AA, Fazekas G & Riley CG (1967) Freezing injury to large blood vessels in dogs. *Surgery* **61**, 748–754.

Gage AA, Guest K, Montes M *et al.* (1985) Effect of varying freezing and thawing rates in experimental cryosurgery. *Cryobiology* **22**, 175–182.

Gilbert JC, Onik GM, Hoddick WK *et al.* (1986) Ultrasound monitored hepatic cryosurgery: longevity study on an animal model. *Cryobiology* **23**, 277–285.

Gill W & Fraser J (1968) A look at cryosurgery. *Scott. Med. J.*, **13**, 268–273.

Gill W, Fraser T & Carter DC (1968) Repeated freeze–thaw cycles in cryosurgery. *Nature* **219**, 410–413.

Gill W, Long W, Fraser J *et al.* (1970a) Cryosurgery for neoplasia. *Br. J. Surg.* **57**, 494–502.

Gill W, Da Costa J & Fraser J (1970b) The control and predictability of a cryolesion. *Cryobiology* **6**, 347–353.

Jacob G, Kurzer MN & Fuller BJ (1985) An assessment of tumor cell viability after *in vitro* freezing. *Cryobiology* **22**, 417–426.

Jacob G, Li AK and Hobbs KE (1984) A comparison of cryodestruction with excision or infarction of an implanted tumor in rat liver. *Cryobiology* **21**, 148–156.

Miya K, Saji S, Morita T *et al.* (1986) Immunological response of regional lymph nodes after tumor cryosurgery: experimental study in rats. *Cryobiology* **23**, 290–295.

Neel HB, Ketcham AS & Hammond WG (1971) Ischemia potentiating cryosurgery of primate liver. *Ann. Surg.* **174**, 309–318.

Onik G, Cooper C, Goldberg HI *et al.* (1984) Ultrasonic characteristics of frozen liver. *Cryobiology* **21**, 321–328.

Onik G, Gilbert J, Hoddick W *et al.* (1985) Sonographic monitoring of hepatic cryosurgery in an experimental animal model. *AJR* **144**, 1043–1047.

Onik G, Kane R, Steele G *et al.* (1986) Monitoring hepatic cryosurgery with sonography. *AJR* **147**, 665–669.

Pusey WA (1907) The use of carbon dioxide snow in the treatment of nevi and other lesions of the skin: a preliminary report. *J.A.M.A.* **49**, 1354–1356.

Rubinsky B, Lee CY, Bastacky J *et al.* (1990) The process of freezing and the mechanisms of damage during hepatic cryosurgery. *Cryobiology* **27**, 85–97.

Schlinkert RT & Chapman TP (1990) Nitrogen embolus as a complication of hepatic cryosurgery. *Arch. Surg.* **125**, 1214.

Stewart GJ, Preketes AP, Horton MD *et al.* (1994) Hepatic cryotherapy: double freeze cycles achieve greater hepatocellular injury in man. *Cryobiology*.

Stone D, Zacarian SA & DiPeri C (1969) Comparative studies of mammalian normal and cancer cells subjected to cryogenic temperatures *in vitro*. *Cryosurgery* **2**, 43–52.

Trump BF, Goldblatt PJ, Griffin CC *et al.* (1964) Effects of freezing and thawing on the ultrastructure of mouse hepatic parenchymal cells. *Lab. Invest.* **13**, 967–1001.

Whittaker DK (1984) Mechanisms of tissue destruction following cryosurgery. *Ann. R. Coll. Surg. Engl.* **66**, 313–318.

Wing MG, Rogers K, Jacob G *et al.* (1988) Characterisation of suppressor cells generated following cryosurgery of an HSV-2 induces fibrosarcoma. *Cancer Immunol. Immunother.* **26**, 169–175.

Zacarian SA (1977) The observation of freeze–thaw cycles upon cancer-cell suspensions. *J. Dermatol. Surg. Oncol.* **3**, 173–174.

Zhou Z-D, Tang Z-Y, Yu Y-Q *et al.* (1988) Clinical evaluation of cryosurgery in the treatment of primary liver cancer. *Cancer* **61**, 1889–1892.

III Cryotherapy: patient selection, perioperative care, results

David L. Morris and Angelo Preketes

The appropriate selection of patients may be divided into exclusion of extrahepatic disease, assessment of liver disease and deciding whether the patient is fit to undergo the procedure.

Extrahepatic disease

We had a significant rate of bone recurrence in our early series and have certainly found and excluded 2 patients since then by routine bone scan. Similarly, chest X-ray is mandatory to exclude lung metastases and it could be argued that pulmonary CT would be more useful. Particular attention to the upper abdominal CT films may reveal basal lung metastases not seen on chest X-ray. Demonstration of locally recurrent intra-abdominal or peritoneal disease is also a contraindication. We do not exclude patients on the basis of enlarged coeliac lymph nodes on CT scans, which are often non-malignant, and we are prepared to treat patients with histologically involved lymph nodes, if these lie within the perfusion territory of our catheter system, but this is controversial and at present part of an evaluation.

Patients with para-aortic or other lymph node involvement are not treated. The preoperative diagnosis of peritoneal disease is often difficult. We have not used laparascopy to identify peritoneal disease because of the dangers and limited access in patients with adhesions due to their previous colorectal surgery but this may well be able to reduce the number of patients who at laparotomy are excluded from cryotherapy or resection.

Liver disease

The boundaries of hepatic cryotherapy have not yet really been accurately defined but clearly there are physical limits to the performance of equipment. Almost all of our experience of the 138 procedures reported here is in colorectal cancer, with the remainder made up by neuroendocrine metastases and primary liver cancer.

Number

Whilst the critical number for results of liver resection is four, this is not yet established for cryotherapy and we certainly have 1 patient who appears disease-free at 1 year who had five lesions. The Pittsburgh group similarly have a disease-free patient who had seven lesions, but clearly it is likely that number of lesions will be predictive of survival.

Volume

We would not advise cryodestruction of more than 50% of liver volume. The sequelae of massive hepatic cryosurgery are probably greater than after a hepatic lobectomy and, whilst we may develop strategies to prevent these problems, they are at present a limiting factor. Results of treatment by hepatic artery chemotherapy appear to relate to volume replacement but the issue of hepatic cytoreduction is controversial. Can cryocytoreduction improve the results of regional chemotherapy? Our data suggest that survival is closely related to percentage reduction in carcinoembyronic antigen so that, even when this is not returned to normal, the percentage reduction predicts outcome. Carcinoembryonic antigen is, in our experience, a very reliable measure of the volume of disease within a single patient – that is, whilst the carcinoembryonic antigen secretion of tumours varies, the values in an individual patient closely parallel the outcome of treatment, at least for hepatic disease (Preketes *et al.* 1994).

Diameter

The maximum diameter of lesion which can be adequately treated is clearly dependent on probe characteristics, including diameter, and the coolant flow rate achieved. Hepatic in-flow occlusion will significantly improve the efficacy of the system (Dilley *et al.* 1993). Position of the lesion in the liver also affects cryotherapy; deep lesions or those adjacent to large vessels are more difficult to treat. The number of probes used will also clearly have a great effect on the diameter of lesions which can be treated. Concurrent multiple probe application achieves very different temperature profiles from serial probe use, and can also significantly shorten procedure time.

A 5 mm probe will produce a 5 cm ice ball in approximately 20 min and little further progress will be achieved thereafter. A 6 cm metastasis will clearly require a bigger probe or several probes. A 1 cm cryomargin around the lesion is currently advised.

Fitness for the procedure

We have rejected very few patients because of other serious medical illnesses, neither has age been a bar to successful outcome, but we accept that very unfit patients are probably not referred. Cryoglobinaemia might be a contraindication to hepatic cryosurgery. We have not treated patients with jaundice.

Perioperative care of cryotherapy patients

For most patients, hepatic cryotherapy will be a morbidity-free procedure with short hospital stay; some care is needed to achieve this and, in less fortunate patients, serious, life-threatening complications will need to be managed appropriately.

Adequate prehydration, intraoperative volume replacement, together with careful monitoring of intra- and postoperative urine output are, in our view, necessary to prevent renal failure. The only 3 patients in our experience of 138 patients with significant renal impairment have had significant intra- or postoperative hypotension. The Pittsburgh group, however, have seen renal impairment in patients as part of the cryoshock phenomenon.

Chest problems are frequent after any upper abdominal operation but pleural effusions are not infrequently seen; 2 were large enough to require aspiration. We believe that this problem is more frequently seen when it has been impossible to prevent freezing of the diaphragm and presumably sometimes the lung above.

Anaesthetic care

Patient temperature can clearly be a cause for concern, although our patients have seldom gone below 33°C (Goodie *et al.*, 1992) and the length of procedure is probably of greater importance than the freezing process. We use a hot air warming device, a ripple heating mat, insulating foils and blankets and occasionally lavage the peritoneum with warm saline.

Prophylaxis for thromboembolism and infection

We recommend prophylactic subcutaneous heparin, graded pressure stockings and intraoperative calf compression devices. Despite the fall in platelet numbers after cryosurgery, which has sometimes made us cease heparin, the risk of pulmonary embolism is a real one; we have had 2 clinically recognized cases. We also use prophylactic antibiotics (cefotaxime 1 g intravenously 8-hourly, 24 h) starting at induction.

Intraoperative problems

Haemorrhage has been the most frequent and difficult to manage intraoperative complication and has almost always been due to cracking (Fig. 12.19). Compression of the mobilized liver will always in our experience control this bleeding, by holding the crack together either manually or by packing. The crack is then managed by a deep running suture using a blunt liver needle (Fig. 12.20). Care is taken not to allow it to cut through when tying. If one can avoid allowing the ice ball on to the surface of the liver at the probe entry site, this will reduce the risk of cracking. This is clearly not possible when the lesion is on or near the surface. Ice balls *must* be allowed to thaw out fully before closing the abdomen as it is impossible to assess haemostasis until then. In soft tumours, considerable care should be used. In one of the two melanomas we have treated, the soft tumour literally shattered and required packing to control bleeding.

Postoperative bleeding

We have had to return 2 of our patients to the operating theatre for control of postoperative bleeding; in 1, we probably achieved inadequate intraoperative control but, in the second, bleeding occurred later due to a disseminated intravascular coagulation-type phenomenon. We have described a considerable fall in postoperative platelet count after cryotherapy (Goodie *et al.*, 1992) and this is greater after twin freeze/thaw cycles than single ones (Stewart *et al.*, 1994). We have recently shown that there is a very close relationship between platelet count fall and serum alaninc scrum

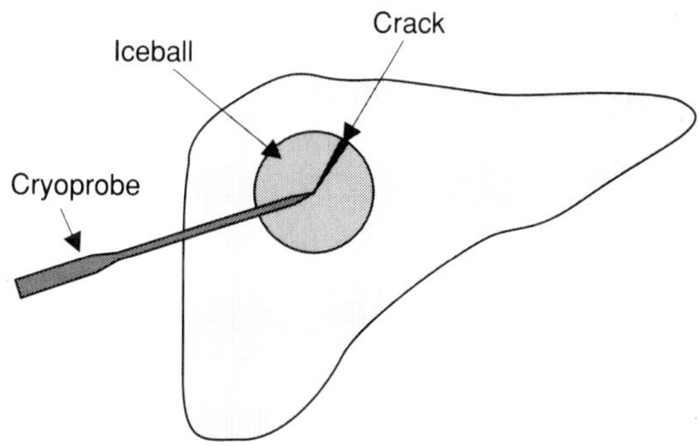

Figure 12.19 Radial crack of hepatic ice ball.

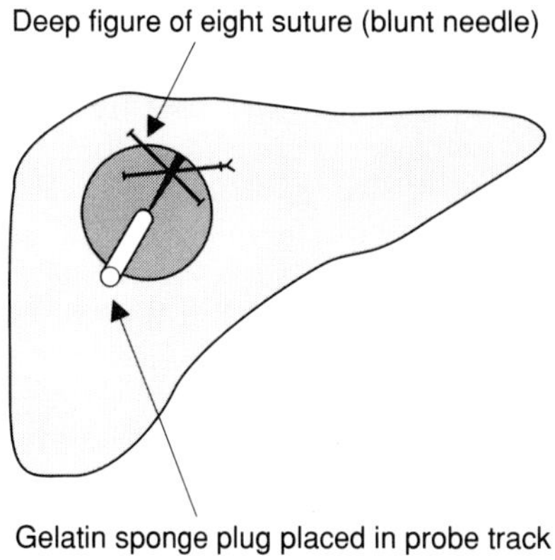

Figure 12.20 Placement of central gelfoam plug, then figure-of-eight suture to control haemorrhage from crack.

transferase, which we presume to be an accurate measure of hepatocellular injury.

Cryoshock phenomenon

The Pittsburgh group have experienced 3 postoperative deaths due to a syndrome of multiorgan failure (renal, pulmonary, hepatic), together with disseminated intravascular coagulation-type blood picture. We believe that we have seen similar but less severe manifestations of this. We have *not* used a complete thaw before refreezing our double freeze/thaw patients; only approximately a 1 cm rim of liver tissue was allowed to thaw. As we have clearly shown that double freeze/thaw produces a much higher alanine serum transferase levels (Fig. 12.21) and greater fall in platelet count we believe that this syndrome may well be similar to the crush syndrome caused by release of cellular debris due to the far greater immediate cell wall disruption of a twin freeze/thaw cycle. In contrast, the major effects of a single freeze/thaw are vascular, producing vascular thrombosis and ischaemic infarction.

Postoperative follow-up

We follow all patients with monthly carcinoembryonic antigen, provided the tumour secretes it, and CT at 3 months. We believe that careful follow-up can be justified for clinical as well as research reasons. We have now reoperated on 7 patients with localized hepatic recurrence with good results: 6 are still alive at a mean follow-up of almost 2 years.

Adjuvant hepatic artery chemotherapy

There are six controlled trials of hepatic artery chemotherapy, two of which show survival benefit (Rougier *et al.*, 1972; Hunt *et al.*, 1990) – the latter only found an advantage in patients with less than 50% hepatic replacement. We have used adjuvant hepatic artery chemotherapy in the majority of our cryotherapy patients.

Results: morbidity

We have no operative or 30-day mortality but lost one 79-year-old lady with a hepatic abscess at 10 weeks: she had undergone concurrent colonic resection. Significant morbidity has been infrequent: we have had 2 patients with pulmonary embolism. One also had a myocardial infarct. We have experienced 3 perioperative arrhythmias: 1 of these was in the patient with myocardial infarction, the other 2 of ventricular tachycardia during thawing of a pericaval freeze. Our subsequent animal work has indicated that this is likely to be due to transient hyperkalaemia (Ross *et al.*, 1995).

The median hospital stay is 6 days, some patients being discharged on day 3.

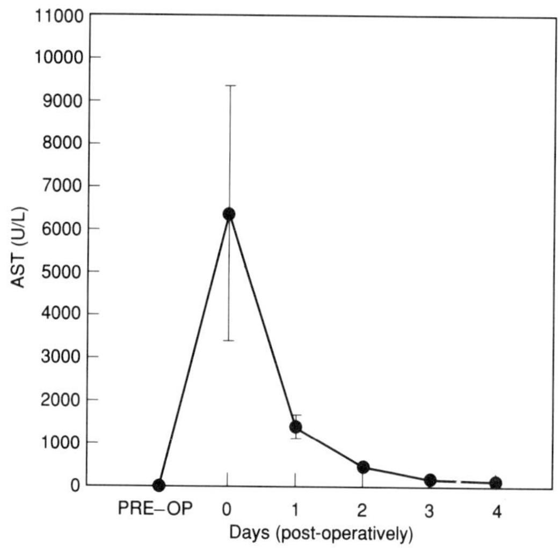

Figure 12.21 Daily serum alanine serum transferase (AST) in 8 patients following hepatic cryotherapy with a double freeze–thaw cycle.

Results cryotherapy for hepatic tumours

There is currently quite little published experience but over 500 patients have probably now been treated. Zhou *et al.* (1988) reported the results of treating 60 patients with primary liver cancer by hepatic cryotherapy using mostly a single freeze/thaw technique. There was no mortality and no serious morbidity. Overall survival and that of patients with lesions less than 5 cm in diameter is given in Table 12.2.

Table 12.2 Survival of patients with hepatocellular carcinoma after cryotherapy (Zhou *et al.*)

	Survival (%)	
Years	All	<5 cm
1	52	76
2	34	62
3	21	50
4	15	41
5	11	37

There is now considerable experience of cryotherapy treatment of hepatic metastases. Early results have been reported by several groups (Ravikumar *et al.*, 1987; Charnley *et al.*, 1991; Onik *et al.*, 1991). Our own series of 138 procedures is also without operative or 30-day mortality. Overall survival is plotted in Figure 12.22.

Quality of life had been excellent until patients develop symptomatic recurrent disease. Survival of our colorectal cancer patients

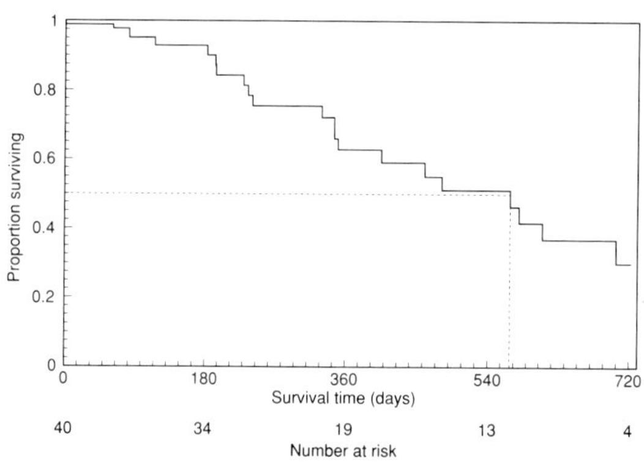

Figure 12.22 Survival posthepatic cryotherapy – all patients (Kaplan–Meier survival curve).

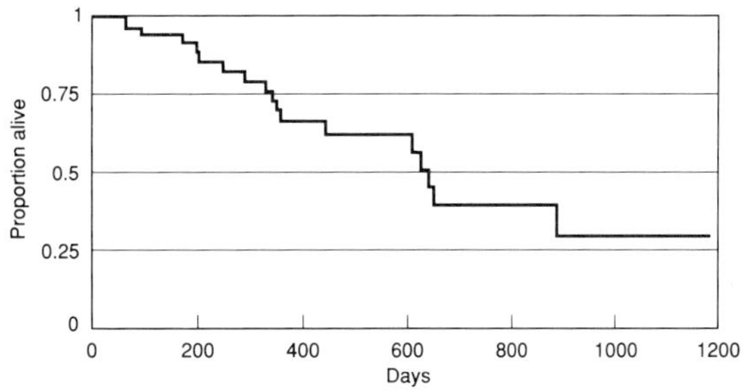

Figure 12.23 Survival posthepatic cryotherapy for colorectal cancer metastases (Kaplan–Meier survival curve).

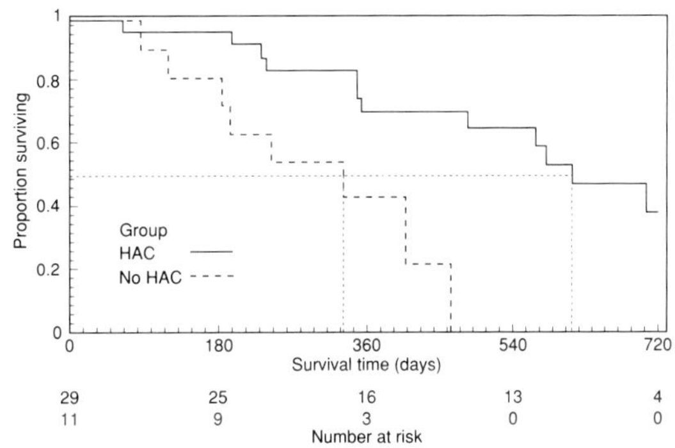

Figure 12.24 Survival after hepatic cryotherapy for colorectal metastases. Comparison of cryotherapy alone and cryotherapy with hepatic arterial chemotherapy (HAC).

treated in Sydney is illustrated in Figure 12.23. The patients who received adjuvant hepatic artery chemotherapy are compared with those who did not in Figure 12.24. The reasons for the latter group were physician non-compliance, system failure or toxicity. Whilst these treatment groups are not randomly allocated, there is a survival advantage to adjuvant hepatic artery chemotherapy after cryotherapy.

Carcinoembryonic antigen

The serum carcinoembryonic antigen is usually considerably increased immediately after surgery and this falls rapidly. The maximum mean percentage reduction seen was 64% and in 17% of patients the carcinoembryonic antigen returned to the normal range. Clearly, such patients might be expected to have a better

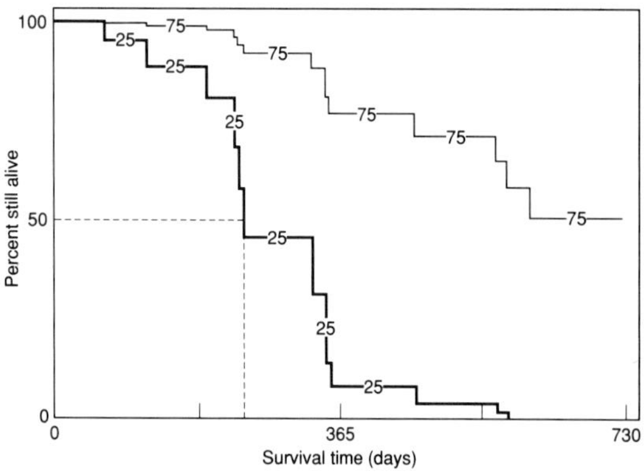

Figure 12.25 Survival following hepatic cryotherapy for colorectal cancer liver metastases. Comparison of patients with 25–50% and 75–100% reduction in carcinoembryonic antigen (Cox regression model).

prognosis. What was more surprising to us is that the percentage reduction in carcinoembryonic antigen is prognostic. Figure 12.25 shows the survival of two groups of patients, those with 25–50% and 75–100% reduction, of carcinoembryonic antigen. The survival of these two groups is significantly different and is, perhaps, the first piece of evidence that cytoreduction of hepatic metastatic disease by cryotherapy, at least when combined with hepatic artery chemotherapy, will improve survival even when not all the malignancy is destroyed.

Long-term complications

We have seen one late liver abscess (Stewart *et al.*, 1993) in a patient almost 2 years after hepatic cryosurgery. Catheter-related problems of thrombosis, leakage or fistula into biliary or gastrointestinal tracts have been seen. We have not seen any biliary sclerosis or hepatocellular problems from our chemotherapy regime. We have one, probably benign, left hepatic duct stricture as a result of cryotherapy, where we did not use a bile duct warming device.

References

Charnley RM, Thomas M & Morris DL (1991) Effect of hepatic cryotherapy on serum CEA concentration in patients with multiple inoperable hepatic metastases from colorectal cancer. *Aust. N.Z. J. Surg.* **61**, 55–58.

Dilley AV, Dy DY, Warlters A *et al.* (1993) Laboratory and animal model evaluation of the Cryotech LCS 2000 in hepatic cryotherapy. *Cryobiology* **30**, 74–85.

Goodie DB, Horton MDA, Morris R *et al.* (1992) The anaesthetic experience with hepatic cryotherapy for metastatic colonic carcinoma. *Anaesth. Intensive Care* **20**, 491–496.

Hunt TM, Flowerdew ADS, Birch ST *et al.* (1990) Prospective randomised controlled trial of hepatic arterial embolisation or infusion chemotherapy with 5-fluorouacil and degradable starch microspheres for colorectal liver metastases. *Br. J. Surg.* **77**, 779–782.

Onik G, Rubinsky B, Zemel R *et al.* (1991) Ultrasound guided hepatic cryosurgery in the treatment of metastatic colon carcinoma. Preliminary results. *Cancer* **67**, 901–907.

Preketes AP, King J, Caplehorn JRM, Clingan PR, *et al.* (1994) CEA reduction after cryotherapy for liver metastases from colon cancer predicts survival. *Aust. N.Z. J. Surg.* **64**, 612–614.

Ravikumar TS, Kane R, Cady B *et al.* (1987) Hepatic cryosurgery with intraoperative monitoring for metastatic colon carcinoma. *Arch. Surg.* **122**, 403–409.

Ross WB, Horton M, Bertolino P & Morris DL (1995) Cryotherapy of liver tumours – a practical guide. *HPB Surgery* **8**, 167–173.

Rougier PH, Laplanche A, Huguier MM *et al.* (1972) Hepatic arterial infusion of floxuridine in patients with liver metastases from colorectal carcinoma. Long term results of a prospective randomised trial. *Clin. Oncol.* **10**, 1112–1118.

Stewart GJ, Preketes A, Horton M *et al.* (1995) Hepatic cryotherapy: double freeze cycles achieve greater hepatocellular injury in man. *Cryobiology* **32**, 215–219.

Stewart GJ, Glenn D & Morris DL (1993) Late hepatic abscess following cryotherapy and regional cytotoxic perfusion. *Reg. Cancer Treat.* **3**, 144–145.

Zhou ZD, Tang ZY, Yu YQ. *et al.* (1988) Clinical evaluation of cryosurgery in the treatment of primary liver cancer. Report of 60 cases. *Cancer* **61**, 1889–1892.

13

Physical methods of imaging-controlled destruction: percutaneous ethanol injections for hepatic metastases

Tito Livraghi and Claudio Vettori

Alcohol enters the cell by diffusion and produces immediate coagulation necrosis followed by the formation of granulation tissue and fibrosis and by partial or complete thrombosis of small vessels. These phenomena are the outcome of cellular dehydration and protein denaturation.

Percutaneous ethanol injection (PEI) under ultrasound (US) guidance was developed a few years ago for the treatment of small hepatic cell carcinoma (HCC) (Livraghi *et al.*, 1986; Sheu *et al.*, 1987; Shiina *et al.*, 1987). Very high 3-year survival rates, possibly higher even than for surgery, have recently been reported, although this may reflect selection bias, and so it has been proposed that PEI is an appropriate therapeutic option (Ebara *et al.*, 1990; Shiina *et al.*, 1990; Livraghi *et al.*, 1992). The rationale for using PEI in HCC includes the following:

1. HCCs initially grow regionally.
2. US screening of cirrhotic patients allows detection of HCC at this stage.
3. Alcohol diffuses selectively in the HCC, whose consistency is softer than that of the surrounding cirrhotic tissue.
4. PEI involves no loss of cirrhotic tissue, as does surgery (an important point because in these patients liver function is compromised and any intervention that makes it worse further hastens the onset of terminal liver failure).
5. PEI has no major complications, whereas surgery is associated with morbidity and mortality.

In the PEI treatment of hepatic metastases there are two basic limitations:

1. Metastatic disease differs markedly from HCC in its natural course, and PEI is only a local therapy.
2. The ethanol distribution inside the metastatic tissue is less good than in HCC, because the neoplastic vascular supply is lower and the tissue around is usually not harder. (Livraghi *et al.*, 1990, 1993).

The rationale for PEI in the treatment of liver metastases is based on the assumption that by the reduction of the neoplastic volume, survival can be improved.

Method

Equipment

To perform PEI we use a US scanner with 3.5 MHz real-time probe with a guide device. The alcohol is sterile ethanol 95% (SALF, Bergamo, Italy). We use two kinds of needle: a 22-gauge spinal needle (Becton-Dickinson, Rutherford, NJ, USA) for lesions smaller than

2–3 cm, and a 21-gauge multihole needle (Hakko, Tokyo, Japan) for the others.

As a rule, treatment is given in the outpatient department. Local anaesthetics are not given. Alcohol is injected in a dose of 1–8 ml per session, with one or more injections in the same session, depending on lesion size and mode of perfusion. The injection site is chosen before each session to ensure perfusion of areas considered not to have been treated. To monitor the treatment, we record the areas treated on a simple graph and on a personal videotape. The area perfused is easily recognized as a hyperechogenic patch (Fig. 13.1). At the end of the injection the needle is left in place for about 20 s and then slowly withdrawn to prevent reflux of the alcohol into the peritoneal cavity, which can cause pain. Patients experiencing severe pain receive analgesic drugs before subsequent sessions: buprenorphine (Temgesic) 0.2 mg sublingually and/or diclofenac (Voltaren) 200 mg rectally.

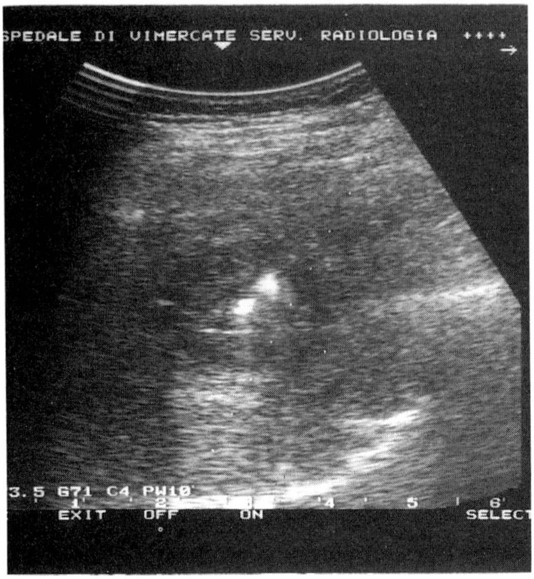

Figure 13.1 Intercostal ultrasound sections in a patient with hypoechogenic metastasis (3.2 cm) from cancer of the colon. (a) Before percutaneous ethanol injection, the tip of the needle is recognizable at the centre of the lesion.

Treatment is performed at the rate of 1–2 sessions per week. We treat lesions under 2 cm for 3–6 sessions, lesions of 2–3.5 cm for 10 session and lesions 3.5–5 cm for 12–15 sessions. More recently, when the lesions are several, or more than 3 cm, we perform PEI under general anaesthesia (one-shot technique) (Livraghi *et al.*, 1993). This technique presents some advantages:

1. *Ad libitum* administration of ethanol, because there is no pain.
2. Shorter treatment time.
3. Better patient compliance.

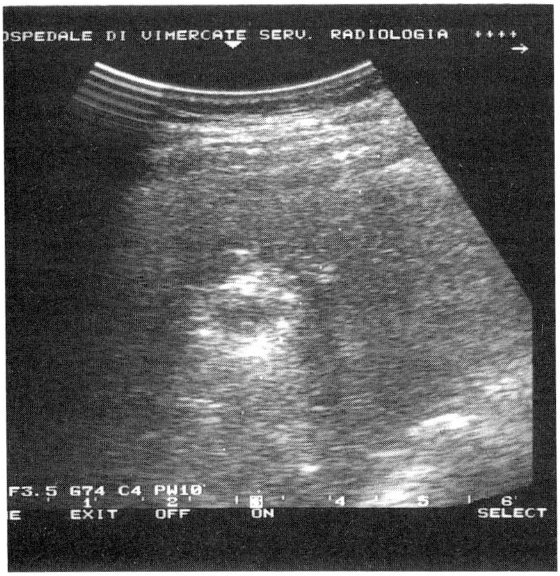

Figure 13.1(b) Just after the treatment, there is good diffusion of the ethanol, recognizable as a hyperechogenic area, inside the lesion.

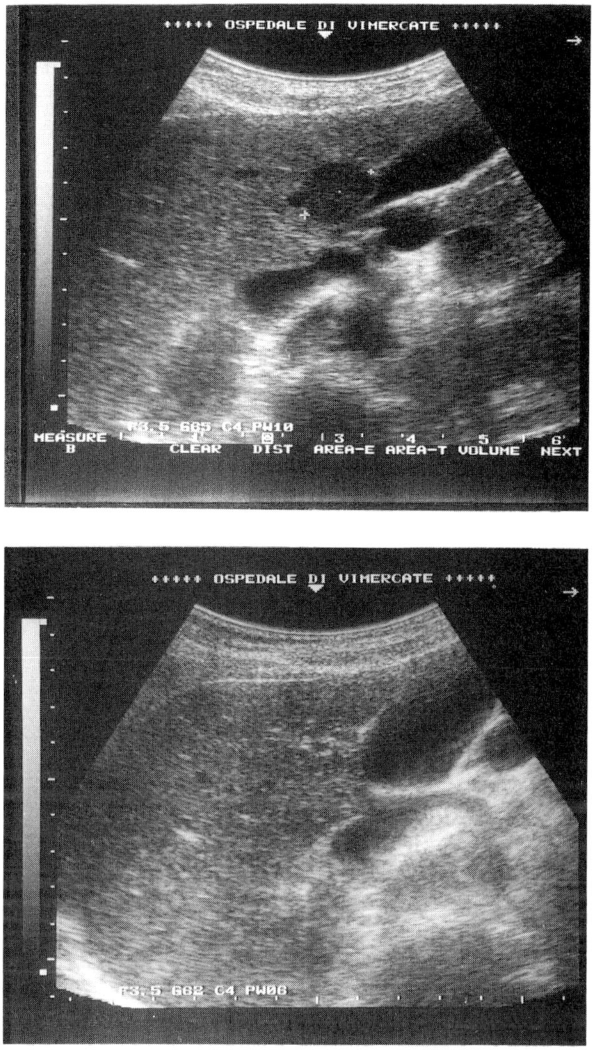

a

b

Figure 13.2 Oblique subcostal ultrasound sections in a patient with single hypoechogenic metastasis (2.1 cm) from the breast, located beside the gallbladder. (a) Before treatment. (b) One month after treatment, the lesion was undetectable (no chemotherapy was given during this period).

At present, the greatest amount of ethanol administered was 165 ml with 22 injections in a patient with around 40% of liver tissue involved by metastases from colon cancer.

Pre- and posttreatment investigations

In the pretreatment work-up, patients have US measurements of the two greatest diameters of the lesions, plain and dynamic computed tomography (CT) in the arterial and portal phases, and carcinoembryonic antigen (CEA) or other tumour markers in relation to the origin. The same examinations are used as parameters of therapeutic efficacy 1 month after the last treatment. In a single lesion, where the goal is complete necrosis, if CT does not definitely show the absence of residual neoplastic tissue, fine-needle biopsy (FNAB) is done; if CT or FNAB reveals the presence of residual neoplastic tissue, additional treatments are administered. Follow-up includes US and tumour marker screening every 4 months and CT every 8 months.

Results

We treated 28 patients, 27 of them carriers of 46 focal lesions and 1 with around 40% of the liver involved by metastases. Primary cancer was of the colon/rectum in 18, stomach in 4, breast in 2, abdominal leiomyosarcoma in 1, endocrine in 3 (1 bronchi, 2 of unknown origin). Size of the lesions ranged from 1.1 to 10 cm. Table 13.1 shows imaging response and follow-up. Complete response was considered on imaging examinations and when absence of growth was proved during the follow-up (Fig. 13.1); partial response included when the rate of necrosis was more than 50% and the growth of the lesion was stopped for some time, while progressive disease was assessed when in spite of some rate of necrosis, the lesion increased in size. Table 13.2 shows CEA modifications in patients with pathological baseline values. In all these patients, the decrease in CEA values lasted for 2–6 months; subsequent elevations were attributed to regrowth of the treated lesion, recurrence of the primary tumour, extrahepatic metastases or new liver metastases. All endocrine metastases were associated with complete response; this was because of their small size (maximum 2.1 cm), slow growth and hypervascularity. The longest follow-up of complete response is 4 years, in a patient with three metastases from gastrinoma of unknown origin. PEI was not associated with noteworthy complications.

Table 13.1 Percutaneous ethanol injection in hepatic metastases: response

Diameter	Complete response	Partial response	Progressive disease	Total
<2 cm	13	2	0	15
2–3 cm	4	7	4	15
3–4 cm	1	4	4	9
>4 cm	0	0	7	7
Total	18	20	8	46

Table 13.2 Percutaneous ethanol injection in hepatic metastases: carcinoembryonic antigen modifications

No.	Diameter (cm)	Before treatment	After 1 month
1	3.7	>200	170
2	3.8	30	4
3	2.3	18	11
4	2.7	190	40
5	3.2/2.6	60	28
6	2.1	23	12
7	2.4	17	4
8	10.0	25	5
9	3.1/2.8/1.5	35	18
10	6.8/2.0	30	21
11	6.8/2.1	48	11
12	2.8	18	8
13	40%	1396	560
14	1.4	20	17
15	3.2/2.9/2.1	188	108
16	4.6	70	8

Conclusions

Since the one-shot technique started, the range of indications has become wider. At the moment those of our patients with inoperable metastases, whether multiple or single greater than 4 cm without extrahepatic spread receive the one-shot treatment while those with single metachronous lesions <3–4 cm are still treated by the traditional procedure. Clearly, it is difficult to establish whether, how much, and in which cases patient survival is lengthened, and the controlled trials would be biased because of the variety of factors which can modify the prognosis. Arguably, the same prognostic factors that are applied in the selection of candidates for surgical resection play an important rule in PEI patients, too. Because the procedure has proved safe and cheap, when palliative purpose is requested in our centre, it is hard to deny treatment to an inoperable patient with disease which is not advanced. However, in a recent article, an increase in survival was reported for patients in whom a complete response was obtained (38 versus 21 months; $P < 0.04$; Giovannini & Seitz, 1994).

References

Ebara M, Ohto M, Sugiura N *et al.* (1990) Percutaneous ethanol injection for the treatment of small hepatocellular carcinoma. Study of 95 patients. *J. Gastroenterol. Hepatol.* **5**, 616–626.

Giovannini M & Seitz UF (1994) Ultrasound guided percutaneous alcohol injection of small liver metastases. *Cancer* **73**, 294–297.

Livraghi T & Solbiati L (1993) Percutaneous ethanol injection in liver cancer: methods and results. *Semin. Intervent. Radiol.* **32**, 69–77.

Livraghi T, Festi D, Monti F *et al.* (1986) US-guided percutaneous alcohol injection of small hepatic and abdominal tumors. *Radiology* **161**, 309–312.

Livraghi T, Vettori C & Lazzaroni S (1991) Liver metastases: results of percutaneous ethanol injection in 14 patients. *Radiology* **179**, 709–712.

Livraghi T, Bolondi L, Lazzaroni S *et al.* (1992) Percutaneous ethanol injection in the treatment of hepatocellular carcinoma in cirrhosis. Study on 207 patients. *Cancer* **68**, 926–929.

Livraghi T, Lazzaroni S, Pellicano S *et al.* (1993) Percutaneous ethanol injection of hepatic tumours: single session therapy with general anesthesia. *AJR* **161**, 1065–1069.

Sheu JC, Sung JL, Huang GT *et al.* (1987) Intratumor injection of absolute ethanol under ultrasound guidance for the treatment of small hepatocellular carcinoma. *Hepato-Gastroenterology* **34**, 255–261.

Shiina S, Yasuda H, Muto H *et al.* (1987) Percutaneous ethanol injection in the treatment of liver neoplasms. *AJR* **149**, 949–952.

Shiina S, Tagawa K, Unuma T *et al.* (1990) Percutaneous ethanol injection therapy of hepatocellular carcinoma: analysis of 77 patients. *AJR* **155**, 1221–1226.

14

Laser treatment of metastases

Zahir Amin and Stephen G. Bown

Lasers are playing an increasingly important role in a wide variety of clinical applications. They deliver light energy to tissue with great precision, and can produce a range of tissue effects. Clinically, the most important laser tissue effects are thermal and include tissue vaporization, necrosis and coagulation (Brown, 1991). In endoluminal tumour therapy, with the laser fibre a few millimetres above the target area, high powers (50–80 W) are used for 1–2 s to vaporize the surface layers and recanalize advanced obstructing cancers (Bown *et al.*, 1986, 1987). Using very low powers (1–2 W) over a long time (500–1000 s), with a thin flexible laser fibre buried within the tissue, tumours in the centre of solid organs can be necrosed *in situ* – this is called interstitial laser photocoagulation (ILP).

Lasers

A laser is a sophisticated light source which produces a coherent, monochromatic and highly collimated beam. These properties allow laser light of appropriate wavelength to be delivered in a precise, controlled and predictable manner to a very small area. The laser light is transmitted by thin flexible optical fibres, and the effects produced are limited to the desired target area with greater accuracy than is possible with other techniques (Carruth & McKenzie, 1986).

There are several types of lasers, each producing light of a specific wavelength in the electromagnetic spectrum. The most suitable laser for ILP is thought to be neodymium: yttrium aluminium garnet (Nd:YAG) laser, which has a wavelength of 1064 nm in the near infrared region of the electromagnetic spectrum. A new Nd-YAG laser is capable of producing a beam with a wavelength of 1320 nm, which may be suitable for ILP (Stokes *et al.*, 1981). Another recent development is a portable semiconductor diode laser, capable of delivering powers of up to 25 W. The light from this laser has a wavelength of 805 nm and its thermal effects also appear suitable for ILP (Jacques *et al.* 1992a).

Principles of ILP

The concept of ILP was first described by Brown in 1983. Instead of delivering light from a non-contact fibre or by a fibretip in contact with the tissue surface, the fibre is inserted directly into the target organ (interstitial placement). This results in maximum response at the desired site within the organ, with minimal surface effects, apart from the small hole required for fibre insertion. This does create the problem of assessing the results of treatment by any immediate visual effects. Therefore, it is essential to be able to predict or monitor carefully the nature, extent and healing of the tissue damage that given laser parameters produce, by using imaging techniques such as ultrasound (US), computed tomography (CT) and magnetic resonance imaging (MRI).

When the fibretip is buried in tissue, the response occurs in a very confined space. If the energy is delivered too fast, the result can be drastic; an excessive amount of tissue water is vaporized and, since there is nowhere for this to go, local pressure disruption of tissue may occur. Also the fibretip can be damaged if it gets too hot while in contact with biological material. Thus, interstitial therapy is best carried out at very low laser powers (around 2 W).

Laser–tissue interactions

The absorption of laser light in tissue is highly dependent on its wavelength (Stokes *et al.*, 1981; Bown, 1983, 1991; Blanc & Colles, 1990; Jacques *et al.*, 1992a). It is the absorbed energy which produces a biological effect, but reflection, transmission and scattering determine where the light goes, and consequently the volume of tissue in which it is absorbed. During ILP, the laser beam exits from the fibretip and undergoes multiple scatterings in the surrounding tissue, so that the light becomes distributed in an almost spherical pattern around the fibretip (Matthewson, 1991). The size of the spherical distribution depends on the optical penetration of the light into the tissue, which in turn depends on the wavelength of the light and the optical properties of the tissue (Svaasand, 1989; Blanc & Colles, 1990). The Nd:YAG laser has excellent tissue-penetrating qualities and is highly scattered, compared with other medical lasers used for their thermal effects, such as the carbon dioxide laser (wavelength 10 600 nm) and the argon laser (wavelength 488 and 514 nm; Bown, 1983). Hence, the Nd:YAG laser gives the largest volumes of necrosis (Svaasand, 1989) and this, combined with the ability of Nd:YAG laser light to be transmitted down thin, flexible optical fibres, makes it the most suitable laser for ILP.

The principal biological effect of the absorbed light during ILP is a thermal one and dependent on the tissue temperature reached. At temperatures below 45°C tissue effects are only produced over a long time (30 min to several hours) and are often reversible (Okumura & Reinhold, 1978). At 45–99°C there is irreversible denaturation of tissue proteins and coagulation occurs, the extent of which is dependent on the exposure time (Priebe *et al.*, 1975). At 100°C tissue water boils; the conversion of water to steam results in a thousandfold expansion and the cell walls rupture, allowing steam to escape (Brackett *et al.*, 1986; Carruth & McKenzie, 1986). During ILP, with the heating occurring in a closed space, the steam escapes along tissue planes and into any adjacent blood vessels. Once the water around the fibretip has dried, the temperature will rapidly rise to 300–400°C, with subsequent tissue blackening, carbonization and smoke production (Carruth & McKenzie, 1986; Matthewson, 1991).

Experimental studies of ILP on normal liver

The best documented work is by Matthewson *et al.* (1987) in rat liver. They inserted a 0.4 mm diameter fibre from an Nd:YAG laser directly into the centre of a lobe of liver exposed at laparatomy in Wistar rats. Power settings of 0.5–2 W and exposure times of 50–2400 s were used to give well-defined lesions of coagulative necrosis with sharp boundaries between normal and necrotic liver. The size of the necrotic zone increased with increasing laser energy (power × time), but there was a plateau effect above 600 J and also above 1 W of power. The maximum diameter of the necrotic zone was 16 mm. Histologically, there was a small area of vacuolation where the fibretip had been, which was surrounded by a thin layer of carbonization. Around this was a zone of coagulative necrosis. By the fourth day following ILP, there was an inflammatory infiltrate at the margin of the necrotic lesion. Healing was by laying down of granulation tissue, followed by fibrosis and regeneration. Two months later, a small fibrous nodule was all that remained.

In order to produce larger volumes of necrosis, Steger *et al.* (1992a) used a 1 × 4 fibreoptic coupling system to split the input beam into four output fibres which could be fired simultaneously. With the four fibres spaced 1.5 cm apart, in dog liver, and using 1.5 W for 670 s, necrotic lesions up to 4 cm in maximum diameter were produced.

Ultrasound monitoring of ILP has been performed *in vivo* using dog (Steger *et al.* 1992b) and pig (Dachman *et al.*, 1990) liver. This shows the formation of a coalescing echogenic zone around the fibretips, with good correlation between the US appearances suggestive of thermal damage and histopathological findings of necrosis. The echogenic zone is due to the boiling of tissue water and the formation of steam bubbles, induced by the high thermal energies (Brackett *et al.* 1986).

Rationale for treating liver tumours with ILP

The liver is a large and easily accessible organ by percutaneous puncture since it lies just under and adjacent to the anterior and lateral abdominal wall. It is well-imaged by US, CT and MRI, and vital structures can be seen and avoided during guided percutaneous puncture. The size of the liver and its vascularity mean that there is sufficient normal tissue around most hepatic tumours which are being considered for ILP. This acts as a heat sink and protects the remaining liver parenchyma and other nearby structures from any adverse effects of the laser light and absorbed heat energy.

Secondary liver tumours present a common clinical problem worldwide and have a poor prognosis (Pommier *et al.*, 1987). Colorectal cancer is also common (Boring *et al.*, 1991; Cancer Research Campaign, 1991), with over 50% of patients developing liver metastases (Ward *et al.*, 1989). The survival time of patients with secondary hepatic tumours is rarely more than 1 year (Jaffe *et al.*, 1968). Surgical resection is the only real hope of a cure. However, only 5–10% of patients with colorectal liver secondaries are suitable for surgery (Steele & Ravikumar, 1989), with a resulting 5-year survival of 10–60% depending on the type and extent of tumour (Adson *et al.*, 1984; August *et al.*, 1985; Butler *et al.*, 1986; Hughes *et al.*, 1988; Franco, 1990). Surgery also carries a small mortality and morbidity. Thus, a minimally invasive method which avoids the need for a laparotomy and destroys the tumour *in situ* could improve the survival of a large number of patients. ILP has the potential for fulfilling this role, and may be of particular use in completely destroying two or three small tumours in different parts of the liver which may be unsuitable for surgical resection.

Alternative interstitial techniques for destroying liver tumours all have limitations (Masters *et al.*, 1991). Cryotherapy requires a laparotomy (Ravikumar *et al.*, 1987); percutaneous intrahepatic alcohol injection gives imprecise and poorly defined areas of necrosis (Livraghi *et al.*, 1991); interstitial radiotherapy cannot be effectively monitored (Dritschilo *et al.*, 1986). ILP is minimally invasive, gives precise and well-defined areas of tumour necrosis, and the changes during treatment can be monitored with US.

Clinical studies on ILP of liver tumours

The first reported clinical work was by Hashimoto *et al.* (1985), who used a modified diffuser fibretip to deliver 1000 J of energy from an Nd:YAG laser set at 5 W. Two cases of hepatocellular carcinoma (HCC) and 8 cases of liver metastases were treated at laparotomy, under ultrasound guidance, with a subsequent marked drop in serum α-fetoprotein (AFP) and carcinoembryonic antigen (CEA), respectively. Schroder and Hahl (1989) treated 4 patients with liver tumours, again at laparotomy, using a sapphire fibretip at higher powers (15–20 W). CT follow-up at 1 and 2 weeks showed areas of necrosis at the treatment sites; however, 1 patient developed an infection in a necrotic area and another died from an air embolus attributed to the use of coaxial gas to cool the sapphire fibretip.

More recently, an US-guided percutaneous approach for ILP of liver tumours has been used (Steger *et al.*, 1989; Huang *et al.*, 1991; Dachman *et al.*, 1992). Huang *et al.* (1991) used a diffuser fibretip with a relatively large outer diameter (1.8 mm), and a power setting of 2–3 W for 20–30 min. They treated 5 patients with small HCCs. Guided biopsies were taken from 4 patients following treatment, and all showed evidence of necrosis. In 1 patient there was no recurrence after 16 months of follow-up, 3 patients had recurrent disease after 5, 12 and 18 months, and 1 patient died of liver failure after 2.5 months which was not thought to be related to the treatment. In 3 patients who had a raised AFP, only in 1 case was there a fall following ILP. Steger *et al.* (1989) and Dachman *et al.* (1992) used a 1 × 4 fibre-splitter (four output fibres fired simultaneously) to achieve larger areas of necrosis during ILP. Masters *et al.* (1992) have recently reported a pilot study of ILP in 10 patients with 18 liver metastases, and found an overall response rate of 44% as assessed by enhanced CT and guided biopsies.

We have treated 26 patients with ILP using a four-fibre system and bare fibretips (Amin *et al.*, 1993). The methods and results are presented below.

Technique

The 26 patients had ILP performed on 70 liver metastases (median 3 per patient, range 1–10), measuring 1–15 cm (median 2.5 cm) in maximum diameter. Primary sites were colorectal in 21 patients, 1 gastric, 1 oesophageal, 1 renal, 1 small bowel carcinoid and 1 pancreatic islet cell.

Immediately prior to the procedure patients received sedation, analgesia and antibiotic cover. After localization of the liver tumour with US, the abdominal wall and liver capsule were infiltrated with lignocaine (1%), and four hollow 19 G needles inserted into the tumour at the site of intended necrosis. The needle tips were positioned about 1–1.5 cm apart in the deepest part of the tumour. A freshly cleaved, sterile 0.2 mm optical fibre from a 1 × 4 star coupler (Canstar, Canada) was inserted down each needle, and the needle withdrawn slightly, so that 3–4 mm of bare fibretip lay within the tumour. This was then irradiated with laser light (wavelength 1064 nm) from a continuous-wave Nd:YAG laser (Flexilase, Living Technology, Glasgow) at a power of 2 W per fibre for 500 s (total energy 4000 J). The ensuing tissue changes were monitored during treatment with US. The needles and fibretips were then carefully adjusted by withdrawing them approximately 1.5 cm and the treatment repeated. This was done up to four times at one session, depending on the size of the tumour and the thermal changes seen on US. For tumours larger than 4 cm, in order to achieve greater areas of necrosis, the needles had to be withdrawn and replaced in a different part of the tumour.

Dynamic CT scanning, performed before and after ILP, was used to evaluate laser-induced necrosis, which was differentiated from spontaneous tumour necrosis by looking for new areas of non-enhancement on the posttreatment scan. Areas of the lesion which still enhanced were assumed to indicate residual viable tumour. Treatment effects as seen on CT were graded as follows: grade I necrosis – 100% of tumour avascularized; grade II necrosis – greater than 50% of tumour avascularized; grade III necrosis – less than 50% of tumour avascularized.

Biopsies of previously treated areas were frequently undertaken, using an 18 G Tru-cut needle under US guidance to check histologically for the presence of necrotic tissue or residual tumour.

Results

Each patient had 1–8 treatment sessions (median 3), and there were 99 tumour treatments (since some tumours were treated several times). The total energy used at each session varied from 5000 to 34 000 J (median 15 000 J).

During treatment, US showed an expanding and coalescing hyperechoic zone around each fibretip, gradually encompassing the tumour (Fig. 14.1; Steger *et al.*, 1992). One week or more later, the treated areas often appeared brightly echogenic, sometimes casting an acoustic shadow, but there were no distinctive features differentiating necrotic tissue from viable tumour. This is in contrast to dynamic CT which differentiates treated from untreated areas very well (Fig. 14.2).

Figure 14.3 shows a tumour before and after ILP, demonstrating a grade I necrosis. The sites of the fibretips are frequently recognized as very small areas of vacuolation on CT, which are presumably due to a small area of tissue vaporization and/or charring at the fibretip.

All the tumours treated had some evidence of necrosis of at least 10% by volume. Grade I necrosis occurred in 37 (53%) tumours, grade II in 23 (33%) and grade III in 10 (14%). Tumours which had grade I or II necrosis were smaller than those with a grade III necrosis (median sizes 2, 3 and 5.5 cm, respectively) and required fewer treatments (medians 1 versus 2.5 for grades I and III, respectively). Overall, 16 out of 26 patients (61%) had a reduction in their tumour volume of greater than 50% at the end of the ILP treatments.

Most of the tumours which had a grade I necrosis have remained fairly well-defined avascular lesions, with no definite evidence of recurrent tumour. These lesions gradually decreased in size over several months, and in 3 cases they completely disappeared. However, patients in whom a grade II or III necrosis had

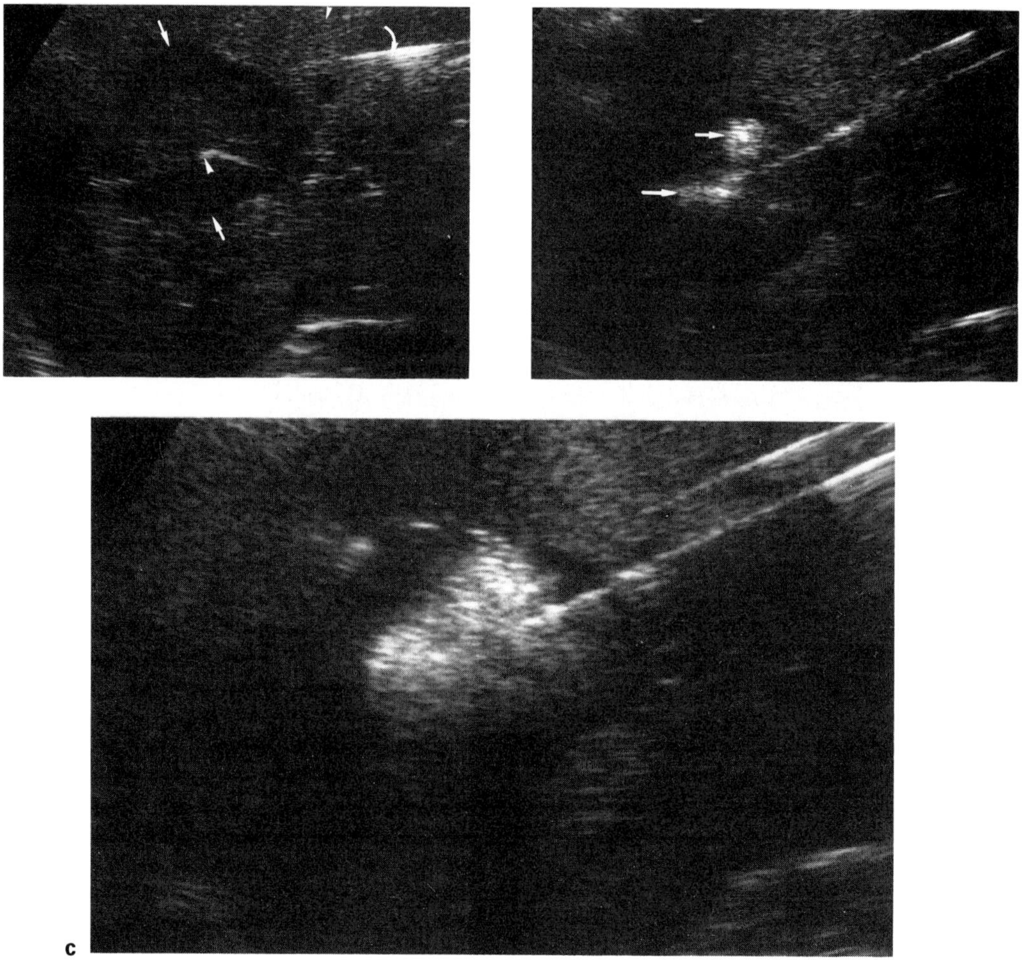

Figure 14.1 (a) Ultrasound scan of liver with a 3 cm hypoechoic metastasis (arrowed) prior to ILP. The echogenic spot (arrowhead) represents a needle-tip within the tumour. The linear track of another needle is also seen (curved arrow). (b) After 300 s of ILP, there are enlarging echogenic zones around the needle-tips (arrows). (c) After 500 s of ILP, the echogenic zones have coalesced, and occupy a large part of the tumour.

been achieved invariably had tumour progression in a 2- or 3-month interval, although evidence of treatment-induced necrosis was still seen.

Biopsies of treated avascular areas on CT have confirmed the presence of necrosis and absence of viable tumour in several cases.

Twelve of the patients with colorectal metastases who had an initially raised serum CEA had serial levels performed after each ILP treatment. In 6 patients there was a fall in CEA, but 4 of these had also had chemotherapy, and in only 2 cases was the decrease in tumour marker demonstrated to be a direct result of ILP. In these latter two cases the CEA fell after ILP from 16 to 2 ng/l and from 40 to 10 ng/l (normal range 0–5 ng/l). Both patients had single liver metastases measuring 2.5 and 3.5 cm in diameter, requiring one or two ILP treatment sessions respectively; complete tumour necrosis (grade I) had been achieved on dynamic CT criteria following ILP.

Ten patients who were followed up for 14 months or longer had evidence of disease progression, with increased liver tumour (5 patients), lung metastases (4 patients) or local colonic recurrence (1 patient). Sixteen patients have evidence of overall tumour reduction, but

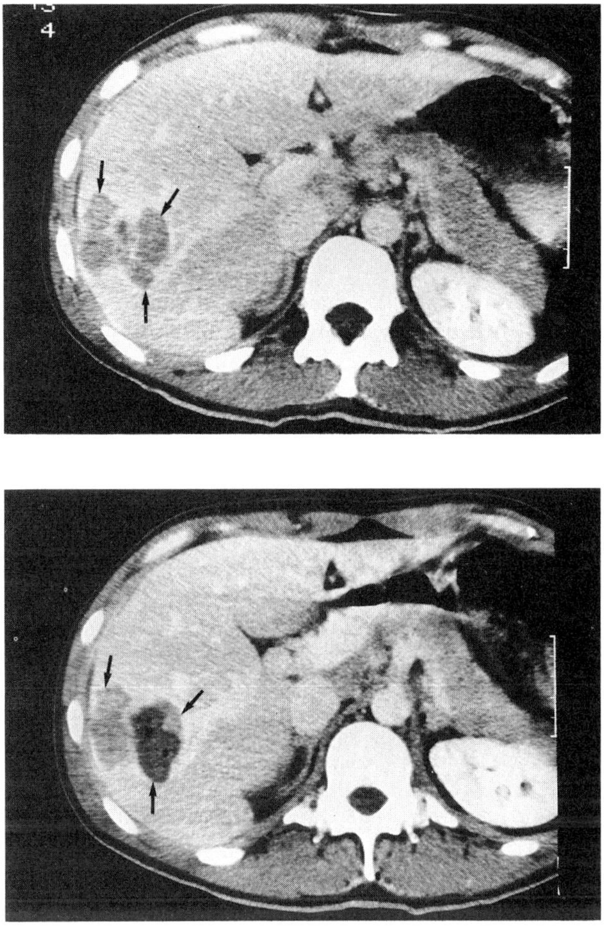

a

b

Figure 14.2 (a) Dynamic computed tomographic (CT) scan showing a 5 cm low-density metastasis (arrows) in the right lobe of the liver before treatment. (b) One day after interstitial laser photocoagulation (ILP), there is a well-defined area of avascularity (arrow) which represents ILP-induced necrosis. Residual untreated tumour lying medially and laterally (arrowheads) continues to enhance.

their follow-up has so far been less than 1 year (median 4 months). Three of these patients have had their only metastases (1 or 2) completely avascularized on CT, and there has been no evidence of recurrence at 4-, 6- and 9-month follow-up.

Of the 26 patients treated over the past 4 years, 8 have died (median survival 21.5 months), and 18 are still alive (median follow-up 6 months). Figure 14.4 shows the life survival curve of our data. The longest survivor died 3 years and 4 months after ILP. The estimated 1-year survival is 82%, and estimated 2-year survival 70%.

Complications

Most patients complained of mild abdominal discomfort during treatment and for 24–48 h afterwards. Additional analgesia was often required for lesions just under the liver capsule, either for shoulder pain due to diaphragmatic irritation or abdominal/back pain thought to be due to heat conduction to nearby peritoneum or retroperitoneum. In some cases the pain results in shortening of the treatment time, to intermittent bouts of 100 s, rather than continuous 500 s. A marked bradycardia occurred in 1 patient during treatment of a lesion in

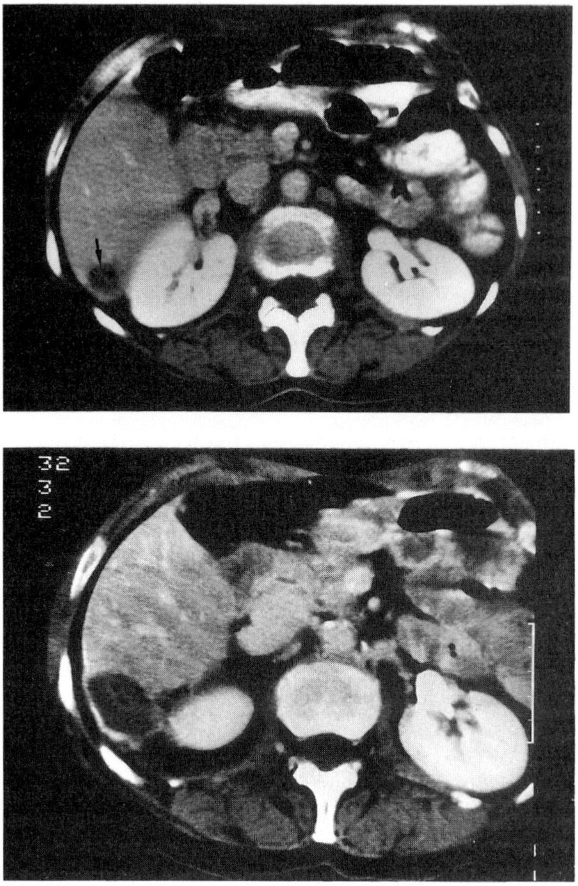

a

b

Figure 14.3 (a) Dynamic computed tomographic (CT) scan showing a 2 cm low-density metastasis (arrow) in the right lobe of the liver, adjacent to the right kidney, before treatment. (b) One day after interstitial laser photocoagulation, the whole tumour, together with a margin of normal liver, has been avascularized.

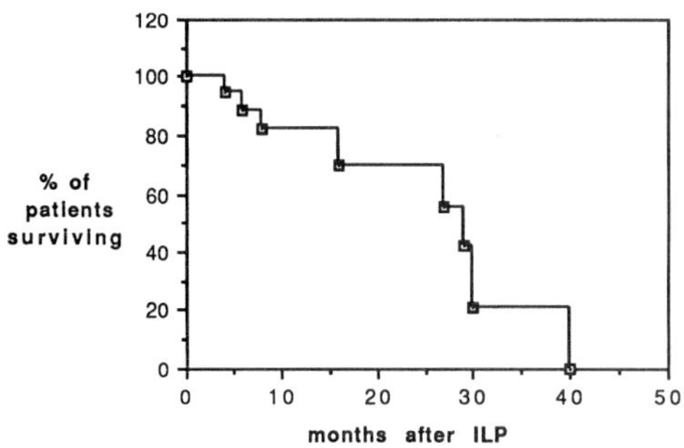

Figure 14.4 Life survival curve based on life-table analysis of 26 patients treated with interstitial laser photocoagulation (ILP) using the Kaplan–Meier method of estimating life survival.

the tip of the left lobe, and was thought to be due to stimulation of vagal branches in adjacent stomach wall. All patients were haemodynamically stable in the 24 h post-ILP, but the subsequent CT scan did demonstrate subcapsular haematomas in 4 cases, and in 1 case there was a drop in haemoglobin by 2 g/dl after 2 treatments 1 week apart. Serum liver function tests demonstrated a transient two- to threefold rise in transaminases following ILP in several cases. Small pleural effusions were seen on post-ILP CT scans in 6 cases after treating lesions close to the diaphragm, but there were no respiratory symptoms and the effusions resolved within a month. All patients were discharged at 24 h post-ILP, and on 11 occasions patients required oral analgesia for up to 10 days. A transient and mild elevation of temperature was observed in several cases 24-72 h posttreatment.

Discussion

Tumour necrosis

This study showed evidence of laser-induced tumour necrosis in all 70 liver metastases treated by ILP, and greater than 50% reduction in tumour volume in 61% of patients. A grade I tumour necrosis (indicating 100% avascularity on CT) was achieved by encompassing the whole tumour by an echogenic zone on US as well as a margin of surrounding normal tissue of about 1 cm thickness in order to destroy any surrounding micrometastases. A grade I necrosis implies an assumption that the avascularity (or non-enhancement) on CT is indicative of necrosis with non-viable tumour. Although this can only be proven by detailed histological correlation with a resected specimen, it is a logical assumption for three reasons:

1. Experimental work on normal liver, using the same laser parameters, confirms a well-defined area of coagulative necrosis which corresponds with arteriographic evidence of loss of all small and some large vessels in the treated area (Matthewson *et al.*, 1987; Steger *et al.*, 1992).
2. The temperatures reached at the fibretip are over 100°C, and 8 mm away are over 50°C (Matthewson *et al.*, 1987), making it highly unlikely that tumour cells can survive these temperatures for the treatment time of 500 s.
3. Needle-core biopsies from non-enhancing areas on CT have confirmed necrosis.

Also, Takayasu et al. (1984) correlated CT images of liver tumours treated by chemoembolization with pathological specimens after surgical resection, and found non-enhancing areas to correspond well with treatment-induced necrosis.

The maximum tumour size in which complete (grade I) necrosis was achieved was 3.5 cm (median size 2 cm). It was not possible to achieve complete necrosis in larger lesions, despite several treatment sessions. The main reason for this is that the differentiation between treated and untreated tumour is not clear on US, especially with larger lesions which appear as a heterogeneous mass after ILP. Since US is the primary modality for needle-fibretip placement, tumours greater than 3.5 cm were at best debulked. If the objective is to destroy all tumour completely, then patients with tumour larger than 3.5 cm should not be treated by ILP at present. An exception is patients with endocrine secondaries who may benefit from debulking of liver tumours.

Laser parameters and optical fibres

The mechanism of ILP was originally thought to be predominantly due to the scattering and diffusion of the laser light over as wide an area as possible, followed by absorption and thermal necrosis (Bown, 1983). This led to the design of various diffuser fibretips (Fujii *et al.*, 1984; Daikuzono & Joffe, 1985) to maximize the volume in which the light is absorbed. However, these modified fibretips are either too large (sapphire tips) for safe percutaneous use or easily damaged (etched tips), and have no significant advantage over bare fibretips (Van Eeden *et al.*, 1988). It is now becoming apparent that, using the same laser power, larger necrotic lesions occur when there is charring at the fibretip (Wyman *et al.*, 1992), indicating that some charring is desirable to maximize the zone of necrosis. Steger (1991) has proposed that the laser light is initially transmitted through tissue but after 20–30 s coagulation of blood and then charring occur. Light is then strongly absorbed in this area, so that it acts like a point heat source. Charring is more likely to occur if there is debris on the fibretip, and also at higher laser powers. Different light wavelengths, such as 805 and 1320 nm, have greater absorption and decreased penetration in tissue (Stokes *et al.*, 1981; Jacques *et al.*, 1992b); this leads to higher temperatures around the fibretip than with the 1064 nm, and increased charring. Hence, these wavelengths would be expected to give larger areas of necrosis, and may be more suitable for ILP. Higher powers (up to 100 W) have been used experimentally for ILP (Godlewski *et al.*, 1988), but there is rapid build-up of pressure and tissue disruption; during tumour treatment this is likely to lead to embolization of viable tumour cells. With lower powers, there is slow 'cooking' of the tumour, with a gradual build-up and release of pressure via escaping microbubbles. These microbubbles are likely to have a temperature over 100°C, and any associated tumour cells will therefore be non-viable. Development of a 1 × 8 or 1 × 12 fibre-splitter would allow larger tumours to be treated in a shorter time, but technical problems with this type of system include excessive heating of the coupler and very low power outputs at each fibretip.

Ultrasound

US plays a useful role in the ILP of liver tumours: it allows evaluation of the size and location of the liver tumours and may detect lesions not seen on the pretreatment CT scan; it enables accurate guided placement of needles into the appropriate part of the tumour; real-time imaging of the treated area as a developing and enlarging echogenic zone has been reliable in predicting the extent of necrosis when treating some smaller (less than 3 cm) metastases (Masters *et al.*, 1992). However, the echogenic zone is often poorly defined with very irregular margins and linear streaks radiating from it. This distorts the image with subsequent difficulty in clearly identifying remaining tumour as well as in seeing the needle tips. This could result in areas of tumour escaping treatment. US is also unhelpful in evaluating lesions post-treatment, since the echogenic area rapidly becomes heterogeneous (within minutes). Follow-up US shows brightly echogenic ellipsoid zones with acoustic shadowing in the treatment area; they are likely to be due to charred tissue along the tracks of the fibretip. This appearance makes the treatment area look very heterogeneous, and as a result any residual tumour cannot be clearly distinguished.

Computed tomography

Precontrast, dynamic and delayed CT is used to define the number and sizes of metastases prior to ILP. Dynamic CT shows the results of ILP very clearly as well-defined, non-enhancing areas, and easily distinguishes these from untreated enhancing tumour. The optimal time to perform the post-ILP CT assessment is after 1–4 days, which corresponds well with the time at which experimentally induced necrotic lesions have their maximum size (Matthewson *et al.*, 1987). Dynamic CT scans have been found to be more useful than precontrast or delayed scans in evaluating treatment-induced necrosis. An enhancing rim often appears at the margins of a treated area between 1 week and several months post-ILP. This may be due to inflammatory change, regenerating liver or recurrent tumour, but CT cannot differentiate these. Histological studies on lesions resected after ILP are required to establish what this enhancing rim means. Tumours that are difficult to locate on US can be treated using CT-guided needle placement. Real-time CT monitoring could allow immediate depiction of untreated tumour, enabling planning and retreatment of the remaining tumour at the same session, and so allowing complete tumour necrosis to be more reliably achieved after a single session.

Magnetic resonance imaging

This has recently been used to evaluate lesions after ILP. With standard spin-echo sequences, T1-weighted images demonstrate a decrease in signal intensity of the lesions following ILP; after gadolinium, an enhancing rim is seen around the necrotic lesion. On T2-weighted images, the treated lesion become heterogeneous, with areas of high and low signal intensity. Using these sequences, the lesion-to-liver contrast is not as good as with dynamic-enhanced CT. This may be improved by trying different MRI parameters to optimize the sequences and maximize contrast between the treated area and surrounding normal liver. New contrast agents may improve MRI of laser-induced changes in liver (Saini *et al.*, 1987; Elizondo *et al.*, 1991).

Carcinoembryogenic antigen

Monitoring of the biological marker, CEA, in patients with colorectal liver metastases showed ILP treatment-related decrease in only 6 out of 12 patients with initially raised tumour marker. All of these patients had a Dukes C colorectal carcinoma at operative resection of their primary tumour, and most patients had significant tumour volume when referred for ILP. Although CT scans of the abdomen and pelvis and a chest X-ray showed no gross extrahepatic disease, this could not definitely be excluded, and is likely in patients with a Dukes C carcinoma. Also, in only 3 patients (2 with colorectal primaries and 1 with a renal primary) was complete tumour avascularization achieved on CT criteria. Treating some lesions invariably meant progression of others in the treatment interval. These factors may account for the continued rise in CEA in 6 of the patients. What is needed is careful monitoring of patients who have surgically resectable disease but are unfit for surgery or refuse an operation, and in whom ILP is performed to give complete tumour avascularization.

Survival

Survival analysis is limited by the small number of patients and relatively short follow-up time. Of the 21 patients with colorectal metastases 6 have died (median survival 28 months, range 4–40 months) and 15 are still alive (follow-up 3–30 months, median 6 months). The 1-year survival of untreated patients with colorectal liver metastases varies from 2 to 27%, depending on the degree of hepatic involvement (Bengmark & Hafstrom, 1969; Wood *et al.*, 1976). Following surgical resection the median 1-year survival from eight studies was 80%, and the mean 3-year survival 55% (Taylor, 1985). Longer follow-up of our patients will give more valid data. The other problem is that many of our patients have received chemotherapy either before or after ILP, which may well have some effect on survival, although chemotherapy alone has not been shown to have any convincing survival benefit (Cunningham, 1989). This makes reliable survival analysis very difficult, and the only way to make valid comments on this is from a long-term controlled trial, with patients receiving either ILP or chemotherapy or both.

Future of ILP

If ILP is to become an accepted form of treatment of liver metastases, there must be a way of monitoring treatment delivery in real time, and of accurately predicting when the extent of thermal damage has matched the tumour volume. The echogenic changes seen during real-time US are only sometimes helpful in this respect. Real-time CT, using a multiple-fibre system, and faster scanners (helical scanners being capable of 30 scans per minute) may allow immediate thermal changes to be detected. MRI has great potential for real-time monitoring of laser–tissue interactions because of the temperature dependence of T1 relaxation time (Jolesz *et al.*, 1988), and the development of temperature-sensitive sequences (Le Bihan *et al.*, 1989). Another way of predicting when ILP has caused sufficient thermal damage to destroy a tumour is by strategically placing microthermocouples at tumour margins in order to monitor tissue temperatures. This set-up can be linked to a computer, and a feedback system can be used to measure the temperature and control the laser energy delivered. By integrating the temperature and time for which that temperature is maintained, the laser power is turned off when the total exceeds that required to produce thermal necrosis (Diakuzono *et al.*, 1987).

Further developments in the imaging methods include better mapping of the tumour distribution in three dimensions – this can be achieved by three dimensional reconstruction of CT, MRI or US images, and will help in delineating the exact extent of the tumour and its relationship to other structures, prior to ILP. US and/or CT stereotactic methods can be used to improve the accuracy of needle, and hence fibretip, placement. For tumours larger than 3–4 cm, placing eight needles prior to starting ILP will allow much more effective necrosis – four needles are used initially, then the fibres are passed down the other four needles which are already accurately placed, thus avoiding the difficult task of resiting needles in an echogenic field (due to treatment).

Selecting patients with limited disease will increase the likelihood of complete tumour ablation, and is more likely to have a positive effect on patient survival. The high chance of extrahepatic and microscopic disease in patients with liver metastases suggests that chemotherapy in combination with ILP would be more effective than ILP alone. ILP could be used to debulk macroscopic hepatic metastases significantly and chemotherapy used to destroy residual, microscopic and extrahepatic disease. A combination of 5-fluorouracil and ILP has been shown to be more effective than 5-fluorouracil or ILP alone in experimentally induced gastric cancer in mice (Narumi *et al.*, 1990). One could also argue for the potential benefits of a continuous-infusion chemotherapy regime during ILP, to take advantage of increased tumour sensitivity to chemotherapy during hyperthermia (Storm *et al.*, 1984).

The potential of interstitial photodynamic therapy is also being evaluated for treating liver metastases (Purkiss *et al.*, 1993). This involves the systemic administration of a photosensitizing drug (such as haematoporphyrin derivative) which is taken up by tumour. Subsequent illumination with laser light of an appropriate wavelength (630 nm) causes a photochemical reaction with production of singlet oxygen and other free radicals, resulting in tumour destruction. Purkiss *et al.* (1993) reported treating 10 patients with this technique, at laparotomy and percutaneously. They found a significant reduction in growth of small colorectal liver metastases. Although this technique can be performed with low morbidity, it is unlikely to be capable of complete liver tumour destruction.

Conclusion

Progress in the development of ILP for liver tumour destruction will be made with improvements in the monitoring methods. US has a very useful role to play in targeting the tumours, and in allowing real-time changes to be seen. Dynamic CT clearly shows treated areas as avascular, and can be used for further treatment planning. With appropriate patient selection and further development of monitoring modalities, this technique may offer a safe, practical and minimally invasive alternative to major surgery for eradicating small, deep-seated tumours, and debulking larger ones.

References

Adson MA, Van Heerden JA, Adson HM *et al.* (1984) Resection of hepatic metastases from colorectal cancer. *Arch. Surg.* **119**, 647–651.

Amin Z, Donald JJ, Masters A *et al.* (1993) Interstitial laser hyperthermia of liver metastases: the role of ultrasound and dynamic CT scanning in monitoring treatment. *Radiology* **187**, 339–347.

August DA, Sugarbaker PH, Ottow RT, Gianola FJ & Schneider PD (1985) Hepatic resection for colorectal metastases. *Ann. Surg.* **201**, 210–218.

Bengmark S & Hafstrom L (1969) The natural history of primary and secondary malignant tumours of the liver. *Cancer* **23**, 198–202.

Blanc D & Colles MJ (1990) Transmission measurements on various tissue samples between 1064 and 2000 nm. *Lasers Med Sci.* **5**, 71–75.

Boring CC, Squires TS & Tong T. (1991) Cancer statistics 1991. *CA Cancer J. Clin.* **41**, 19–51.

Bown SG (1983) Phototherapy of tumours. *World J. Surg.* **7**, 700–709.

Bown SG (1991) Laser–tissue interactions. In: Krasner N (ed) *Lasers in Gastroenterology*, pp. 37–50. London: Chapman & Hall Medical.

Bown SG, Barr, H, Matthewson K *et al.* (1986) Endoscopic treatment of inoperable colorectal tumours with the Nd: YAG laser *Br. J. Surg.* **73** 949–952.

Bown SG, Hawes R, Matthewson K *et al.* (1987) Endoscopic laser palliation for advanced malignant dysphagia. *Gut* **28**, 792–798.

Brackett KA, Sankar MY & Joffe SN (1986) Effects of Nd:YAG laser photoradiation on intra-abdominal tissues: a histological study of tissue damage versus power density applied. *Lasers Surg. Med.* **6**, 123–130.

Butler J, Attiyeh FF & Daly JM (1986) Hepatic resection for metastases from the colon and rectum. *Surg. Gynecol. Obstet.* **162**, 109–113.

Carruth JAS & McKenzie AL (1986) *Medical Lasers, Science and Clinical Practice*. Bristol: Adam Hilger.

Cunningham D (1989) Cytotoxic drugs for gastric and colorectal cancer. *Br. Med. J.* **299**, 1479–1480.

Dachman AH, McGehee JA, Beam TE Burris JA & Powell DA (1990) US-guided percutaneous laser ablation of liver tissue in a chronic pig model. *Radiology* **176**, 129–133.

Dachman AH, VanDeMerwe WP, Czege J, Ward FT, Beam TE & Shay SS (1992) Interstitial tumour ablation of hepatic metastases from colorectal carcinoma using Nd:YAG laser; initial clinical experience. *Laser Surg. Med.* (suppl. 4) A131.

Daikuzono N & Joffe SN (1985) An artificial sapphire probe for contact photocoagulation and tissue vaporisation using the Nd:YAG laser. *Med. Instrum.* **19**, 173–178.

Daikuzono N, Joffe SN, Tajiri H *et al.* (1987) Laserthermia: a computer controlled contact Nd:YAG system for interstitial local hyperthermia. *Med. Instrum.* **21**, 275–277.

Dritschilo A, Grant EG, Harter KW *et al.* (1986) Interstitial radiation therapy for hepatic metastases: sonographic guidance for applicator placement. *AJR* **146**, 275–278.

Elizondo G, Fretz CJ, Stark DD *et al.* (1991) Preclinical evalutation of MnDPDP: a new paramagnetic hepatobiliary contrast agent for MRI. *Radiology* **178**, 73–78.

Franco D (1990) Malignancy of the liver. *Curr. Opin. Gastroenterol.* **6**, 447–453.

Fujii H, Asakura T, Jutamulia S, Kaneko S & Tsuru M (1984) Light scattering properties of a rough ended optical fibre. *Opt. Laser Technol.* **16**, 40–44.

Godlewski G, Sambuc P, Eledjam JJ *et al.* (1988) A new device for inducing deep localised vaporization in liver with the Nd:YAG laser. *Lasers Med. Sci.* **3**, 111–117.

Hashimoto D, Takami M & Ideezuki Y (1985) In depth radiation therapy by Nd:YAG laser for malignant

tumours of the liver under ultrasonic imaging. *Gastroenterology* **88**, A1663.
Huang G, Wang T, Sheu J *et al.* (1991) Low-power laserthermia for the treatment of small hepatocellular carcinoma. *Eur. J. Cancer* **27**, 1622–1627.
Hughes K, Simon R, Adson MA *et al.* (1988) Registry of hepatic metastases. Resection of the liver for colorectal carcinoma metastases: a multi-institutional study for indications of resection. *Surgery* **103**, 278–287.
Jacques S, Thomsen S, Schwartz J, Motamedi M, Rasteger S & Mannonen I (1992) Comparing tissue optics and coagulation for a diode laser (805 nm) versus the Nd:YAG laser (1064 nm). *Lasers Surg. Med.* (suppl. 4) A9.
Jacques SL, Rastegar S, Motamedi M *et al.* (1992) Liver photocoagulation with diode laser (805 nm) vs Nd:YAG laser (1064 nm). In: *Proc. SPIE*, 1646, 107–117.
Jaffe BM, Donegan WL, Watson F & Spratt JS (1968) Factors influencing survival in patients with untreated hepatic metastases. *Surg. Gynecol. Obstet.* **127**, 1–11.
Jolesz FA, Bleier AR, Jakab P, Ruenzel PW, Huttl K & Jako GJ (1988) MR imaging of laser–tissue interactions. *Radiology* **168**, 249–253.
Le Bihan D, Delannoy J & Levin RL (1989) Temperature mapping with MR imaging of molecular diffusion: application to hyperthermia. *Radiology* **171**, 853–857.
Livraghi T, Vettori C & Lazzaroni (1991) Liver metastases: results of percutaneous ethanol injection in 14 patients. *Radiology* **179**, 709–712.
Masters A, Steger AC & Bown SG (1991) Role of interstitial therapy in the treatment of cancer. *Br. J. Surg.* **78**, 518–523.
Masters A, Steger AC, Lees WR, Walmsley KM & Bown SG (1992) Interstitial laser hyperthermia: a new approach for treating liver metastases. *Br. J. Cancer* **66**, 581–522.
Matthewson K (1991) Low power laser hyperthermia. In: Krasner N (ed) *Lasers in Gastroenterology*, pp. 281–299. London: Chapman & Hall Medical.
Matthewson K, Coleridge-Smith P, O'Sullivan JP, Northfield TC & Bown SG (1987) Biological effects of intrahepatic neodymium: yttrium–aluminium–garnet laser photocoagulation in rats. *Gastroenterology*, **93**, 550–557.
Narumi H, Suzuki S & Miwa T (1990) A combination of laserthermia and chemotherapy for the treatment of human gastric cancers transplated into nude mice. *Tokai J. Exp. Clin. Med.* **15**, 449–457.
Okumura Y & Reinhold H (1978) Heat sensitivity of rat skin. *Eur. J. Cancer* **14**, 1161–1166.
Pommier RF, Woltering EA, Campbell JR & Fletcher WS (1987) Hepatic resection for primary and secondary neoplasms of the liver. *Am. J. Surg.* **153**, 428–433.
Cancer Research Campaign (1991) *Annual Report.* London: Cancer Research Campaign, p. 26.
Priebe LA, Cain CP & Welch AJ (1975) Temperature rise required for the production of minimal lesions in the *Macaca mulutta* retina. *Am. J. Ophthalmol.* **79**, 405–413.
Purkiss SF, Abulafi M, Allardice JJ, Grahn M & Williams NS (1993) Interstitial photodynamic therapy for patients with colorectal liver metastases. *Lasers Surg. Med.* **13** (suppl. 5), 21.
Ravikumar TS, Kane R, Cady B *et al* (1987) Hepatic crysurgery with intraoperative ultrasound monitoring for metastatic colon carcinoma. *Arch. Surg.* **122**, 403–409.
Saini S, Stark DD, Hahn PF *et al.* (1987) Ferrite particles: a superparamagnetic MR contrast agent for enhanced detection of liver cancer. *Radiology* **162**, 217–222.
Schroder T Hahl J (1989) Laser induced heperthermia in the treatment of liver tumours. *Lasers Surg. Med.* (suppl. 1) A53.
Steele G Jr & Ravikumar TS (1989) Resection of hepatic metastases from colorectal cancer. Biologic perspectives. *Ann. Surg.* **210**, 127–138.
Steger AC (1991) Interstitial laser hyperthermia for the treatment of hepatic and pancreatic tumours. *Photochem. Photobiol.* **53**, 837–844.
Steger AC, Lees WR, Walmsley K & Bown SG (1989) Interstitial laser hyperthermia: a new approach to local destruction of tumours. *Br. Med. J.* **299**, 362–365.
Steger AC, Lees WRL, Shorvon P, Walmsley K & Bown SG (1992a) Multiple-fibre low-power interstitial laser hyperthermia: studies in the normal liver. *Br. J. Surg.* **79**, 139–145.
Steger AC, Lees WR, Walmsley K & Bown SG (1992b) Ultrasound studies in interstitial laser hyperthermia. *Clin. Radiol.* **46**, 88–93.
Stokes LF, Auth DC, Tanaka D *et al.* (1981) Biomedical utility of 1320 nm Nd:YAG laser radiation. *IEEE Trans. Biomed. Eng. BME* **28**, 297–299.
Storm FK, Silberman AW, Ramming KR *et al.* (1984) Clinical thermochemotherapy: a controlled trial in advanced cancer patients. *Cancer* **53**, 863–868.
Svaasand LO (1989) Dosimetry for laser-induced hyperthermia. *Lasers Med. Sci.* **4**, 309–315.
Svaasand LO, Boerslid T & Oeveraason M (1985) Thermal and optical properties of living tissue: application to laser-induced hyperthermia. *Lasers Surg. Med.* **5**, 589–602.
Takayasu K, Moriyama N, Muramatsu Y *et al.* (1984) Hepatic arterial embolisation for hepatocellular carcinoma. *Radiology* **150**, 661–665.
Taylor I (1985) Colorectal metastases – to treat or not to treat. *Br. J. Surg.* **72**, 511–516.
Van Eeden P, Steger AC & Bown SG (1988) Fibre tip considerations for low power insterstitial laser hyperthermia. *Lasers Med. Sci.* **3**.
Ward BA, Miller DL, Frank JA *et al.* (1989) Prospective evaluation of hepatic imaging studies in the detection of colorectal metastases: correlation with surgical findings. *Surgery* **105**, 180–187.
Wood CB, Gillis CR & Blumgart LH (1976) A retrospective study of the natural history of patients with liver metastases from colorectal cancer. *Clin. Oncol.* **2**, 285–288.
Wyman DR, Wilson BC & Malone DE (1992) Medical imaging systems for feedback control of interstitial laser photocoagulation. *Proc. IEEE* **80**, pp. 890–902.

15

Hyperthermia

Mark A. Burton and Bruce N. Gray

The use of regional hyperthermia for the treatment of hepatic metastases has only recently been investigated in the clinical setting. This has resulted from serious technical difficulties in delivering clinically applicable levels of temperature (in excess of 42°C) into a substantial proportion of a tumour load deep within the body. It is only in the past 5–10 years that the development of heating devices has enabled the deposition of a sufficient heat load into the liver to promote hyperthermia as a potential adjuvant modality with either radiotherapy or chemotherapy. This reliance on the efficiency of the heating device is central to all hyperthermia treatments. The mode of heat induction and the physical characteristics of the device must be purpose-matched to the site of the tumour (whether superficial or deep) for practical heating.

The most common heating modalities used in hyperthermia generally include ultrasound, capacitively coupled and inductive radiofrequency techniques, microwave antennas, Currie point implants and, to a lesser extent, whole-body hyperthermia (Valdaghi, 1990). This list excludes laser therapy, described previously, which used heat for single-modality ablation rather than as an adjuvant to other forms of treatment (Masters & Brown, 1990). Hyperthermia of the liver is primarily delivered in combination with chemotherapy rather than radiotherapy, since the latter has limited value in terms of objective response rates. Tumour imaging is central to the use of any form of regional heating to enable concentration of the deposition of energy as close to the tumour as possible to prevent normal tissue damage. Demonstrably the most effective current form of hyperthermia for regional liver disease utilizes radiofrequency hyperthermia in conjunction with the fluorinated pyrimidines; however, there are a number of promising new hyperthermia programmes currently undergoing preclinical evaluation which will be described.

Capacitive radiofrequency hyperthermia

In the clinical setting, the most frequently reported heating modality for the liver has been capacitive radiofrequency hyperthermia. In general, this form of heating utilizes 500–1300 W of radiofrequency energy with a frequency of approximately 8–14 MHz delivered to the patient through planar electrodes on opposing sides of the upper abdomen (LeVeen *et al.*, 1976; Moffat *et al.*, 1983a; Abe *et al.*, 1986). The electrodes are coupled to the body surface through bolus bags of cooled water (5–10°C) to reduce surface fat and skin heating. Invariably, the hyperthermia treatments are combined with chemotherapy such as doxorubicin for primary disease or 5-fluorouracil for metastatic disease.

Preliminary reports have described high partial response rates (66.7%) for hepatic metastases treated with radiofrequency hyperthermia combined with primarily intrahepatic arterial infusion chemotherapy of 5-fluorouracil and mitomycin (Moffat *et al.*, 1983b, 1985). These studies, using reasonable patient numbers (up to 137), demonstrated a cumulative survival at 1 year of approximately 80% and at least partial tumour regression in about 80% of patients. Response rates were found to be lower (44%) for patients who had previous treatment. Interestingly, the high response rates were achieved despite the inability of the heating device to produce high temperatures in the tumour. While the core body temperature in a subset of patients was shown to rise by less than 1°C, the mean maximum tumour temperature reached only about 40°C. The therapeutic result could therefore be expected to be improved by providing higher temperatures. Because of the low temperatures, the side-effects related to the hyperthermia were minor and occurred in fewer than 10% of patients. They included partial-thickness skin burns at the site of the electrodes and subcutaneous fat necrosis.

The majority of the more recent clinical studies with this heating technique have been performed by Japanese groups using an 8 MHz radiofrequency device. Nagata and co-workers (1990) reported thermal distributions using copper-constantin microthermocouples and therapeutic responses in 20 patients with metastatic liver disease and 47 patients with primary liver cancers. They found that the highest average minimum tumour temperatures and the highest mean maximum temperatures occur in metastatic tumours (41.0 and 42.7°C respectively) rather than primaries. The most beneficial hyperthermia protocol utilized administration of heat for at least 40 min twice a week for a total of 8 times. Combination treatments with the hyperthermia included transcatheter arterial embolization with gelatin sponge particles or starch microspheres, fractionated radiotherapy to 50–60 Gy or doxorubicin chemotherapy. Complete plus partial response rate for patients with metastatic liver tumours was 54% and was found to be greatest for the transcatheter embolization combination (86%). The low number of patients in these subsets precludes an accurate appraisal of the response and it is difficult to evaluate how much of the benefit was due to embolization and to hyperthermia, but the study did demonstrate that clinically applicable temperatures can be readily achieved in metastatic liver tumours.

A similar multi-institutional study with hyperthermia in combination with either radiotherapy or chemotherapy against a variety of deep-seated cancers has been reported (Kakehi *et al.*, 1990). Although all 18 cases treated in this study were hepatocellular carcinomas rather than metastatic cancer, the results deserve special comment. All cases were treated twice weekly with 40–50 min of hyperthermia immediately preceded by chemoembolization with starch microspheres and doxorubicin. The complete plus partial response rate was 56%. However, the authors also described a control study of 26 patients with chemoembolization alone, which resulted in a response rate of 42%. This indicates a clear improvement in response to chemotherapy with the addition of hyperthermia over the single modality. Similarly, the 1-year survival rate was 83% for the thermochemotherapy but only 58% for the chemotherapy alone. Temperatures were measured during treatment of 9 patients to assess the impact of vascular embolization with the starch microspheres in reducing the cooling effect of blood influx to the tumour. This was demonstrated by the mean maximum intratumour temperature, which was 41.5°C for heating alone but rose to 42.4°C during embolization.

Further recent trials have followed the concept of using degradable starch microspheres to prevent or slow the heat dissipation due to tumour blood flow in the liver. Akuta and coworkers (1991) reported on 26 patients, of whom 6 had metastatic disease, treated with intra-arterial starch microspheres of sufficient number to cause temporary blockade of the hepatic artery. This was followed by 20–60 min of heating with an 8 MHz capacitive radiofrequency system. No chemotherapy was used. In the metastatic cancers intratumoral temperatures increased by approximately 4°C during heating alone but the increase was almost 7°C when heating was administered during embolization. Under both circumstances the mean increase was higher for metastatic tumours compared to primary tumours. Response rate for the metastatic cancers was low (33%, though in only 3 evaluable cases) reflecting the absolute requirement to combine chemotherapy or at least some form of supportive treatment with hyperthermia. Another combination treatment that has been reported used transcatheter hepatic arterial injection of doxorubicin and styrene maleic anhydride neocarzinostatin

(SMANCS) in lipiodol with starch microsphere embolization during hyperthermia for hepatocellular carcinoma (Yumoto *et al.*, 1991). The response rates for this treatment were also low (40%) compared to previously described studies, but this was twice the response for chemotherapy alone.

Radiative electromagnetic applicators

One of the early devices used for deep-body hyperthermia was the BSD-1000 annular phased array system (Turner, 1983), which has been used for treating hepatic metastases (Petrovich *et al.*, 1989a, 1989b). The annular phased array is a couch arrangement on which the patient lies within a cylindrical set of eight radiofrequency applicators. A large water bolus bag envelops the patient's upper abdomen and variations in power deposition can be applied through the bolus to the deep regions of the body, such as the liver. The frequency used is variable but is generally around 55 MHz, with a mean power of 780 W. In one study 49 patients with 'massive' metastatic liver disease were to be treated with hyperthermia at 42.5°C for 30 min, in combination with radiotherapy, chemotherapy or both. The desired hyperthermic temperatures could be achieved in fewer than 60% of the patients because of technical difficulties and patient pain. The overall objective response rate was only 12%; however, several important points were demonstrated by the study. Combining treatments will always improve the therapeutic outcome. Response rates for patients receiving hyperthermia alone was 0; for those receiving hyperthermia plus chemotherapy (primarily 5-fluorouracil) it was 7%; for hyperthermia plus radiotherapy (mean of 24 Gy) it was 18%, and for those receiving a combination of all three treatments it was 50%. It was also demonstrated that response was primarily related to thermal dose and to radiation dose received. Clinical studies are currently underway on a second-generation BSD-2000 annular phased array system (BSD, Utah, USA), which should provide better control over energy deposition and thus temperature in tumour tissue; further new phased array microwave devices are being developed (Tianquan *et al.*, 1991). These systems are also being supplemented by the incorporation of computer-controlled treatment planning where digitized body tissue mapping from diagnostic scans will determine the phasing of the power from the applicators to provide more efficient heating.

Perfusion hyperthermia

Hyperthermia can be induced in the liver by the surgical technique of isolated perfusion. This process has been described in use for some time using hyperthermia alone (Quebbeman *et al.*, 1984) and also by combining the heat with 5-fluorouracil chemotherapy (Pugner *et al.*, 1982). Generally, the technique isolates the liver vasculature by cannulating the hepatic artery, the portal vein and the inferior vena cava and then occluding the suprahepatic vena cava and the proximal hepatic artery. The liver is then perfused with a variable flow (1500–1800 ml/min) and temperature probes placed in the hepatic parenchyma and the liver metastases. The perfusate is warmed to 43.0–44.0°C with a resultant liver and tumour temperature of approximately 42.5°C. In both reported studies either histological or radiological evidence of tumour necrosis or cessation of tumour growth was demonstrated.

A further study reported on toxicity and responses to isolated hepatic perfusion of metastatic disease in 8 patients (Skibba & Quebbeman, 1986). During the isolated perfusion lactate levels and pyruvate levels increased significantly in both blood and perfusate. Immediately following the operation serum aspartate aminotransferase and lactate phosphatase levels were elevated. There was also a transient elevation in serum bilirubin and evidence of thrombocytopenia and hypokalaemia. Despite these relatively minor signs of adverse liver function, 2 of the treated patients died postoperatively from hepatic failure. Of the 6 surviving patients, 5 had objective responses to treatment as measured by computed tomographic scans. It was suggested that a better response may be possible by combining treatment with chemotherapy or radiotherapy.

Whole-body hyperthermia

Whole-body hyperthermia, as opposed to regional or local heating of tumours, has been examined for the treatment of disseminated deep tumours and can be achieved by a variety of different methods. These include paraffin wax, hot air, radiofrequency devices, water-perfused blankets or suits or by extracorporeal heated circuits. Some partial responses have been described, when hyperthermia is accompanied by radiotherapy or chemotherapy, but essentially none of these techniques has produced good results with either primary liver disease or metastases (Van der Zee *et al.*, 1983; Maeta *et al.*, 1987). Most importantly, the side-effects of the treatments have proven to be extremely severe and include significant hepatic necrosis or insufficiency causing postoperative death or, in almost all patients, intense gastrointestinal problems such as diarrhoea and vomiting.

Targeted treatment

The future for hyperthermia of the liver is likely to be centred on new technologies that have the potential to target the treatment to tumour tissue selectively, since the limiting factor in most modalities is the normal tissue damage caused by the treatment medium. There are a number of interesting new approaches to targeting either the heat or the combination radiotherapy or chemotherapy. One central concept utilizes intra-arterially injected microspheres (as described in Chapter 11) to transport the antitumour agent directly to the tumour tissue where they embolize the tumour vasculature and localize the agent to the tumour. The addition of hyperthermia to this treatment has the potential to promote a synergistic or additive effect on the tumour which is localized, which in turn may allow increases in dosimetry because of the relative sparing of normal tissue.

This form of treatment has been reported. Grady and coworkers (1983) first combined regional hyperthermia with targeted radiotherapy using yttrium 90 microspheres in 15 patients being treated for secondary liver cancer. The use of internal radiation therapy for liver metastases with microspheres was originated by this group in 1960 and they had endeavoured to improve this treatment by adding heat, which is more effective against areas of poor blood supply, anoxia and low pH, as in tumour tissue. The study reported regression or control of liver disease in half of the patients and subjective palliation in the others. The hyperthermia used was relatively crude and temperatures were not measured, so the efficiency of the heating is questionable. However, heating techniques have been significantly improved since this report and there is thus a need to re-examine this combination.

Along similar lines, preclinical studies have demonstrated the potential efficacy of combining hyperthermia with targeted chemotherapy. The use of microspheres for the transport of anticancer drugs has focused primarily on doxorubicin because of its chemical structure, which is suited to incorporation into resin or protein matrices and has been shown to act in an additive fashion, in combination with heat in liver tumour models (Burton *et al.*, 1991). This has opened the possibility of targeted therapy, particularly for primary liver cancer, but also for metastatic disease and again may be utilized in combination with hyperthermia. Animal studies have demonstrated significant improvement in therapeutic response for targeted microsphere chemotherapy in conjunction with regional hyperthermia compared to either treatment alone (Burton *et al.*, 1992).

These combinations of treatments show particular promise since they are complementary in action and site of influence. Hyperthermia is a potent drug sensitizer acting through several potential mechanisms. Heat can increase cell membrane permeability to drugs or, in some case, reduce efflux of drug from the cell as well as inhibit repair mechanisms. Thus, the direct action of heat on tissue is combined with an improved potential for response to chemotherapy. Drugs or radiation can be delivered preferentially to hepatic tumour tissue on intravascular microspheres by virtue of the high blood supply to the vascular growing edge (Burton *et al.*, 1989). As a secondary effect the microspheres embolize the tumour vasculature, promoting ischaemic damage and reducing any cooling effects from influx of blood to the tissue is being heated. Additionally, the effects of the hyperthermia are most pronounced in the central semiavascular areas of the tumour where drugs have difficulty permeating and which are generally hypoxic and radioresistant, while radioactive or chemotherapeutic microspheres lodge in the vascular growing edge. The result is complementary treatment of both the central and the peripheral areas of the tumour.

The above treatment options all utilize basically regional hyperthermia to treat the liver. In this way normal tissue is also being heated and there is thus a strong likelihood that treatments will be limited by patient compliance, where large areas of the visceral mass being heated may cause abdominal pain. It is therefore favourable to be able to target the heat as well as the combination treatment, which may allow increases in the levels of combinations being used because of less general or regional toxicity. Such systems are available and will reach clinical significance in the near future. The principal technique utilizes scanned focused ultrasound (Hand *et al.*, 1992). Scanning with a focused point of high-energy ultrasound may be achieved either by mechanical means or by electronic switching, but the result is the ability to be able to deposit large amounts of heat energy in targeted areas of tumour tissue of almost any size or shape.

Scanned focused ultrasound as a true regional or local form of hyperthermia is very dependent on imaging of the tumour to provide information on exactly where to deposit the heat energy and in what pattern. The imaging and heating components of the treatment have been combined in a device developed by a group at the University of Arizona (Hynynen *et al.*, 1987) and an Australian company (Ausonics, Sydney, Australia). The concept has been adapted and varied by others but is basically an array of six to eight 1 MHz ultrasound heating transducers located around a central 3.5 MHz imaging transducer. This system allows the imaging transducer to record the size, shape and location of a tumour and have the information integrated into a computerized treatment program that essentially controls the heating process administered through the heating transducers almost at the same time. This form of localizing the hyperthermia has such fine control that it is now being developed from just heating the tumour to 42–44°C to complete ablation of the tissue using the focused ultrasound, guided by either ultrasound imaging or magnetic resonance imaging (Hynynen *et al.*, 1992).

In conclusion, there is little doubt that hyperthermia can provide an enhanced response to conventional treatment for liver metastases. The limiting factor for treatment of this deep-seated organ has historically been the efficiency of heating devices in depositing sufficient energy in the region of the tumour. Such devices are now becoming commercially available and techniques for targeting heat and radiotherapy or chemotherapy in combination have been developed. What is now required is the accumulation of more controlled clinical data examining the therapeutic responses to different treatment parameters, and heating devices being employed to promote general acceptance of this emerging modality.

References

Abe M, Hiraoka M, Takahashi M *et al.* (1986) Multi-institutional studies on hyperthermia using an 8 MHz radiofrequency capacitive heating device Thermotron RF-8 in combination with radiation for cancer therapy. *Cancer* **58**, 1589–1595.

Aigner K, Walther H, Tonn JC *et al.* (1982) Die isolioerte leberperfusion mit 5-Fluorouracil (5FU) beim menschen. *Chirurgica* **53**, 571–573.

Akuta K, Abe M, Kondo M *et al.* (1991) Combined effects of hepatic arterial embolisation using degradable starch microspheres (DSM) in hyperthermia for liver cancer. *Int. J. Hyperthermia* **7**, 231–242.

Burton MA, Gray BN, Klemp PF *et al.* (1989) Selective internal radiation therapy: distribution of radiation in the liver. *Eur. J. Cancer Clin. Oncol.* **25**, 1487–1491.

Burton MA, Kelleher DK, Gray BN *et al.* (1991) Low dose systemic doxorubicin in combination with regional hepatic hyperthermia. *Reg. Cancer Ther.* **3**, 26–30.

Burton MA, Chen Y, Atkinson H *et al.* (1992) *In vitro* and *in vivo* responses of doxorubicin ion exchange microspheres to hyperthermia. *Int. J. Hyperthermia* **8**, 485–494.

Grady ED, McLaren J, Auda SP *et al.* (1983) Combination of internal radiation therapy and hyperthermia to treat liver cancer. *South. Med. J. (Ga)* **76**, 1101–1105.

Hand JW, Vernon CC & Prior MV (1992) Early experience of a commercial scanned focused ultrasound hyperthermia system. *Int. J. Hyperthermia* **8**, 587–608.

Hynynen K, Roemer RB, Anhalt D *et al.* (1987) A scanned focused, multiple transducer ultrasonic system for localised hyperthermia treatments. *Int. J. Hyperthermia* **3**, 21–35.

Hynynen K, Damianou C, Darkazanli A *et al.* (1992) On-line MRI monitored noninvasive ultrasound surgery. In: Morucci JP *et al.* (eds) *Proceedings of the 14th International Conference IEEE Engineering in Medicine and Biology Society*, vol. **14**. New York: IEEE, pp. 350–351.

Kakehi M, Ueda K, Mukojima T *et al.* (1990) Multi institutional clinical studies on hyperthermia combined with radiotherapy or chemotherapy in advanced cancer of deep-seated organs. *Int. J. Hyperthermia* **6**, 719–740.

LeVeen HH, Wapnick S, Piccone V *et al.* (1976) Tumour eradication by radiofrequency therapy. *J.A.M.A* **235**, 2198–2002.

Maeta M, Koga S, Wada J *et al.* (1987) Clinical evaluation of total body hyperthermia combined with anticancer chemotherapy for far advanced miscellaneous cancer in Japan. *Cancer* **59**, 1101–1106.

Masters A & Brown SG (1990) Interstitial laser hyperthermia in tumour therapy. *Ann. Chir. Gynaecol.* **79**, 244–251.

Moffat FL, Falk RE, Calhoun K *et al.* (1983a) The effect of radiofrequency hyperthermia and chemotherapy on primary and secondary liver neoplasms when used with adjuvant metronidazole. *Surgery* **94**, 536–542.

Moffat FL, Falk RE, Calhoun K *et al.* (1983b) The effect of radiofrequency hyperthermia and chemotherapy on primary and secondary liver neoplasms when used with adjuvant metronidazole. *Surgery* **94**, 536–542.

Moffat FL, Gilas T, Calhoun K *et al.* (1985) Further experience with regional radiofrequency hyperthermia and cytotoxic chemotherapy for unresectable hepatic neoplasia. *Cancer* **55**, 1291–1295.

Nagata Y, Hiraoka M, Akuta K *et al.* (1990) Radiofrequency thermotherapy for malignant liver tumours. *Cancer* **65**, 1730–1736.

Petrovich Z, Langholz B, Gibbs FA *et al.* (1989a) Regional hyperthermia for advanced tumours: a clinical study of 353 patients. *J. Radiat. Oncol. Biol. Phys.* **16**, 601--607.

Petrovich Z, Langholz B, Kapp DS *et al.* (1989b) Deep regional hyperthermia of the liver. *Am. J. Oncol.* **12**, 378–383.

Quebbeman EJ, Skibba JL and Petroff RJ (1984) A technique for isolated hyperthermic liver perfusion. *J. Surg. Oncol.* **27**, 141–145.

Skibba JL & Quebbeman EJ (1986) Tumoricidal effects and patient survival after hyperthermia liver perfusion. *Arch. Surg.* **121**, 1266–1271.

Tianquan D, Zheng L & Wei R (1991) Theoretical analysis of H-horn annular phased array system for heating deep seated tumors. *J. Microwave Power Electromag. Energy* **26**, 100–106.

Turner PF (1983) Regional hyperthermia with annular phased array. *IEEE Trans. Biomed. Eng.* **31**, 106–114.

Valdagni R (1990) International consensus meeting on hyperthermia: final report. *Int. J. Hyperthermia* **6**, 839–877.

Van der Zee J, Van Rhoon G, Wike-Hooley L *et al.* (1983) Whole body hyperthermia in cancer therapy: a report of a phase I-II study. *Eur. J. Cancer Clin. Oncol.* **9**, 1189–1200.

Yumoto Y, Jinno K, Tokuyama K *et al.* (1991) Transcatheter hepatic arterial injection of lipiodol soluble anticancer agents SMANCS and ADR suspension in lipiodol combined with arterial embolisation and local hyperthermia for treatment of hepatocellular carcinoma. *Int. J. Hyperthermia* **7**, 7–17.

16

Non-cytotoxic control of liver metastases from colon cancer

David L. Morris

The role of growth factors and other biological therapies in the formation and subsequent progression of hepatic metastases has received relatively little attention. This chapter reviews current progress and prospects for the future.

Somatostatin

Somatostatin is a naturally occurring tetradecapeptide growth regulator which profoundly inhibits the release or action of gastrointestinal hormones. It has been shown to control growth of experimental pancreatic cancer, prostate cancer (Bensaid *et al.*, 1992), small cell lung cancer and osteosarcoma (Schally, 1988).

The use of somatostatin for tumour is best established for endocrine tumours – carcinoid, insulinoma, glucagonoma, gastrinoma and vasoactive intestinal peptide tumours. There is some possibility of therapeutic benefit in breast cancer.

We and others have shown that a proportion of colorectal cancers have somatostatin receptors (Iftikhar *et al.*, 1992) and that SMS 201.995 (Sandostatin, Sandoz) produced significant inhibition of *in vitro* growth of two of four human colorectal cancer cell lines, as well as significantly inhibiting both cancer cell lines that were grown as xenografts (Dy *et al.*, 1992). Qin *et al.*, (1991), working with RC160, showed significant inhibition of a rat colonic adenocarcinoma.

We have also recently reported (Stewart *et al.*, 1994) that SMS 201.995 or Sandostatin can very significantly reduce the number and size of metastases developing in nude mice given an intrasplenic injection of human colon cancer cells (C170). In our experiment, the animals treated with SMS by minipump 50 μg/kg per day developed 7.7 (2.9) liver metastases, compared with 20.7 (4.3) in controls. Tumour weight, percentage replacement and serum carcinoembryonic antigen were similarly affected. This finding is similar to that of Qin *et al.* (1992) using RC160, a similar somatostatin analogue, where a reduction in growth of hepatic metastases of a rat colon cancer cell line was achieved. Human colon cancer xenografts of 320 DM or WidR cell lines in nude mice were also significantly inhibited by 4 weeks of RC160 administration. No clinical trials looking at the effect of somatostatin administration on liver metastases have yet been reported.

The possible mechanism of effect of SMS on liver metastases are several: SMS reduces liver blood flow (Hemingway *et al.*, 1992), has direct inhibitory effects on colon cancer cells and can be shown to stimulate the hepatic reticuloendothelial system. Somatostatin also blocks intracellular secondary messengers. SMS also reduced synthesis or release of the growth factors, including insulin-like growth factor 1 and the trophic hormones gastrin, cholecystokinin and bombesin (Townsend *et al.*, 1986; Schally, 1988).

Growth factor antagonists

Gastrin

There is good *in vitro* and animal evidence of stimulation of colorectal cancers by gastrin (Karlin *et al.*, 1985; Tanaka *et al.*, 1986; Winsett *et al.*, 1986; McGregor *et al.*, 1989). There is evidence that patients with colorectal cancer have a significantly higher serum gastrin than controls – or perhaps that a subpopulation do (Smith *et al.*, 1989). There is some evidence that both colorectal cancers and gastric cancers synthesize gastrin or progastrin (Hoosein *et al.*, 1990; Watson *et al.*, 1991a).

Gastrin antagonists have not yet been adequately investigated in colorectal cancer. In *in vitro* culture and animal models there is evidence of inhibition of gastrin-stimulated growth and inhibition of basal growth of some cell lines (Watson *et al.*, 1991b). Whether these can be translated into clinical benefit is not yet clear. We have reported a pilot clinical study with proglumide in human colorectal cancer with no evidence of regression (Morris *et al.*, 1990), but this was a small study in advanced disease and much larger studies, including adjuvant trials (Harrison *et al.*, 1990), are needed. Much more potent receptor antagonists are available: whilst a concentration of 10^{-3} mol/l proglumide is required to achieve inhibition of gastrin-stimulated growth, some of the newer antagonists can inhibit growth at concentrations of 10^{-10} mol/l (Romani & Morris, 1994). If an autocrine or intracrine mechanism is really involved in colon cancer, we may see regression rather than just control of growth. The use of gastrin receptor antagonists for hepatic metastases from colorectal cancer has not yet been researched.

Histamine and antagonists

The established effects of cimetidine and ranitidine on immune function are a possible reason for the proven survival advantage in patients with gastric cancer treated with cimetidine (Tonneson *et al.*, 1988; Nielsen *et al.*, 1989) and the occasional regression of other tumours. We have recently reported preservation of perioperative immune function in cimetidine-treated patients in a control trial of patients with colorectal cancer (Adams *et al.*, 1994).

We believe, however, that histamine may be an important growth factor for colon cancer. Histamine stimulates *in vitro* and *in vivo* growth of some human colonic cancer cell lines. Cimetidine inhibits all these effects. Cimetidine also inhibits growth of xenografts and carcinogen-induced tumours and histamine-stimulated cyclic adenosine monophosphate release of cells (Adams *et al.*, 1993, 1994; Warlters *et al.*, 1993).

Whilst the histamine content of several tumour types is known to be high, the source of this histamine is not yet clear. Whether this is tumour produced or released by the infiltrating mast cells now known to be prognostic is not yet clear.

H_2-receptor antagonists may well be of value in patients with colorectal cancer, including those with liver metastases. Clinical and animal studies are already in hand. A very preliminary study from Nielsen in Copenhagen reports a survival advantage in patients with liver metastases from colorectal cancer treated with ranitidine (H. J. Nielsen, 1993, personal communication).

Prostaglandins

Prostaglandins can produce very considerable inhibition of early growth of colorectal cancer xenografts (Lawson *et al.*, 1994), but their possible effects on liver metastases have not been investigated.

Sex steroids

Whilst a proportion of colorectal cancers have oestrogen receptors as measured estrogen receptor related protein clone D5 (ERD5), this is not prognostic, in contrast to gastric cancer (Harrison *et al.*, 1989; Robertson *et al.*, 1991).In gastric cancer, tamoxifen failed to improve survival and, in oestrogen receptor-positive tumours, significantly worsened it (Harrison *et al.*, 1989b) – a finding which was later reproduced in the laboratory (Harrison *et al.*, 1989c).

Androgen receptors also appear to be of importance and may explain sex differences in the incidence of colon cancer (Singh *et al.*, 1993). This has not been explored in any therapeutic model of liver cancer.

Gene therapy

The insertion of new genetic material into target cells to produce a new cellular phenotype could clearly be used in cancer. Multiple genetic abnormalities exist in most cancers but correction of even one of these may be therapeutically valuable. Genetic loss in colon cancer has been demonstrated on chromosomes 5q, 17p and 18q. Delivery of genes to the cancer cell can be achieved by disabled retroviruses which selectively enter proliferating cells. Dramatic reduction in cancer cell proliferation has been achieved by such approaches (Roth, 1993). Genes can also be transferred by microinjection, or by chemically mediated transfer.

Tumour vaccines

Cancer vaccines have used autologous major histocompatibility complex (MHC)-matched or allogeneic (MHC-mismatched) tumour cells or tumour cell-derived preparations with an adjuvant. We do not have purified tumour antigens of known efficacy, so tumour cells have been the most appropriate method to date. As yet, generally disappointing results have been reported but occasionally responses have been seen (Marx, 1989; Knuth *et al.*, 1991; Oettgen & Old, 1991).

A sialomucin antigen present in epithelial cancer cells is being trialled as the basis of a vaccine in colorectal cancer (O'Boyle *et al.*, 1992).

There are several other possible methods, including the production of loss of major histocompatibility complex antigens, alteration of tumour cells to make them express cytokines to increase immunogeneity and gene correction therapy.

Cytokines

Three cytokines have been extensively studied: IL-2 interleukin 2 (IL-2), tumour necrosis factor (TNF) and interferon-α (IFN-α). IL-2 induces proliferation and activation of lymphokine-activated killer (LAK) cells, and cytotoxic T lymphocytes (CTL) from natural killer (NK) cells. Clinical use of IL-2 has been limited by systemic toxicity, fever, rigors, nausea, vomiting, diarrhoea, hypotension, arrhythmias, fluid retention, hepatic and renal dysfunction (Foon, 1989). IL-2 activation of LAK cells has, however, been associated with significant response in disseminated renal carcinoma and malignant melanoma.

The discovery of the T-cell growth factor IL-2 provided the ability to expand T cells both *in vitro* and *in vivo*. Tumour regression and dense lymphoid infiltration of the tumour were seen with IL-2 therapy. Tumour-infiltrating lymphocytes and lymphokine killer cells can be recovered from tumours, expanded and reinjected, with occasional spectacular regression but with associated severe toxicity. Tumour-infiltrating lymphocyte cells have achieved good response rates in advanced melanoma (Rosenberg *et al.*, 1987).

TNF is a polypeptide made by monocytes and has antitumour activity. The TNF molecule is responsible for the changes of endotoxic shock. Systemic delivery is associated with toxicity. Regional perfusion to date does not seem to be either effective or safe.

Regional biological therapy

The proven benefit of higher response rates, reduced toxicity and survival advantage seen with regional as opposed to systemic administration of 5-fluorouracil (5-FU) or fluorodeoxyuridine (FUDR) makes this route of administration clearly attractive for biological therapy. The systemic administration of recombinant human TNF can be associated with severe hypotension, central nervous system dysfunction, thromboembolic and cardiopulmonary phenomena. High concentrations of recombinant TNF and prolonged exposure are needed to improve chances of response (Frei & Spriggs, 1989). Preliminary dog work with hepatic arterial infusion (Ohkawa *et al.*, 1989) has led on to a clinical trial of 5-day intra-arterial infusion of recombinant human TNF through radiologically placed catheters in 22 patients with hepatic metastases, including 14 from colorectal cancer who had failed chemotherapy. Seven of these 14 achieved a carcinoembryonic antigen fall of >25%, 2 had objective response and 3 additional patients had minor responses (Mavligit *et al.*, 1992). The patients tolerated approximately six times the maximum tolerated systemic dose. There may well be a further possibility for improved response with longer administration times, alterations in liver blood flow and concurrent use of other compounds.

Some work has been done on the intrasplenic delivery of IL-2 in order to enhance LAK cell activity. Recombinant IL-2 was given to 31 patients with advanced metastatic malignant melanoma. The first dose was given intrasplenically, then four intravenous doses were given in a course which was repeated where possible. Four of the 31 patients had partial tumour responses: the authors concluded that this technique could be of use and did not require intensive care facilities (Thatcher *et al.*, 1989).

Non-cytotoxic control of the growth of hepatic metastases is an exciting research area which may well yield clinical benefit.

References

Adams WJ, Lawson JA & Morris DL (1994) Cimetidine inhibits *in vivo* growth of human colon cancer and reverses histamine stimulated *in vitro* and *in vivo* growth. *Gut* **35**, 1632–1636.

Adams WJ, Lawson JA, Nicholson SE *et al.* (1993) The growth of carcinogen induced colon cancer in rats is inhibited by cimetidine. *Eur. J. Surg. Oncol.* **19**, 332–335.

Bensaid M, Tahiri-Jouti N, Cambillau C *et al.* (1992) Basic fibroblast growth factor induces proliferation of a rat pancreatic cancer cell line. Inhibition by somatostatin. *Int. J. Cancer* **50**, 796–799.

Dy DY, Whitehead RH & Morris DL (1992) SMS 201.995 inhibits *in vitro* and *in vivo* growth of human colon cancer. *Cancer Res.* **52**, 917–923.

Foon KA (1989) Biological response modifiers: the new immunotherapy. *Cancer Res.* **49**, 1621–1639.

Frei E III & Spriggs D (1989) Tumor necrosis factor: still a promising agent. *J. Clin. Oncol.* **7**, 291–294.

Harrison JD, Watson SA & Morris DL (1989a) The effect of sex hormones and tamoxifen on the growth of human gastric and colorectal cancer cell lines. *Cancer* **65**, 2148–2151.

Harrison JD, Morris DL, Jones JA *et al.* (1989b) The effect of tamoxifen and estrogen receptor status on survival in gastric carcinoma. *Cancer* **64**, 1007–1010.

Harrison JD, Watson SA & Morris DL (1989c) The effect of sex hormones and tamoxifen on the growth of human gastric and colorectal cancer cell lines. *Cancer* **63**, 2148–2151.

Harrison JA, Jones JA & Morris DL (1990) The effect of the gastrin receptor antagonist proglumide on survival in gastric carcinoma. *Cancer* **66**, 1449–1452.

Hemingway DM, Jenkins SA & Cooke TG (1992) The effects of sandostatin (octreotide, SMS 201.995) infusion on splanchnic and hepatic blood flow in an experimental model of hepatic metastases. *Br. J. Cancer* **65**, 396–398.

Hoosein NM, Kiener PA, Curry RC *et al.* (1990) Evidence for autocrine growth stimulation of cultured colon tumor cells by a gastrin/cholecystokinin-like peptide. *Exp. Cell Res.* **186**, 15–21.

Iftikhar SY, Thomas WM, Rooney PS *et al.* (1992) Somatostatin receptor status in human colorectal cancer. *Eur. J. Surg. Oncol.* **18**, 27–30.

Karlin DA, McBath M, Jones RD *et al.* (1985) Hypergastrinaemia and colorectal carcinogenesis in the rat. *Cancer Lett.* **29**, 73–78.

Knuth A, Wolfel T & Meyer zum Buschenfelde K-H (1991) Cellular and humoral immune responses against cancer: implications for cancer vaccines. *Curr. Opin. Immunol.* **3**, 659–664.

Lawson JA, Adams, WJ & Morris DL (1994) The effect of Misoprostol on colon cancer. *Aust. N.Z. J. Surg.* **64**, 197–201.

McGregor DB, Morriss LL, Manalo PB *et al.* (1989) Pentagastrin stimulation of human colon carcinoma. *Arch. Surg.* **124**, 470–472.

Marx JL (1989) Cancer vaccines show promise at last. *Science* **245**, 813–815.

Mavligit GM, Zukiwski AA, Charnsangavej C *et al.* (1992) Regional biologic therapy: hepatic arterial induction of recombinant human tumor necrosis factor in patients with liver metastases. *Cancer* **69**, 557–561.

Morris DL, Charnley RM, Ballantyne KC *et al.* (1990) A pilot randomized control trial of proglumide (a gastrin receptor antagonist) in advanced colorectal cancer. *Eur. J. Clin. Oncol.* **16**, 423–425.

Nielson HJ, Moesgaard F & Kehlet H (1989) Ranitidine for prevention of postoperative suppression of delayed hypersensitivity. *Am. J. Surg.* **157**, 291–294.

O'Boyle KP, Zamore R, Adluri S *et al.* (1992) Immunisation of colorectal cancer patients with modified ovine submaxillary gland mucin and adjuvants induces IgM and IgG antibodies to sialylated Tn[1]. *Cancer Res.* **52**, 5663–5667.

Oettgen HF & Old LJ (1991) The history of cancer immunotherapy. In: DeVita VT, Hellman S & Rosenberg SA (eds) *Biologic Therapy of Cancer*, pp. 87–119. Philadelphia, Pa: JB Lippincott.

Ohkawa SI, Wright KC, Manajan H *et al.* (1989) Hepatic arterial infusion of human recombinant tumor necrosis factor-alpha. An experimental study in dogs. *Cancer* **63**, 2096–2102.

Qin Y, Schally AV & Willems G (1991) Somatostatin analogue RC-160 inhibits the growth of transplanted colon cancer in rats. *Int. J. Cancer* **47**, 765–770.

Qin Y, Schally AV & Willems G (1992) Treatment of liver metastases of human colon cancers in nude mice with somatostatin analogue RC-160. *Int. J. Cancer* **52**, 791–796.

Robertson JF, Morris DL, Ellis IO *et al.* (1991) The prognostic value of the monoclonal antibody (D5) detected protein p29 in primary colorectal carcinoma. *Br. J. Cancer* **64**, 379–380.

Romani R & Morris DL (1994) New potent gastrin receptor antagonists (GRAs) inhibit basal *in vitro* growth of human colon cancer. *Aust. N.Z. J. Surg.* **64(5)**, 362–363.

Rosenberg SA, Lotze MT, Muul LM *et al.* (1987) A progress report on the treatment of 157 patients with advanced cancer using lymphokine-activated killer cells and interleukin-2 or high dose interleukin-2 alone. *N. Engl. J. Med.* **316**, 889–897.

Roth JA (1993) Molecular surgery for cancer. *Arch. Surg.* **127**, 1298–1302.

Schally AV (1988) Oncological applications of somatostatin analogues. *Cancer Res.* **48**, 6977–6985.

Singh S, Sheppard MC & Langman MJS (1993) Sex differences in the incidence of colorectal cancer: an exploration of oestrogen and progesterone receptors. *Gut* **34**, 611–615.

Smith JP, Wood JG & Solomon TG (1989) Elevated gastrin levels in patients with colon cancer or adenomatous polyps. *Dig. Dis. Sci.* **34**, 171–174.

Stewart GJ, Lawson JA & Morris DL (1994) Octreotide, in a nude mouse model, significantly inhibits hepatic metastases from human colon cancer. *Aust. N.Z. J. Surg.*

Tanaka J, Yamaguchi T, Takahashi T *et al.* (1986) Regulatory effects of gastrin and secretin on carcinomas of the stomach and colon. *Tohoku J. Exp. Med.* **148**, 459–460.

Thatcher N, Dazzi H, Johnson RJ *et al.* (1989) Recombinant interleukin-2 (ril-2) given intrasplenically and intravenously for advanced malignant melanoma. A phase I and II study. *Br. J. Cancer* **60**, 770–774.

Tonneson H, Bulow S, Fischerman K *et al.* (1988) Effect of cimetidine on survival after gastric cancer. *Lancet* **2**, 990–992.

Townsend CM, Singh P & Thompson JC (1986) Gastrointestinal hormones and gastrointestinal and pancreatic carcinomas. *Gastroenterology* **91**, 1002–1006.

Warlters A & Morris DL (1993) Reversible stimulation by histamine of *in vitro* proliferation in a human tubulovillous colorectal adenoma. *Aust. N.Z. J. Surg.* **63**, A379.

Watson SA, Durrant LG, Wencyk PM *et al.* (1991a) Intracellular gastrin in human gastrointestinal tumor cells. *J. Natl Cancer Inst.* **83**, 866–871.

Watson SA, Durrant L, Elston P *et al.* (1991b) Inhibitory effects of the gastrin receptor antagonist L365-260 on gastrointestinal tumor cells. *Cancer* **68**, 1255–1260.

Winsett OE, Townsend CM, Glass EJ *et al.* (1986) Gastrin stimulates growth of colon cancer. *Surgery* **99**, 302–307.

Index

Activity-time curve, of liver, 34 (fig.)
Adenocarcinoma,
  colon, 61
  rectum, 61
Adenoma–carcinoma sequence, genetic changes, 12–14
Adenomatous polyposis col: (APC), 13
Adriamycin,
  microspheres in cytotoxic therapy, 87
  plasma concentrations, 87 (table)
  weight of tumour following treatment, 88 (table)
Alanine serum transferase (AST), following cryotherapy, 140 (fig.)
Albumin microspheres, in cytotoxic therapy, 87
Allelic losses, 16
  and candidate tumour suppressor genes, 12
Allelotypes, chromosomal loss from tumour, 12
Aloka 650 unit, cryosurgery, 119
Anaesthetic, care in cryotherapy, 139
Angiogenesis, molecular basis of metastasis, 9
Angiogram, digital subtraction selective hepatic, 68 (fig.)
Angiography, 21–3
  coeliac axis, 23
  before CT angio-portography (CTAP), 22
  imaging hepatic metastases, 21
  intra-arterial chemotherapy, 70
  preoperative preparation for resection, 46
Angiotensin II,
  effect of, 88 (fig.)
  increase of HPI value, 35
  infusion, 88
  intra-arterial, effects of, 88 (fig.)
Annular phased array, hyperthermia, 162
Anoxia, cellular, 130
Antibiotics, prophylactic, in cryotherapy, 139
Antibody, targeting, in radiotherapy, 112
Anticoagulants, reduction in organ colonization, 8
Antigen-1, lymphocyte function-associated, 6
Antioncogenes, 11
Arteriography,
  demonstration of tumour blood vessels, 67
  preoperative preparation for resection, 46
Artery, ligation, combined with portal vein infusion, 99
Aspartic acid, *N*-phospho-acetyl-L-aspartate, 79
Autocrine motility factor (AMF), 7

Back pain, following ILP, 153
Bile duct, 48
  access to, 53 (fig.)
Biloma, complication of resection, 63
Biological therapy, regional, 168–9
Blood,
  caval, in isolated liver perfusion, 101
  dual supply, in intra-arterial chemotherapy, 70
  flow,
    changes caused by tumours, 33
  portal supply, 96–7
Bowel cancer, molecular basis, 1–19
BSD-1000/2000 annular phased array systems, 162
Buprenorphine, percutaneous ethanol injections, 144

Cadherins, 6–7
Calot's triangle, 49
Cannulation, of gastroduodenal artery, 106
Cantlie's line, 47, 48
Carcinoembryonic antigen (CEA),

in cryosurgery, 141–2
functioning as cell adhesion molecule, 6
in ILP,
clinical studies, 150, 152
monitoring, 156–7
metachronous metastases, 45
percutaneous ethanol injections, 146 (table)
pretreatment, 145
reduction, by cryotherapy, 133
Cardiorespiratory function, preoperative preparation for resection, 46
Cascade theory, 2
CD44 gene, 15
Cefotaxime, prophylactic antibiotics, cryotherapy, 139
Cell adhesion molecules (CAMs), role in tumour progression, 5–6
Cellular anoxia, freezing protocol, 130
Chemoembolization,
isolated liver perfusion, 105
preceding hyperthermia, 161
Chemoperfusion, hepatic arterial, 58
Chemosensitivity,
response to therapy dependent on, 102
testing, 103
Chemotherapy,
combination, 80
future of hyperthermia, 163
systemic, *see* Systemic chemotherapy
Cholangiogram, left hepatectomy, 54 (fig.)
Cholangiography, resection, operative procedures, 46
Cholecystectomy, 49, 51, 68
Cholecystitis, chemical, in intra-arterial chemotherapy, 68
Chromosome 5, 13
Chromosome 17, 12–13
Chromosome 18, 13
Cimetidine,
effects on immune function, 167
suppressor lymphocytes, 136
Cis-platinum, and 5–fluorourcil, 81
Clonal dominance, 9–10
Coagulation, preoperative preparation for resection, 46
Collagen, type IV, 5
Colorectal cancer,
cryotherapy, 137–42
systemic chemotherapy, 103
Combination chemotherapy, for colorectal cancer, 80
Computed tomography (CT), 24 (fig.), 120
angio-portography, 22–30
advantages, 26
artefacts, 27 (fig.)
disadvantages, 26
increased detection of lesions, 33
preoperative preparation for resection, 46
surgical decision-making with, 28–30
dynamic, 21–2
delayed, 26
detection of occult metastases, 33
differential diagnosis
adenomata, 30–1
focal nodular hyperplasia, 30–1
differential diagnosis of colorectal metastases, 30–1
haemangioma, 30
hepatocellular carcinoma, 30
dynamic, role in ILP, 151, 153 (fig.), 154 (fig.), 158
in extrahepatic disease, 26
cardio-oesophageal junction, 28 (fig.)
cupping, 29 (fig.)
pericardial node, 29 (fig.)
portocaval node, 28 (fig.)
interpretation, 26
interstitial laser photocoagulation, 148
percutaneous ethanol injections, 145
precontrast, dynamic and delayed, use in ILP, 156
post operative, cryosurgery, 130
preoperative investigations, 45
real-time, use in ILP, 157
scanning protocols, 21–2
selection of patients for cryotherapy, 138
Convex array probes, ultrasound transducer, 119 (fig.)
Cryoablation, and resection, 66
Cryodestruction, volume, 138
Cryogen, 128–9
Cryoglobinaemia, contraindication to cryosurgery, 138
Cryopreservation, of tissues, 129–30
Cryoprobe(s), 128
design, 126
diameter and temperature, 134
freezing tip, 128
introduction system, 125 (fig.)
number of, dependent on blood flow, 129
placement of, 118 (fig.)
accuracy of, and success of cryosurgery, 132
biplane transrectal ultrasound probe, 122–4
large multiple probes, 124
Seldinger technique, 124

planned route of, 121
selection, 126–31
shapes, 129
ultrasound scans during freezing, 131 (fig.)
vacuum insulated shaft, 128
Cryoshock, 140
Cryosurgery,
ablation compared with resection, 65
angle of needle placement, 125 (fig.)
in animals, increased survival, 116
compared with resection, 116
equipment, 126
impact of residual disease, 65 (fig.)
importance of technical details, 132
intraoperative ultrasound, 115
introduction system, 124–6, 125 (fig.)
outcome, 116 (fig.)
patient selection, 115–18
technical considerations, 115–32
Cryosurgical margin, 126
success of cryosurgery, 132
Cryotherapy, 115–42
adjuvant hepatic artery chemotherapy, 140
alanine serum transferase (AST), 140 (fig.)
as alternative to interstitial laser photocoagulation, 150
in animals, 134
carcinoembryonic antigen reduction, 133
for colorectal cancer, 137–42
extrahepatic disease, 137–8
factors affecting speed and effect of, 134
gelfoam plug controlling haemorrhage, 140 (fig.)
immunological aspects of, 136
improved survival following, 142
intra- and extracellular ice crystal formation, 133 (fig.)
intraoperative problems, 139
large vessels and bile ducts, 136
long-term complications, 142
mechanisms of tissue destruction, 133
morbidity, 140
perioperative care, 139
physics of, 134
postoperative bleeding, 139–40
postoperative follow-up, 140
radial crack of ice ball, 139 (fig.)
survival following, 141 (fig.), 142 (fig.)
technique,
environment, 135
margin and freeze-thaw, 135
osmolality, 135
probe design, 135–6
time, 134–5
tumour cell viability following, 134
ultrasound-controlled, 136
CT *see* Computed tomography
Cyst, ultrasound scan in cryosurgery, 121
Cytotoxic therapy,
deaths, 92 (table)
drug targeting, 85
theory of, 85 (fig.)
physical characteristics of patients, 91 (table)
predicted survival, 92 (fig.)
recurrence, 92 (table)
regional, 85–93
concept of, 90 (fig.)
response rates, 92 (table)
tissue damage, 105
toxicity, 92 (table)

DCC (deleted in colorectal cancer) gene, 6, 13, 18
DCDS, *see* Duplex/colour Doppler sonography
Diaphragm, resection, 49
Diasonics Spectra scanner, 36
Diclofenac, percutaneous ethanol injections, 144
Dihydrofluorouracil dehydrogenase, 74
Dipyridamole, altering 5–FU metabolism, 79
Dissemination,
portal venous, 95
tumour cell, 7–9
Doppler flow ratio (DFR), 36
Doppler perfusion index (DPI), 36–43, 40 (fig.), 42 (fig.)
analogy to HPI, 36
detection of occult metastases, 43
relationship with PHR, 40 (fig.)
specificity of, 41–2
technique of measurement, 36–7
Doppler sonography, duplex colour, *see* Duplex/colour Doppler sonography
Double-balloon catheter, 101, 103, 104 (fig.), 106
Double-lumen perfusion catheter, liver isolation, 101
Doxorubicin,
chemotherapy and hyperthermia, 163
combined with hyperthermia treatment, 160, 161
Drug application, regional, investigation of benefits, 106
Drug exposure,
local, response to therapy dependent on, 102

optimal, prerequisites for, 102–103
Duplex/colour Doppler sonography (DCDS), 36–43
blood flow measurements, 38 (fig.)
cytotoxic therapy, 88
detection of occult metastases, 43
important role in detection of metastases, 43
in vitro tests, 37–9
in vivo tests, 37–9
measurement of Doppler perfusion index, 42
more sensitive than conventional CT scan, 42
more sensitive than intraoperative ultrasound, 42
reproducibility tests, 37–9
Dynamic scintigraphy,
deficiency of, 41–2
hepatic perfusion index, 33–6
indirect method of flow measurement, 36

Echogenicity, of lesion, 121
Electrocardiogram, preoperative preparation for resection, 46
Electrocautery, hemihepatectomy, 50
Electromagnetic applicators, radiative, 162
Embolization, transcatheter arterial, combined with hyperthermia, 161
Endoscopy, intra-arterial chemotherapy, 71
Enzymes, proteolytic, 7
Ethanol, percutaneous injections, *see* Percutaneous ethanol injections
Excision, local, 56
Extracellular matrix (ECM), 5
Extravasation, and invasion, 5–7

Familial adenomatous polyposis (FAP), 11
Femoral artery, 103
α-fetoprotein, clinical studies of ILP, 150
Fibrin, 8
Fibronectin, 5
Fine-needle biopsy (FNAB), 145
Fluorodeoxyuridine (FUDR), regional biological therapy, 168
5–fluorodeoxyuridine, 86
5–fluorourcil,
clearance from plasma, 86 (fig.)
combined with,
biomodulators, 78–9, 80 (table), 81–2,
cis-platinum, 81
folinic acid, 77, 78 (table), 91 (fig.)
hyperthermia treatment, 160, 162
interferon, 82 (table)
levamisole, 43
mitomycin, 43
portal vein chemotherapy, 97
determinants of response to, 75 (table)
factors affecting resistance to, 75 (table)
infusion of, 75–7
intraportal chemotherapy, 99
maximum tolerated dosage, 77 (table)
metabolic fate of, 74 (fig.)
pharmacology, 74–5
portal vein infusion, randomized trials, 98 (table)
regional biological therapy, 168
regional vs systemic therapy, 86 (fig.)
response rate, 76 (table), 85
single-agent, 75
toxicity, 76 (table), 91 (fig.)
tumour response to, 58
Folinic acid,
combined with 5–fluorourcil, 77, 78 (table), 91 (fig.)
increased response rate in cytotoxic therapy, 89
plasma levels of, 91 (fig.)
trials with, 82
Freeze/thaw cycle, cryosurgery, 129–31
Freezing cycle, 129–31
monitoring, 131–2
FuDR, tumour response to, 58

Gardner's syndrome, 11
Gastrin, stimulation of colorectal cancers, 167
Gastroduodenal artery, cannulation of, 106
Gastrointestinal tract, primary tumours in, radiotherapy, 108
Gene(s),
CD44, 15
metastasis-associated, 14–15
ras, 12
neo, clonal dominance in primary tumours, 10
Gene therapy, non-cytotoxic control of metastases, 168
Genetic mapping, of locus predisposing to HNPCC, 13–14
Genetics, molecular, *see* Molecular genetics
Glycosaminoglycans, molecular basis of metastasis, 5

Haemoglobin, preoperative, resection, 46
Helium, liquid, as cryogen, 129
Hemicolectomy, left, preparation for, 54 (fig.)
Hemihepatectomy,
left, 53–5

right, 49–52
Heparin,
and portal vein 5–FU, 98
prophylactic subcutaneous, 139
thromboembolism as complication of resection, 46
Hepatectomy, 52, 53, 55 (fig.)
Hepatic arterial resistive index (HARI), 36–7
Hepatic perfusion index (HPI), 33–6, 34 (fig.)
deficiency of dynamic scintigraphy, 41–2
Doppler perfusion index as analogy of, 36
sensitivity of, 35
value of
increased by angiotensin H, 35
reduced by intrahepatic portosystemic shunting, 35
Hepatitis, radiotherapy, 108
Hepatocellular carcinoma
following cryotherapy, 141 (fig.)
resectable, 59
Hepatocyte growth factor, 7
Hepatoduodenal ligament, lymph nodes in, 47
Hereditary non-polyposis colorectal cancer (HNPCC), 11, 13–14
Hilar plate, extended right hepatectomy, 52
Hilum, hemihepatectomy, 51
Hydrochloride, papaverine, 23
Hyperfractionation, 109
Hyperthermia, 160–5
capacitive radiofrequency, 160–62
combined with,
chemotherapy, 160
radiotherapy, 111
future for, 163
perfusion, 162
preceded by chemoembolization, 161
whole-body, 162–3
Hypoechoic mctastases, 118 (fig.)

Ice ball, radial crack of, 139 (fig.)
Ice crystals, cryotherapy, 133, 134
Imaging-controlled destruction, physical methods of, 143–7
Immunoglobulin, superfamily, 6
In-plane biopsy guide, deficiencies of, 124 (fig.)
Infusaid, hepatic arterial chemoperfusion, 58
Infusion,
hepatic arterial, 59, 103, 105 (fig.)
portal vein, *see* Portal vein infusion
Infusional therapy, 5–fluorouracil, *see* 5–fluorouracil
Inplane biopsy, placement of cryoprobes, 122
Integrins, 6
Intercellular adhesion molecule 1 (ICAM-1), 6
Interferon, 168
inhibition of thymidilate synthetase, 81
trials with, 82
with fluorouracil, 81, 82 (table)
Interleukin 2 (IL-2), 168
stimulating lymphocyte activity, 136
Interstitial laser photocoagulation (ILP), 148
clinical studies of, 150–5
combined with chemotherapy, 157–8
compared with other techniques, 150
complications, 153–5
experimental studies of, 149–50
future of, 157–8
laser-induced tumour necrosis, 155
potential of, 158
principles of, 148–9
rationale for using, 150
role of dynamic CT, 158
role of MRI, 156
role of ultrasound, 152 (fig.), 156, 158
survival rates, 154 (fig.), 157 (fig.)
technique, 151
Interstitial placement, 148
Intra-arterial chemotherapy
blocked catheter, 71 (fig.)
methyl blue injection, 70 (fig.)
normal anatomy, 68 (fig.)
postoperative complications, 70–2
surgical approach, 67–72
trifurcation, 68 (fig.)
Intrahepatic portosystemic shunting, 35
Intraoperative ultrasound, *see* Ultrasound
Invasion,
and extravasation, 5–7
vascular, 96
venous, 95–6
incidence of, 96 (table)
Isolated-target metastases, 66
Isolation perfusion, *see* Perfusion

Jaundice, unsuitability for cryosurgery, 138
Jeule Thompson effect, gas cryogen cryoprobes, 128

Karyotypic analysis, of primary tumours, 10

Laminin, molecular basis of metastasis, 5
Laparotomy,
confirmation of resection, 46
elevated HPI values, 34
obviation of, 65
required by cryotherapy, 150

Lasers, 148–59
  Nd:YAG,
    clinical studies of ILP, 148, 150
    ILP technique, 151
    tissue-penetrating qualities, 149
  parameters and optical fibres, 155–6
  portable semiconductor diode, 148
  thermal effects, 149
  tissue interaction, 149
  tumour necrosis induced by, 155
Leidenfrost boiling effect, 128
Lesion(s),
  adjacent to hepatic veins, 116 (fig.)
  approach to, placement of cryoprobes, 123 (fig.)
  diameter, cryotherapy treatment dependent on, 138
  extrahepatic, following liver perfusion, 105 (fig.)
  multiple, cryosurgery, 116
  path through, ultrasound probe, 122 (fig.)
  planning route to, cryosurgery, 121
  postoperative scans, 117 (fig.)
Levamisole, combined with 5–fluorourcil, 43, 97
Lignocaine, clinical studies of ILP, 151
Linear array transducer, 119
Lipiodol,
  during hyperthermia treatment, 162
  iodine-labelled, 112, 131
Lung-derived growth factor (LDGF-1), stimulation of mitogenesis, 9
Lymph nodes, resection, operative procedure, 47
Lymphocyte, proliferation, following cryotherapy, 136
Lymphocyte function-associated antigen-1 (LFA-1), 6
Lymphokine-activated killer (LAK) cells, 168
Lynch syndromes, 11

MCC (mutated in colorectal cancer) gene, 13
Magnetic resonance imaging (MRI), 31–2, 120
  in colorectal metastatic disease, 32
  contrast-enhanced, increasing detection of lesions, 33
  diagnosis limitation, 33
  imaging hepatic metastases, 21
  interstitial laser photocoagulation, 148
  localization of hyperthermia, 164
  potential in ILP, 157
  role in ILP, 156
Mesenteric node, disease in non-resected patients, 62
Metachronous disease, 62
  resection, 45
Methotrexate, and 5–fluorourcil, 78–9
Microemboli, biodegradable, drug targeting in cytotoxic therapy, 87
Microspheres,
  adriamycin-loaded albumin, 87
  biodegradable albumin, 89
  radiolabelled, 87 (table)
  starch,
    chemoembolization preceding hyperthermia, 161
    drug targeting in cytotoxic therapy, 87
  yttrium-90, 89, 163
Microthermocouples, hyperthermia treatment, 161
Mitomycin,
  in colorectal cancer, 79–80
  combined with,
    5–fluorourcil, 43, 98
    hyperthermia treatment, 160
  ethylcellulose microencapsulated, 89
  isolated liver perfusion, 103
Molecular basis of metastasis, 1–19
  animal models, 3
  cascade theory, 2
  seed and soil hypothesis, 1–2
Molecular genetics,
  of large bowel cancer progression, 10–14
  progress in, 11
Monosegmentectomy, resection, 56
Motility, of cell, 7
MRI, *see* Magnetic resonance imaging
mts-1 gene, 14–15
Multihole needle, percutaneous ethanol injections, 144
Multistep theory, 4–5

Natural killer (NK) cells, 8–9, 168
Nd:YAG laser, *see under* Lasers
Needles, for percutaneous ethanol injections, 143–4
Neodymium: yttrium aluminium garnet (Nd:YAG) laser, *see under* Lasers
Nitrogen, liquid, cryosurgery, 128
NK cells, *see* Natural killer cells
nm23 gene, 14–15

Occult metastases, detection of, 33–43
  clinical results, 39(table), 39–41
  computed tomography, 33
  follow-up results, 41

one-year follow-up, 41 (fig.)
ultrasound, 33
Omeprazole, complicating intra-arterial chemotherapy, 71 (fig.)
Oncogenes,
metastasis-associated genes, 14
molecular genetics of cancer progression, 11
Optical fibres, and laser parameters, ILP, 155–6

PALA, *see* N-phospho-acetyl-L-aspartate aspartic acid
Papaverine hydrochloride, 23
Parenchymal transection, 53
Percentage hepatic replacement (PHR), 37, 40 (fig.)
Percutaneous ethanol injections (PEI), 143–7
in carcinoembryonic antigen, 146 (table)
equipment, 143–5
one-shot technique, 144, 146
pre and posttreatment investigations, 145, 146
response, 146 (table)
ultrasound sections, 144 (fig.), 145 (fig.)
Percutaneous intrahepatic alcohol injection, 150
Perfusion,
circuit, 102 (fig.)
compared with radiation, 110
double-lumen catheter, 101
hepatic arterial, 67
isolated, 101–7
candidates for, 106
clinical cases, 103–5
double-balloon vena cava catheter, 104 (fig.)
extrahepatic lesions, 105 (fig.)
hyperthermia, 162
side effects, 105
simplification of techniques, 106
technique, 101–102
Periaortic node, disease in non-resected patients, 62
Periportal node, disease in non-resected patients, 62
N-phospho-acetyl-L-aspartate aspartic acid (PALA)
optimum scheduling of, 82
modulating agent for 5–FU, 79
Phosphoribosylpyrophosphate (PRPP), 78
Platelets, contribution to metastatic process, 8
Polysaccharides, 5
Poral venous congestive index (PVCI), 42 (fig.)
Portal blood supply, 96–7
Portal vein, 48
chemotherapy, 95–9
dormant liver metastases, 96
clamping of, 106
cytotoxic infusion, combined with artery ligation, 99
dissemination, 95
infusion,
clinical trials of, 97–9
conclusions, 99
as prophylaxis, 97
randomized trials, 98 (table)
treatment of established metastases, 99
Probes, *see* Cryoprobes; Ultrasound probes
Prophylaxis,
H2, reduced gastroduodenal ulceration, 70
portal vein infusion as, 97
cryotherapy for thromboembolism and infection, 139
Prostaglandins, inhibition of cancer growth, 167
Proteolytic enzymes, 7
Proto-oncogenes, molecular genetics of cancer progression, 11

Quadrate lobe, 52

Radiation, high, inability to target, 112
Radioactive seeds, direct implantation of, 112
Radionuclides,
detection of occult metastases, 34 (fig.)
measuring HPI, 35
Radiotherapy, 108–14
adjuvant, in high-risk patients, 110–11
combined with,
chemotherapy, 109–12
hyperthermia, 111, 162, 161, 163
compared with perfusion, 110
criteria for selecting patients, 108
external-beam, 109, 112
internal, 111–12
selective targeting, 112
symptom control, 111
whole-liver, plus razoxane, 110
Ranitidine, effects on immune function, 167
Ras gene, 12, 14
Razoxane, plus whole-liver radiation, 110
Regional therapy, outcome analysis, 59
Resection, 45–55
abdominal incision, 46 (fig.)
access to bile duct, 53 (fig.)

anatomy, 47–9
colorectal cancer, natural history series, 59 (table)
compared with cryosurgery, 116
completed, 52 (fig.)
and cryoablation, 66
dissection of hepatic vein, 50 (fig.)
dissection of hilum, 49 (fig.)
division into hemilivers, 47
division of peritoneal reflections, 48 (fig.)
extended left hepatectomy, 55
hemiliver, right, 51
hepatic artery and portal vein, 49 (fig.)
right hepatectomy, 53
inferior vena cava ligament, 50 (fig.)
metachronous metastases, 62
operative cholangiogram, 54 (fig.)
operative procedures, 46
postoperative management, 56
preoperative preparation, 46
preoperative vs surgical staging, 64 (table)
preparation for left hemicolectomy, 54 (fig.)
registry of hepatic metastases, 61 (fig.)
results, 57–66
right hepatic duct, 51 (fig.)
right hepatic vein, 50 (fig.)
right lobe, 51 (fig.)
disease in, 62
segmental, 55–6
single institutional series, 63 (table)
surgical morbidity, 62
survival following, 60 (fig.), 61 (fig.), 64–5
cumulative, 61 (fig.)
disease-free, 61 (fig.)
synchronous metastases, 62
thromboembolism as complication, 46
transverse, 47 (fig.)
Resistive indexes,
hepatic arterial, 36–7
superior mesenteric arterial, 37

Sandostatin, 166
Scatter factor, 7
Scintigraphy, dynamic, hepatic perfusion index, 33–6
Seed and soil hypothesis, 1–2
Segmentectomy, 56
Seldinger technique, cryoprobe placement, 124
Sex steroids, 167–8
Shoulder, pain following ILP, 153
Single-agent chemotherapy, response of colorectal cancer, 80 (fig.)
Single-organ metastases, 66
SMS 201.995, 166
Somatostatin, 166
Spinal needle, for percutaneous ethanol injections, 143
Spirometry, preoperative preparation for resection, 46
Steroids, sex, 167–8
Stochastic theory, 4–5
Stopflow, isolation perfusion technique, 106
Styrene maleic anhydride neocarzinostatin (SMANCS), 161–2
Superior mesenteric arterial resistive index (SMARI), 36–7
Synchronous disease, 62
resection, 45
Systemic chemotherapy,
kinetics of colorectal cancer, 73 (table)
results of, 73–82

Three-dimensional treatment, radiotherapy, 109
Thromboembolism,
complicating resection, 46
cryotherapy prophylaxis for, 139
Thymidylate synthetase
inhibition by alpha-Interferon, 81
reaction of 5–FU and folinic acid, 77
Time-activity curve, 34 (fig.)
TIMPS (tissue inhibitors of metalloproteinases), 7, 16
Transcatheter arterioal embolization, 161
Transducers, ultrasound,
longitudinal linear array, 125 (fig.)
5 MHz linear array, 119
success of cryosurgery, 132
Transection, parenchymal, 53
Trifurcation, intra-arterial chemotherapy, 68
Tumorigenesis, colorectal, genetic model for, 12
Tumour necrosis factor (TNF), 168

Ultrasound,
compared with CT scan, 46
detection of occult metastases, 33
during ILP treatment, 151
in cryosurgery, 115, 118–21, 131–2(figs.)
cyst scan, 121 (fig.)
heating transducers, 164
in ILP, 148, 156, 158
in imaging metastases, 21, 31
inadequate resolution capacity, 62
intraoperative (IOUS), 31, 116–17 (fig.)
cryosurgery, 115, 118–21, 131–2(figs.)
increased detection of lesions, 33

resection, 47, 57, 65
percutaneous ethanol injection, 143
pre- and post chemotherapy treatment, 90 (fig.)
preoperative assessment, 31
probes,
biplane transrectal, 120 (fig.), 122–4, 123
safe placement of, 122 (fig.)
scanned focused, 164
transducers, *see* Transducers, ultrasound
Uridine, oral, combined with 5–FU and PALA, 79

Vaccines, tumour, 168
Vascular pedicle, early ligation of, 97
Vascularization, tumour, response to therapy dependent on, 102
Vena cava, inferior, 48
double-balloon technique, 106
hemihepatectomy, 51
lesions on, suitability for cryosurgery, 117
isolated liver perfusion, 101

X-rays,
preoperative investigations, 45
selection of patients for cryotherapy, 138

Yttrium 90 microspheres, 89
radiotherapy and hyperthermia, 163